The Perioperative Medicine Handbook

The Perioperative Medicine Handbook

Edited by Lana Rogers

hayle medical

New York

Hayle Medical,
750 Third Avenue, 9th Floor,
New York, NY 10017, USA

Visit us on the World Wide Web at:
www.haylemedical.com

ISBN: 978-1-63241-861-6

Cataloging-in-Publication Data

The perioperative medicine handbook / edited by Lana Rogers.
p. cm.
Includes bibliographical references and index.
ISBN 978-1-63241-861-6
1. Preoperative care. 2. Postoperative care. 3. Therapeutics, Surgical. I. Rogers, Lana.
RD50 .P47 2020
617.919 2--dc23

Table of Contents

Preface

The purpose of the book is to provide a glimpse into the dynamics and to present opinions and studies of some of the scientists engaged in the development of new ideas in the field from very different standpoints. This book will prove useful to students and researchers owing to its high content quality.

Perioperative medicine refers to the medical care provided to patients preparing for surgery, undergoing surgery or recuperating from a surgery. Managing operative risks, complications and medical illnesses are the main objectives of perioperative medicine. Various professionals such as anesthesiologists, surgeons, medical consultants and intensivists work in concert in this practice. Many interventions for reducing the adverse outcomes of surgery may be adopted. These may include packages of care for enhanced recovery and maintenance of normothermia. The importance of handling complications in a timely and effective manner as they develop is an important focus of perioperative medicine. This book discusses the fundamentals as well as modern approaches of perioperative medicine. While understanding the long-term perspectives of the topics, it makes an effort in highlighting their impact as a modern tool for the growth of the discipline. With state-of-the-art inputs by acclaimed experts of this field, this book targets students and professionals.

At the end, I would like to appreciate all the efforts made by the authors in completing their chapters professionally. I express my deepest gratitude to all of them for contributing to this book by sharing their valuable works. A special thanks to my family and friends for their constant support in this journey.

Editor

1

Measuring outcomes after major abdominal surgery during hospitalization: reliability and validity of the Postoperative Morbidity Survey

Simon J Davies[1*], James Francis[1], Jonathan Dilley[1], R Jonathan T Wilson[1], Simon J Howell[2] and Victoria Allgar[3]

Abstract

Background: Measurement of outcomes after major abdominal surgery has traditionally focused on mortality, however the low incidence in elective surgery makes this measure a poor comparator. The Postoperative Morbidity Survey (POMS) prospectively assesses short-term morbidity, and may have clinical utility both as a core outcome measure in clinical trials and quality of care. The POMS has been shown to be a valid outcome measure in a mixed surgical population, however it has not been studied in patients undergoing major abdominal surgery. This study assessed the inter-rater reliability and validity of the POMS in patients undergoing major abdominal surgery.

Methods: Patients undergoing elective major abdominal surgery were visited on postoperative day 1 until discharge by two novice observers who administered the POMS in order to assess inter-rater reliability. Subjects who had previously had the POMS performed prospectively on postoperative days 3 and 5 were identified from a database. The pattern and prevalence of morbidity was analyzed against hospital length of stay (LOS) in order to validate the POMS in this patient group.

Results: Fifty one patients were recruited to the inter-rater reliability study giving a total of 263 POMS assessments. Inter-rater reliability showed a 97.7% agreement with a κ coefficient of 0.912 (95% CI: 0.842 to 0.982). On domain analysis percentage agreement was lowest in the gastrointestinal domain (87.5%), whilst correlation was lowest in the wound (κ: 0.04; 95% CI: −1.0 to 1.0) and hematological domains (κ: 0.378; 95% CI: 0.035 to 0.722). All other domains showed at least substantial agreement. POMS assessments were analyzed for postoperative days 3 (n = 258) and 5 (n = 362). The absence or presence of morbidity as measured by the POMS was associated with a hospital LOS of 6 (IQR: 4 to 7) *vs.* 11 (IQR: 8 to 15) days on postoperative day 3 (P <0.0001), and 7 (IQR: 6 to 10) *vs.* 13 (IQR: 9 to 19) days on postoperative day 5 (P <0.0001). The presence of any morbidity on postoperative day 5 conferred an odds ratio for a prolonged hospital LOS of 11.9 (95% CI: 5.02 to 11.92).

Conclusions: This study shows that the POMS is both a reliable and valid measure of short-term postoperative morbidity in patients undergoing major abdominal surgery.

Keywords: Major surgery, Morbidity, Postoperative morbidity survey, Postoperative outcome

Background

Measurement of patient outcomes after major abdominal surgery has traditionally focused on mortality; however, the relatively low event rate for the majority of elective surgical procedures makes this a poor discriminator of both the quality of care between institutions and the effectiveness of interventions. Although absolute in terms of an outcome measure, the use of mortality as a clinical end-point is not without its discrepancies. The temporal variation in reporting, ranging from in hospital mortality to up to 1 year mortality, means that it is a difficult and poor comparator, and the loss of patients to long-term follow-up is an additional confounder. It has been suggested that 30-day mortality may underestimate short-term patient outcomes following major abdominal surgery, with a significant increase in mortality seen at 90 days [1].

* Correspondence: simon.davies@york.nhs.uk
[1]Department of Anaesthesia, York Hospitals NHS Foundation Trust, Wigginton Road, York YO31 8HE, UK
Full list of author information is available at the end of the article

Morbidity is a more frequent occurrence after major surgery, particularly in the higher risk patient. The importance of complications in the immediate postoperative period is clear, however perioperative complications may have long-term implications for both the quality and quantity of an individual's life with an associated reduction in median survival [1,2]. The measurement and reporting of outcomes following major surgery is a fundamental process to improving the quality and safety of care that a health system provides, both in terms of the health framework and delivery of care by institutions and the individual clinicians themselves [3,4]. It is theoretically desirable to have a core set of outcomes measured and reported as a minimum in clinical research, allowing differing interventions to be compared and contrasted with greater ease and reducing the risk of outcome reporting bias.

The postoperative morbidity survey (POMS) is a nine-domain system that prospectively identifies short-term mortality after surgery [5]. For each of the nine domains morbidity is recorded on the presence or absence of preset criteria and it appears to accurately describe the pattern and prevalence of morbidity in the postoperative setting.

The purpose of this study was firstly to ascertain whether it is feasible to use the POMS as a core outcome measure for reporting in clinical trials by assessing the inter-rater reliability of two novice observers, and secondly to evaluate its validity as an outcome measure in terms of its prediction of hospital length of stay (LOS).

Methods

The protocol was approved by the Local Research Ethics Committee of York Hospital NHS Trust. A member of the research team screened patients for eligibility, and written informed consent was obtained from patients prior to surgery. The study was performed in 2 parts, a prospective analysis of the inter-rater agreement of the POMS, and a retrospective analysis of data to assess its validity.

Inter-rater agreement of the POMS

Inclusion criteria

Patients undergoing elective major abdominal surgery defined as procedures expected to last more than 2 hours, or with an anticipated blood loss greater than 500 mL, were recruited. This included general surgery (colorectal, pancreatic, gastric surgery), vascular surgery (abdominal aortic aneurysm repair) and urological surgery (cystectomy, prostatectomy and nephrectomy).

Protocol

Two independent and novice researchers, neither of whom had used the POMS previously, visited patients independently on postoperative day 1 and then daily until hospital discharge. The researchers observed and questioned the patient regarding the items defined in the POMS (Table 1), and also reviewed patient notes, charts and pathology results in order to complete the POMS accurately.

Statistical analysis

Inter-rater reliability of the individual components of the POMS (absence or presence of individual domain morbidities) and the occurrence of any morbidity in any domain was assessed using the κ coefficient, which assesses agreement beyond that expected by chance alone. Non-parametric data was analyzed using the Mann–Whitney U-test. Incidences were calculated using the χ^2

Table 1 The Postoperative Morbidity Survey (POMS) showing morbidity types, definitions and source data

Morbidity type	Criteria	Source data
Pulmonary	*De novo* requirement for supplemental oxygen or other respiratory support (e.g., CPAP or IPPV)	Patient observation Treatment chart Observation chart
Infectious	Currently on antibiotics or temperature >38°C in the last 24 hrs	Treatment chart Observation chart
Renal	Presence of oliguria (<500 mL/day), increased serum creatinine (>30% from baseline value), or urinary catheter in place for a non-surgical reasons	Patient observation Fluid balance chart Biochemistry results
Gastrointestinal	Unable to tolerate an enteral diet (either by mouth or feeding tube) for any reason, including nausea, vomiting and abdominal distension	Patient questioning Fluid balance chart
Cardiovascular	Diagnostic test or therapy in last 24 hrs for any of the following reasons: *de novo* myocardial infarction or ischemia, hypotension (requiring drug therapy or fluid >200 mL/hr), atrial or ventricular arrhythmia or pulmonary edema	Treatment chart Fluid chart Observation chart Note review
Neurological	Presence of a *de novo* focal deficit, coma or confusion/delirium	Patient questioning Note review
Wound complications	Wound dehiscence requiring surgical exploration or drainage or pus from the wound	Note review Pathology results
Hematological	Requirement for any of the following within last 24 hrs: blood, platelets, fresh frozen plasma or cryoprecipitate	Fluid balance chart
Pain	Surgical wound pain significant enough to require parenteral opiates or regional anesthesia	Treatment chart Patient questioning

test. Relationships between two categorical variables were analyzed by Fisher's exact test, and strength of association calculated. A *P* value less than 0.05 was considered significant. Where appropriate 95% confidence intervals (CI) were calculated. POMS domains that were significant on univariate analysis were entered into a multivariate model for further analysis.

Statistical analysis was performed with GraphPad Prism ver. 5.0b for Mac OS X (GraphPad Software, San Diego, CA, USA) and SPSS ver. 20.0 (SPSS Inc., Chicago, IL, USA).

Validity of the POMS

From a secure research database (Microsoft Access, Microsoft Corporation, Redmond, USA), patients who had POMS assessments on day 3 and 5 postoperatively, and who had undergone elective major abdominal surgery meeting the inclusion criteria above, were identified. POMS data was then analyzed against hospital LOS. This represents the criterion validity of the POMS, with LOS being used as a surrogate for morbidity.

Results

Inter-rater agreement of the POMS

Fifty-one patients were recruited to the study giving a total of 263 individual POMS assessments. Overall the presence or absence of morbidity as defined by the POMS showed a 97.7% agreement between observers, with a κ coefficient of 0.912 (95% CI: 0.842 to 0.982), giving near perfect agreement (Table 2).

The percentage agreements and κ coefficients for individual POMS domain on days 1, 3, 5 and cumulatively, are shown in Table 3. Overall percentage agreement was high for the wound domain at 99.2%. However, there was no evidence of agreement beyond that expected by chance alone, and κ was estimated at near zero. Fair agreement was seen in the hematological domain, substantial agreement in the gastrointestinal and neurological domains, and almost perfect agreement in the remaining 6 domains [6].

Validity of the POMS

POMS assessments were analyzed for postoperative day 3 (n = 258) and postoperative day 5 (n = 362) (Table 4). This data was obtained from the prospective inter-rater reliability study previously described, and three other studies performed in the same institution in which POMS data was prospectively obtained [7,8]. The median LOS for the cohort was 11 days (IQR: 8 to 15 days). The absence or presence of morbidity measured by the POMS was associated with a hospital LOS of 6 (IQR: 4 to 7) *vs.* 11 (IQR: 8 to 15) days when performed on postoperative day 3 (*P* <0.0001), and 7 (IQR: 6 to 10) *vs.* 13 (IQR: 9 to 19) days when performed on postoperative day 5 (*P* <0.0001). Kaplan-Meier analysis for the POMS on postoperative days 3 and 5 and hospital LOS are shown in Figure 1.

The incidence of morbidity in different domains for postoperative days 3 and 5 are shown in Table 5, with renal, pulmonary, gastrointestinal and pain morbidity having the highest incidence on both days.

The relationship between morbidity in individual domains on postoperative days 3 and 5, and median hospital LOS is shown in Figures 2 and 3. On day 3, the presence of morbidity in seven out of the nine domains was associated with a longer hospital LOS, and on day 5 morbidity in all domains, with the exception of hematological morbidity, was also associated with a longer LOS. On multivariate regression analysis only the presence of morbidity in the pulmonary domain on both days 3 and 5 was statistically significant in explaining the variations in hospital LOS (*P* <0.0001).

The presence of any morbidity on postoperative day 5 conferred an OR of 11.9 (95% CI: 5.02 to 28.31) for a prolonged hospital LOS, defined as greater than the 3rd interquartile for the cohort, but no predictive ability was conferred to the same analysis on day 3 (OR: 3.64; 95% CI: 0.83 to 15.92). ROC analysis by domain and day for LOS is shown in Table 6, with significant differences seen in the AUC on days 3 and 5 for the cardiovascular and gastrointestinal domains.

POMS defined morbidity was absent in 9.7% of patients on day 3 and 41.2% of patients on day 5 despite them still receiving inpatient care.

Discussion

This study shows that the POMS is both a reliable and valid measure of short-term postoperative morbidity in patients undergoing major abdominal surgery. The main strength of this paper is that it studies a homogenous group of subjects all of whom underwent major abdominal surgery, and hence could reliably be expected to have a similar pattern of postoperative morbidity. The study also examined the reliability of the survey when

Table 2 Inter-rater correlation and percentage agreement of the presence or absence of morbidity as measured by the POMS

	Day 1 (n = 51)	Day 2 (n = 51)	Day 3 (n = 51)	Day 4 (n = 46)	Day 5 (n = 40)	Total (n = 263)
Percentage agreement (%)	100	100	100	95.7	95	97.7
κ correlation coefficient (95% CI)	N/A	1.0 (1.0-1.0)	1.0 (1.0-1.0)	0.873 (0.760-1.0)	0.895 (0.760-1.0)	0.912 (0.842-0.982)

When observers scored all patients the same the hypothetical probability of chance could not be calculated, and are labeled N/A.

Table 3 Inter-rater correlation and percentage agreement for individual domains of the POMS on days 1, 3, 5 and cumulatively

	Day 1 (n = 51)		Day 3 (n = 51)		Day 5 (n = 40)		Total (n = 263)	
	Percentage agreement	κ	Percentage agreement	κ	Percentage agreement	κ	Percentage agreement	κ
Cardiovascular	94.1	0.876 (0.740-1.0)	100	1.0 (1.0-1.0)	97.5	0.655 (−0.012-1.0)	96.6	0.828 (0.718-0.939)
Gastrointestinal	88.2	0.555 (0.221-0.890)	84.3	0.651 (0.443-0.858)	87.5	0.658 (0.377-0.938)	87.5	0.749 (0.669-0.829)
Hematological	80.4	0.069 (−0.448-0.587)	100	1.0 (1.0-1.0)	100	N/A	95.4	0.378 (0.035-0.722)
Infectious	98.0	0.929 (0.793-1.0)	98.0	0.935 (0.810-1.0)	95.0	0.804 (0.539-1.0)	98.1	0.938 (0.884-0.992)
Neurological	96.1	0.480 (−0.227-1.0)	96.1	0.779 (0.479-1.0)	97.5	0.655 (−0.012-1.0)	97.0	0.717 (0.524-0.910)
Pain	100	1.0 (1.0-1.0)	86.3	0.71 (0.511-0.90)	90.0	0.610 (0.247-0.973)	93.5	0.869 (0.809-0.929)
Pulmonary	100	1.0 (1.0-1.0)	94.1	0.870 (0.727-1.0)	95.0	0.890 (0.742-1.0)	96.2	0.906 (0.852-0.960)
Renal	98.0	0.658 (−0.007-1.0)	96.1	0.897 (0.757-1.0)	92.5	0.845 (0.677-1.0)	95.1	0.869 (0.802-0.936)
Wound	98.0	0.0 (−1.0-1.0)	100	N/A	100	N/A	99.2	−0.004 (−1.0-1.0)

Some κ coefficients could not be calculated as all observations occurred in a single domain, and are labeled N/A.

Table 4 Number and percentage of patients in each surgical specialty analyzed in the assessment of the validity of the POMS

	Day 3	Day 5
	n (%)	n (%)
Colorectal	213 (82.6%)	260 (71.8%)
Vascular	8 (3.1%)	31 (8.6%)
Urology	35 (13.5%)	61 (16.8%)
Upper gastrointestinal	2 (0.8%)	10 (2.8%)
Total	258	362

administered by novice researchers unfamiliar with the POMS, allowing an assessment of its potential use as an outcome measure in both research and clinical practice, where it would be required to be administered by a spectrum of health professionals of varying experience.

Overall the inter-rater reliability of POMS-defined morbidity showed high percentage agreement, and near perfect correlation. Reliability within POMS domains showed varying results, with the lowest percentage agreement seen in the gastrointestinal domain, however the κ correlation coefficient still showed a substantial agreement. A similar result was also shown in the only other validation of the POMS [9], in which the gastrointestinal domain showed the weakest correlation

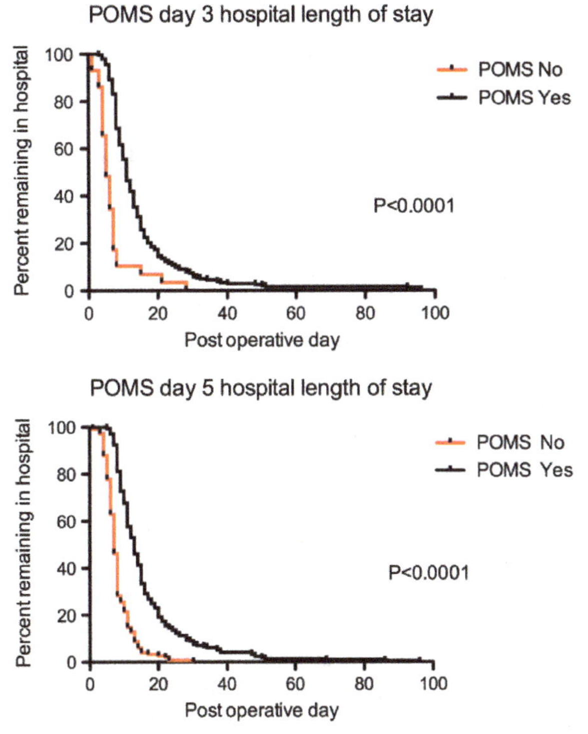

Figure 1 Kaplan-Meier curves for hospital LOS based upon the presence or absence of POMS defined morbidity on postoperative days 3 and 5.

Table 5 Incidence of morbidity by POMS domain on postoperative days 3 and 5

	Incidence of morbidity (%)	
Domain	Day 3	Day 5
Neurological	10.0	3.2
Hematological	3.8	1.2
Pain	70.5	28.7
Gastrointestinal	53.6	31.9
Wound	0	1.2
Cardiovascular	9.2	6.1
Pulmonary	54.7	42.1
Infectious	157	17.4
Renal	46.7	26.3

between observers, suggesting that the criteria may need refining to give it greater clinical utility. In the study by Grocott *et al.* [9] the majority of the items within the POMS domains showed a perfect correlation, however this was not the case in the present study. The reason for the decreased correlation may be due to experienced research nurses having administered the survey in the previous work, whilst we chose specifically to assess the reliability of the POMS when it was administered by novices to its use. Despite this, POMS, as it currently stands, could be used as an outcome measure without specific training in its use.

There are a number of apparent discrepancies in the reliability of individual domains as only fair correlation was seen in the hematological domain, and no correlation was seen in the wound domain despite good percentage agreement between observers. The use of the κ coefficient in this setting unfairly describes the reliability of the POMS as κ is affected by the prevalence of the findings it is describing. When the reported prevalence is low, as was the case in the hematological and wound domains, then κ may not be a reliable measure of correlation as illustrated by the high agreement but poor correlation [10].

As the POMS cannot be used as a scale due to its low internal consistency [9], the presence of any morbidity recorded by the POMS must be associated with an increased hospital LOS in order for it to be valid. The presence of morbidity registered by the POMS at both postoperative days 3 and 5 was associated with a longer hospital LOS, and morbidity at day 5 was associated with an eightfold increase in patients having a prolonged hospital LOS (greater than the 3rd interquartile for the cohort). These observations support the predictive ability of the POMS, but also suggest additional utility for the survey in the context of resource utilization due to its ability to predict those who will remain in hospital for longer.

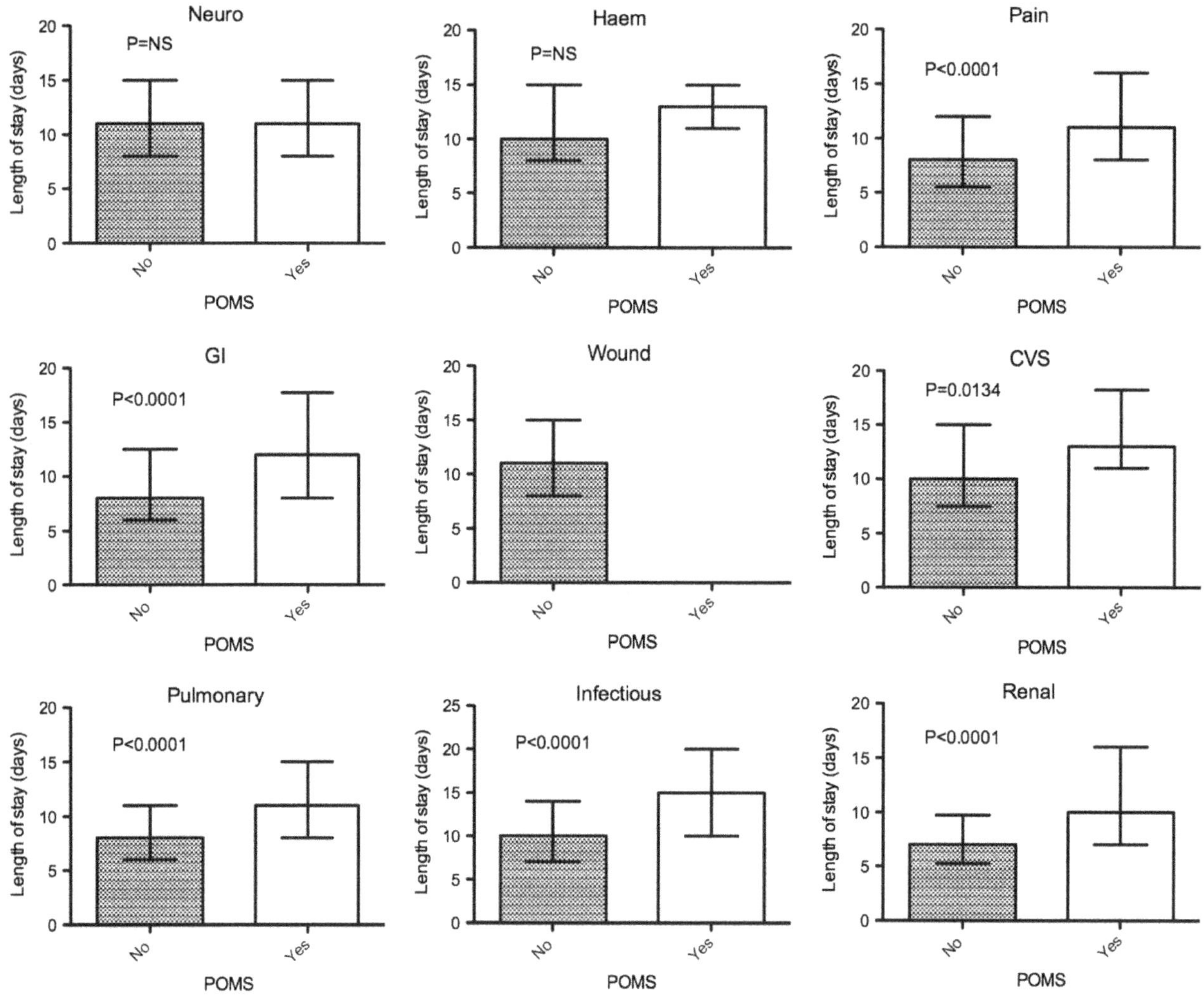

Figure 2 Hospital LOS for the presence or absence of morbidity by individual POMS domain type on postoperative day 3. Data is reported as median with interquartile range.

Grocott *et al.* found that on postoperative day 5 the presence of morbidity within 5 of the 9 domains was associated with a longer hospital LOS; however, we observed this in an additional 3 domains. This may reflect the significant differences in the two populations studied, with the previous cohort consisting of almost two thirds orthopedic patients undergoing peripheral surgery, whilst this study contained a more homogenous cohort all of whom underwent major abdominal surgery. In addition, it also appears that a number of domains are associated with a longer hospital LOS when the POMS is administered earlier at postoperative day 3, allowing a more prompt assessment of significant morbidity that affects hospital LOS and strengthening its validity as an outcome measure.

The pattern of morbidity seen in this study is similar to that previously described [5,9], although higher incidences of pain and pulmonary related morbidity, but lower incidences of gastrointestinal morbidity related morbidity were seen. This is surprising given the nature of the cohort, but a possible explanation for this reduction in gastrointestinal morbidity in a series that has undergone major abdominal surgery may due to differences in postoperative analgesia (epidural *versus* intravenous opiates), or the adoption of enhanced recovery protocols aimed at minimizing morbidity.

There are a number of limitations to this study, primarily the small numbers in the reliability assessment of the POMS; however, the overall number of observations was acceptable. The cohort is not truly homogenous, and although all subjects underwent major abdominal surgery, the inclusion of vascular and urology patients, who may have a different prevalence and pattern of morbidity to those undergoing colorectal surgery, may limit the application of results to this population. In addition we did not assess patients with no POMS defined

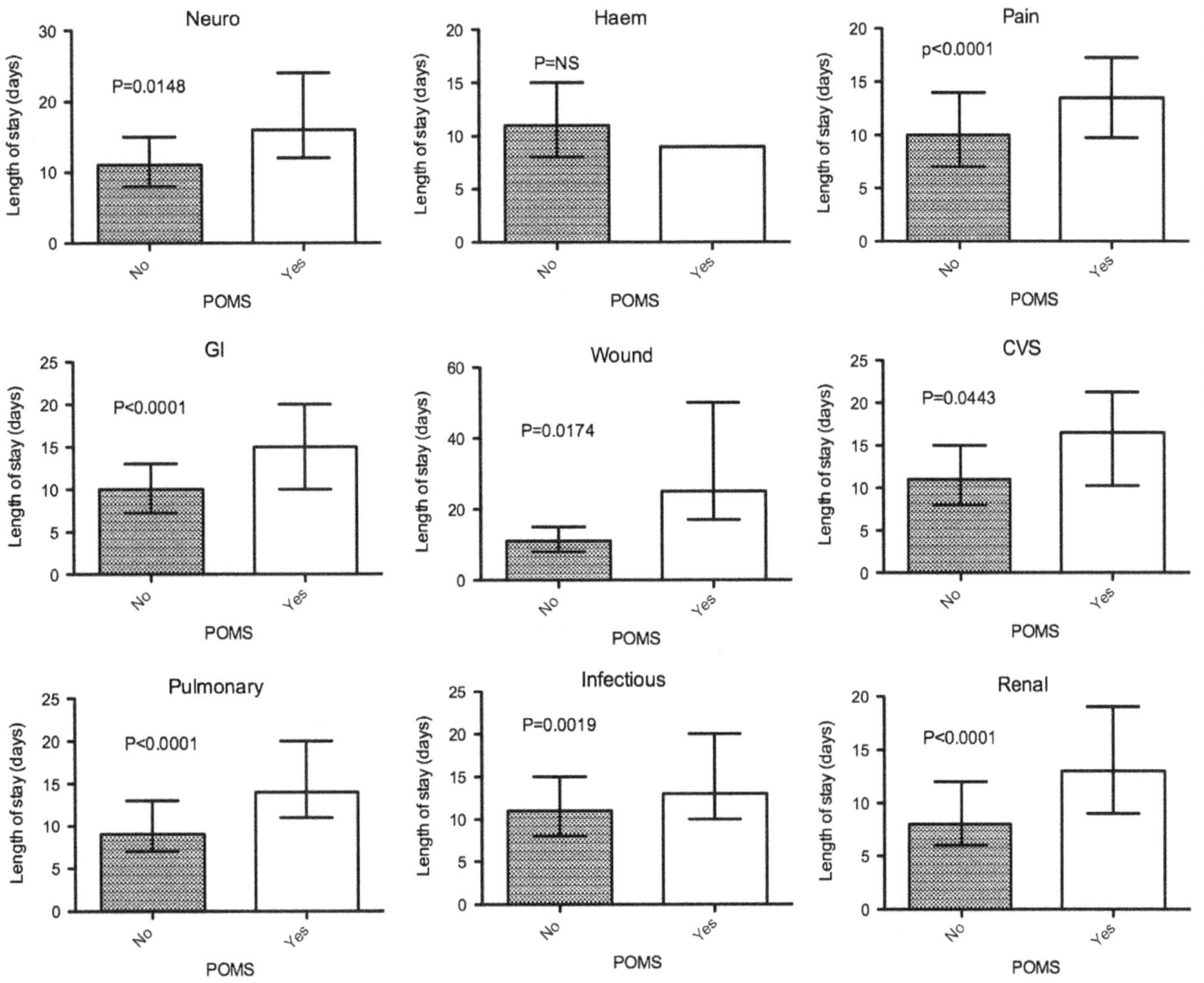

Figure 3 Hospital LOS for the presence or absence of morbidity by individual POMS domain type on postoperative day 5. Data is reported as median with interquartile range.

criteria for potentially important morbidity not captured by the survey. It is possible that this group remained hospitalized due to significant postoperative morbidity rather than social issues or delays in the discharge process. However, it has previously been observed that patients remaining in hospital with no POMS defined morbidity showed no evidence of any other morbidity measured by different means [5,9].

There are also a number of limitations of the POMS itself as many of the domains describe what is considered routine therapy following major surgery (postoperative oxygen, antibiotics, catheterization), however, by postoperative days 3 and 5, these routine therapies should have been ceased, particularly in the context of enhanced recovery programs. The lack of internal consistency of POMS, meaning that it cannot be treated as a scale, only allows the POMS to identify the presence of morbidity but not to measure its severity, a tool that would be inherently useful when measuring postoperative outcomes. Further modification of the POMS may allow the development of a survey that measures a single construct, and hence can be used to measure the severity of morbidity. The validity of the POMS in different and specific surgical cohorts, for example vascular and urology, also needs to be explored as the patterns of morbidity are often different. However, it appears to be both valid and reliable in this group.

Accurate and meaningful reporting of outcomes in clinical trials is essential; however, it has been acknowledged that reporting of surgical adverse events in the health system is inconsistent [11]. The underlying problem remains the lack of standardization of reported outcome measures in terms of timescale, the specific measurement, and the definition of that same measurement. The standardization of a core set of outcome measures would allow for more effective comparison of interventions, allow appropriate outcome measures to be collected and reported in the correct way, aid meta-analysis and sample size calculations, and simplify the design of trials for

Table 6 ROC analysis by POMS domain and postoperative day measured for LOS

Domain	Day	AUC (95% CI)	Z
Cardiovascular	3	0.69 (0.60-0.76)	2.699*
	5	0.46 (0.29-0.60)	
Gastrointestinal	3	0.70 (0.63-0.76)	2.355*
	5	0.58 (0.50-0.65)	
Hematological	3	0.70 (0.60-0.80)	0.307
	5	0.65 (0.33-0.97)	
Infectious	3	0.70 (0.62-0.78)	1.808
	5	0.59 (0.50-0.68)	
Neurological	3	0.60 (0.46-0.73)	1.311
	5	0.73 (0.58-0.87)	
Pain	3	0.73 (0.65-0.80)	1.863
	5	0.63 (0.56-0.70)	
Pulmonary	3	0.75 (0.69-0.81)	0.814
	5	0.71 (0.65-0.76)	
Renal	3	0.50 (0.42-0.57)	0.201
	5	0.48 (0.40-0.57)	
Wound	3	N/A	N/A
	5	0.52 (0.37-0.67)	

*Statistically significant difference between the AUC.

researchers. An additional benefit of reporting a set of core outcome measures would be the reduction of outcome reporting bias. Outcome reporting bias can be defined as the selection for publication of a subset of the originally reported outcome variables based on the results [12].

The POMS is essentially a composite outcome measure, consisting of various domains in which those with multiple items can be collapsed so that each domain becomes a binary outcome. The primary outcome measure can then be considered a composite of the binary outcomes for each domain. A composite outcome measure such as the POMS has a number of inherent advantages over a single clinical endpoint, particularly in clinical trials. Major complications as a core outcome measure have a relatively low event rate; however, the composite measure which combines outcomes increasing the overall incidence of events, improves the power of a study for a set number of participants, or reduces the number of participants required to achieve a preset power. The multi-component nature of composite measures allows researchers the opportunity to be able to describe the disease, or its process, more effectively, particularly in complex states that affect multiple systems such as the inflammatory response and the associated morbidity following major abdominal surgery. The components of a composite measure should describe the outcome of interest, and the POMS was designed by clinicians to reflect clinically important issues that caused patients to remain in hospital after major surgery. Ideally the components should have similar frequency, treatment effects and severity [13,14], however, this is practically difficult in complex disease processes, and can be compensated for by modern statistical methodology, which also allows not only an overall treatment effect to be detected from the composite, but also the effect of the treatment on the individual components [15].

Various statistical methodologies are available to clinically utilize the POMS as a core outcome measure following major abdominal surgery. The composite can be collapsed to a single outcome; however, high frequency items are then over-weighted at the expense of less frequently occurring items that may be more clinically important. Alternatively, a count of events may be employed; however, once again, this can be difficult to interpret unless all events are of an equal severity. Multivariate generalized estimating equation (GEE) methods [16,17] are less affected by issues of unequal severity and frequency [15] and can be described in terms of a common effect GEE in which a treatment effect is estimated across all components of the composite, or an average relative effect GEE in which a treatment effect is estimated for each component. In terms of the POMS as the common effect GEE methods are still biased by events that occur with a higher frequency, a situation that arises in this survey with the gastrointestinal and pain domains having a high frequency, whereas morbidity in the wound domain rarely occurs, the average relative effects GEE is the more appropriate statistical tool to utilize as it compensates for this effect. In addition clinically derived weights for the importance of the various domains can be applied to this model increasing its clinical utility, although these must be assigned prior to data analysis.

Further work is required to simplify the POMS, and to determine which domains and items have poor predictive ability, allowing modification of the survey with additional items with the view to constructing a survey that has acceptable internal consistency, and hence can be used as a scale. Additional consideration is also required as to the potential of weighting individual domains based on perceived clinical importance.

Conclusions

The POMS is reliable, easy to use and shows predictive validity when compared to hospital LOS, and also predicts those subjects who will have a prolonged hospitalization. It has the potential not only to be used as a core outcome measure following major surgery, but also as a tool to aid resource utilization.

Abbreviations
GEE: Generalized estimating equation; LOS: Length of stay; POMS: Postoperative Morbidity Survey.

Competing interests
The authors declare that they have no competing interests.

Authors' contributions
SJD contributed to the study design, conduct of study, data analysis and manuscript preparation. JF and JD participated in data analysis, conduct of the study and manuscript preparation. R JTW helped with the study design, data analysis and manuscript preparation. SJH contributed to study design and manuscript preparation. VA helped with data analysis and manuscript preparation. All authors read and approve the final manuscript.

Author details
[1]Department of Anaesthesia, York Hospitals NHS Foundation Trust, Wigginton Road, York YO31 8HE, UK. [2]Academic Unit of Anaesthesia, Leeds General Infirmary, Great George Street, Leeds LS1 3EX, UK. [3]Hull York Medical School, The University of York, Heslington, York YO10 5DD, UK.

References
1. Visser BC, Keegan H, Martin M, Wren SM: **Death after colectomy: it's later than we think.** *Arch Surg* 2009, **144:**1021–1027.
2. Khuri SF, Henderson WG, DePalma RG, Mosca C, Healey NA, Kumbhani DJ: **Determinants of long-term survival after major surgery and the adverse effect of postoperative complications.** *Ann Surg* 2005, **242:**326–341. Discussion 341–323.
3. Hannan EL, Kilburn H Jr, Racz M, Shields E, Chassin MR: **Improving the outcomes of coronary artery bypass surgery in New York State.** *JAMA* 1994, **271:**761–766.
4. Khuri SF, Henderson WG, Daley J, Jonasson O, Jones RS, Campbell DA Jr, Fink AS, Mentzer RM Jr, Neumayer L, Hammermeister K, Mosca C, Healey N: **Principal Investigators of the Patient Safety in Surgery Study: Successful implementation of the Department of Veterans Affairs' National Surgical Quality Improvement Program in the private sector: the patient safety in surgery study.** *Ann Surg* 2008, **248:**329–336.
5. Bennett-Guerrero E, Welsby I, Dunn TJ, Young LR, Wahl TA, Diers TL, Phillips-Bute BG, Newman MF, Mythen MG: **The use of a postoperative morbidity survey to evaluate patients with prolonged hospitalization after routine, moderate-risk, elective surgery.** *Anesth Analg* 1999, **89:**514–519.
6. Landis JR, Koch GG: **The measurement of observer agreement for categorical data.** *Biometrics* 1977, **33:**159–174.
7. Davies SJ, Yates D, Wilson RJ: **Dopexamine has no additional benefit in high-risk patients receiving goal-directed fluid therapy undergoing major abdominal surgery.** *Anesth Analg* 2010, **112:**130–138.
8. Stone MD, Wilson RJ, Cross J, Williams BT: **Effect of adding dopexamine to intraoperative volume expansion in patients undergoing major elective abdominal surgery.** *Br J Anaesth* 2003, **91:**619–624.
9. Grocott MP, Browne JP, Van der Meulen J, Matejowsky C, Mutch M, Hamilton MA, Levett DZ, Emberton M, Haddad FS, Mythen MG: **The postoperative morbidity survey was validated and used to describe morbidity after major surgery.** *J Clin Epidemiol* 2007, **60:**919–928.
10. Viera AJ, Garrett JM: **Understanding interobserver agreement: the kappa statistic.** *Fam Med* 2005, **37:**360–363.
11. Sinha S, Ashby E, Jayaram R, Grocott MP: **Quality of reporting in randomized trials published in high-quality surgical journals.** *J Am Coll Surg* 2009, **209:**565–571.
12. Hutton JLWP: **Bias in meta-analysis due to outcome variable selection within studies.** *Appl Stat* 2000, **49:**359–370.
13. Chi GY: **Some issues with composite endpoints in clinical trials.** *Fundam Clin Pharmacol* 2005, **19:**609–619.
14. Tomlinson G, Detsky AS: **Composite end points in randomized trials: there is no free lunch.** *JAMA* 2010, **303:**267–268.
15. Mascha EJ, Sessler DI: **Statistical grand rounds: design and analysis of studies with binary- event composite endpoints: guidelines for anesthesia research.** *Anesth Analg* 2011, **112:**1461–1471.
16. Liang KY, Zeger SL: **Longitudinal data analysis using generalized linear models.** *Biometrika* 1986, **73:**13–22.
17. Zeger SL, Liang KY: **Longitudinal data analysis for discrete and continuous outcomes.** *Biometrics* 1986, **42:**121–130.

2

Incidence and characteristic analysis of in-hospital falls after anesthesia

Chen-Fuh Lam[1], Shiu-Ying Hsieh[1], Jen-Hung Wang[2], Hui-Shan Pan[1], Xiu-Zhu Liu[1], Yu-Ching Ho[3] and Tsung-Ying Chen[1*]

Abstract

Background: In-hospital falls may result in serious clinical adverse consequences, but the effects of anesthesia in the occurrence of postoperative falls are still undetermined. Anesthesia may theoretically cause postoperative falls due to the residual pharmacologic and neuromuscular blocking effects of anesthetics. We retrospectively reviewed events of in-hospital falls occurred after anesthesia management to identify the incidence and risk factors of postanesthesia falls.

Methods: We reviewed the postanesthesia visit of patients received anesthesia in the Hualien Buddhist Tzu Chi General Hospital from January 2009 to December 2013. Falls happened within 24 h after anesthesia were recorded. The Poisson regression model was used for simultaneous analysis of the association between incidence proportion of postanesthesia falls and the potential risk factors.

Results: A total of 60,796 inpatients received anesthesia management over the past 5 years, and ten patients fell within 24 h after anesthesia. All cases happened in the general wards. Falls occurred more often at the bedside, presence of caregivers, and during the daytime. Patients underwent regional anesthesia, and old age significantly increased the risk of postanesthesia falls, while differences in gender and ASA physical status did not affect the occurrence of postanesthesia falls.

Conclusions: The overall incidence proportion of postanesthesia falls is 1.6 cases per 10,000 patients (95 % CI 0.006 to 0.026 %) over a 24-h observation period. Falls are more commonly happened during the less expected periods after operation and are increased in the elderly and patients received regional anesthesia. This study highlights that more comprehensive clinical practice guidelines for postoperative care should be exercised to prevent the in-hospital falls.

Keywords: Accidental falls, Poisson distribution, Postoperative complications, Regional anesthesia

Background

Postoperative falls are a relatively rare complication that could have been overlooked in clinical anesthesia. In-hospital falls are particularly serious events resulting in bone fracture, traumatic head injury, visceral organ contusion, and skin abrasion. These in-hospital adverse events not only increase the length of hospital stay and cause extraneous medical expense but may also engender unnecessary medical disputes (Bates et al. 1995; Mion et al. 2012). Therefore, the implementation of preventive strategies for in-hospital falls has been an important practical issue in the hospital care (Hempel et al. 2013). However, the investigation of the in-hospital falls during the postoperative period is insufficient (Amador and Loera 2007; Church et al. 2011). The overall incidence of postoperative falls was 1.6–1.8 % in a veteran's medical center with an average time to falling of 12 days after operation (Church et al. 2011). The incidence of postoperative falls may theoretically increase in patients receiving anesthetic management due to the residual pharmacologic and neuromuscular blocking effects of anesthetics. However, the anesthetic

* Correspondence: chenyting@mail.tcu.edu.tw
This work was accepted to present at the European Anaesthesiology Congress, Euroanaesthesia 2016, London, UK in May 2016.
[1]Department of Anesthesiology, Buddhist Tzu Chi General Hospital and Tzu Chi University School of Medicine, No 707, Chung-Yang Road Section 3, Hualien 970, Taiwan, Republic of China
Full list of author information is available at the end of the article

effect on the postoperative falls is hard to identify from these previous studies, and there is currently no study reported the incidence of postanesthesia falls. Therefore, we retrospectively reviewed the postanesthesia records (2009 to 2013) in our department and analyzed the characteristics of in-hospital falls after anesthesia management. Our long-term aim is to identify the risk factors contributing to falls during the postanesthesia period and to promote prevention programs in the surgical patients who carry high risk of in-hospital falls.

Methods

Patient database and study design

This retrospective chart-review study was approved by the ethics committee and the institutional review board (IRB, Approval number IRB103-14-B) of Hualien Buddhist Tzu Chi General Hospital Taiwan, and the requirement for written informed consent was waived by the ethics committee. Our hospital is a tertiary teaching medical center located at Hualien City of Taiwan that consists of 945 beds. In-hospital patients, who received anesthesia management for surgical or other medical interventions from January 2009 to December 2013, were visited at bedside postoperatively by nurse anesthetists. The postoperative visit recorded the pain scores, patient satisfaction to anesthesia service, and anesthesia-related complications. All adverse events after operation recorded by the ward nurses were reviewed. Falls were defined as sudden events which resulted in a person coming to rest inadvertently on the ground or floor or other lower levels (Haines et al. 2013). The medical records of all patients reported of having in-hospital falls within 24 h after operation were reviewed by the staff anesthesiologists to determine the characteristics of falls. Patients who received only regional infiltration of local anesthetics and who were discharged from hospital within 24 h after operation were excluded.

Statistical analysis

The overall incidence proportion of postanesthesia falls over a 24-h observation period was calculated as the number of falls divided by total number of in-hospital surgical patients who received anesthesia management. The potential risk factors included patient demographic and clinical variables, namely patient age groups, genders, American Society of Anesthesiologists (ASA) classifications of physical status, and types of anesthesia. Poisson regression model was adopted to evaluate the association between these risk factors and postanesthesia falls. The model fitted reasonably well as the goodness-of-fit chi-squared test was not statistically significant ($p = 0.995$). Statistical significance was accepted at a level of $P < 0.05$. All statistical analyses were performed by using SAS 9.4 (SAS Institute, Inc., Cary, North Carolina).

Results

Patient characterization

From January 1, 2009 to December 31, 2013, there were a total of 78,064 individuals who received anesthesia management during surgical or other invasive interventions in the Hualien Buddhist Tzu Chi General Hospital, Taiwan, and 60,796 (77.9 %) of these patients were hospitalized for at least 24 h after anesthesia. The demographic characteristics of patients and types of operation are summarized in Table 1. The overall completion rate of in-hospital visit after anesthesia was 98.7 ± 0.5 % over the past 5 years and less than 0.5 % of missing data were found in our electronic data bank.

Postanesthesia falls

Events of falls within 24 h after anesthesia management were recorded in ten patients over the 5-year study period

Table 1 Demographic characteristics of patients received anesthesia management during January 2009 to December 2013 ($n = 78{,}064$)

Patient characteristics	*N* (%)
Age (years old)	
0–10	2051 (2.6)
11–30	8409 (10.7)
31–50	23,143 (27.6)
51–70	31,226 (40.0)
>70	13,235 (16.9)
Gender	
M	39,941 (51.2)
F	38,105 (48.8)
ASA class[a]	
I	16,889 (21.6)
II	38,657 (49.5)
III	20,861 (26.7)
IV	1511 (1.9)
V	133 (0.2)
Emergency operation	3616 (4.7)
Type of anesthesia	
General anesthesia	57,619 (73.8)
Intravenous sedation anesthesia	18,100 (23.2)
Regional and other anesthesia techniques	2345 (3)
Admission after operation	
General wards	63,778 (81.7)
Intensive care units	7026 (9.0)
Discharged from recovery room	7182 (9.2)
Others	78 (0.1)
Completion of postoperative visits (in-hospital)	97.8 %

[a]A total of 13 patients were classed as ASA VI, who were admitted for organ transplant

(Table 2). The incidence proportion of in-hospital falls after anesthesia was 0.016 % (95 % CI 0.006 to 0.026 %) over 24 h of observation. The average time of postoperative falls was 13.3 ± 8.4 (range 2.6–24) hours. All events of postanesthesia falls occurred at the general wards, as no falling events were reported from the special care. Table 3 illustrates the geographic and other characteristics of falling, including timing and location of falls. Most of these events were minor and did not result in prolonged hospital stay, but there were three victims who were more seriously injured who required extraneous medical or surgical attentions (Table 2).

Analysis of risk stratification indicated that gender and the ASA physical status of the patients with falls were not significantly different from the total and other in-hospital patients (Tables 4 and 5). However, age and types of anesthetic techniques were significant and independent risk factors for the occurrence of postanesthesia falls (Tables 4 and 5). Compared with younger ages, patients who were older (40–70, mean age of 65 ± 15 years) carried significantly higher incidence proportion of postanesthesia falls ($P < 0.001$). In addition, higher incidence proportions of postanesthesia falls were also found in patients who received regional anesthesia (neuroaxial blocks) and intravenous sedation anesthesia ($P < 0.001$ and $P = 0.002$, respectively).

Discussion

We present the first clinical report analyzing the incidence and risk factors of in-hospital falls within 24 h after anesthesia management. The overall incidence proportion of postanesthesia falls was at least 1.6 cases per 10,000 patients over a 24-h observation period. Patients with older age and who received regional anesthesia or intravenous sedation anesthesia carried significantly higher incidence proportion of postanesthesia falls. Falls happened more often during the relatively less expected periods and locations after operation, such as at the bedside, presence of caregivers, and during the daytime. Although most of these events did not result in serious consequences, there were considerable proportions of patients (30 %) who required additional medical or surgical attentions.

Successful surgical and anesthesia managements do not necessarily guarantee the avoidance of postoperative complications or adverse events. Therefore, several preoperative risk assessment systems have been developed to reduce the occurrence of postoperative adverse events (Barnett and Moonesinghe 2011; Hariharan and Zbar 2006). However, the identification of the incidence and risk factors of the rare adverse events is more challenging, as the conduction of prospective clinical studies is impractical and could be insensitive to detect the low incidence events. Therefore, the access to a comprehensive medical record of postoperative visit may be an acceptable alternative to prospective trials in the identification of the rare postoperative adverse events.

Postoperative falls are one of the relatively rare complications that could have been overlooked in clinical practice. There is currently very limited information in the study and prevention programs for postoperative falls (Church et al. 2011). Church et al. conducted a comprehensive retrospective study analyzing the occurrence of postoperative falls in patients admitted to a tertiary Veteran hospital for more than 23 h after surgery (Church et al. 2011). They reported that 154 male patients experienced 190 falls in a total of 9625 inpatient surgical procedures over the 5-year study period, thereby yielding an overall incidence of postoperative falls of 1.6 %. The authors found that older age,

Table 2 Characteristics of postanesthesia falls

Patient ID	Gender	Age (years)	ASA class	Type of surgery	Type of anesthesia	Injury after fall	Hours after anesthesia	Outcome
1	M	66	3	Debridement of hip wound	LMA	Scalp laceration	24	Wound repair
2	M	76	2	Herniorrhaphy	SA	NP	9.7	
3	F	64	2	Hemorrhoidectomy	IV sedation	NP	3.3	
4	M	61	2	FESS	ETGA	Scalp laceration	23.3	Wound repair
5	F	36	3	Arteriovenous graft	LMA	Head injury	19.8	Admitted to ICU
6	M	71	3	Endoscopic examination	IVG	NP	2.6	
7	F	52	1	Sling operation	SA	NP	8.5	
8	M	92	3	TURP	SA	Humeral fracture	23.5	ORIF
9	M	83	2	Endoscopic examination	IV sedation	Shoulder contusion	3.6	X-ray examination
10	F	53	2	Knee arthroplasty	LMA + NB	NP	14.6	

FESS functional endoscopic sinus surgery, *IV sedation* intravenous sedation anesthesia, *ICU* intensive care unit, *LMA* laryngeal mask anesthesia, *NB* femoral nerve block for pain control, *NP* nothing in particular, *ORIF* open reduction and internal fixation surgery, *SA* spinal anesthesia, *TUPP* transurethral resection of the prostate

Table 3 Characteristics of postanesthesia falls

Characteristics of fall events	*n* (%)
Time of fall	
Daytime (7:00–18:00)	7 (70)
Nighttime (18:01–06:59)	3 (30)
Place of fall	
Bedside	6 (60)
Washroom	4 (40)
Presence of accompany	
Yes	6 (60)
No	4 (40)
Attempts of getting off bed	
First	4 (40)
>1 attempts	6 (60)

ASA class > III, low albumin level, longer surgical time, and increased blood transfusion were the independent risk factors for postoperative falls. Nevertheless, the effects of anesthesia on the occurrence of postoperative falls are still undetermined and are unable to generalize from these previous studies.

Table 4 Risk stratification for postanesthesia falls

Patient characteristics	All patients (total 78,064) *n* (%)	In-hospital patients (total 60,796) *n* (%)	Postanesthesia falls (total 10) *n* (%)
Age (years old)			
0–10	2051 (2.6)	1385 (2.3)	0 (0)
11–30	8409 (10.7)	7544 (12.4)	0 (0)
31–50	23,143 (27.6)	17,498 (28.8)	1 (10)
51–70	31,226 (40.0)	22,594 (37.2)	5 (50)
>70	13,235 (16.9)	11,775 (19.3)	4 (40)
Gender			
Male	39,941 (51.2)	33,391 (54.9)	6 (60)
Female	38,105 (48.8)	27,405 (45.1)	4 (40)
ASA classification[a]			
I	16,889 (21.6)	9597 (15.8)	1 (10)
II	38,657 (49.5)	29,733 (46.0)	5 (50)
III	20,861 (26.7)	19,821 (32.6)	4 (40)
IV	1511 (1.9)	1500 (2.5)	0 (0)
V	133 (0.2)	132 (0.2)	0 (0)
Types of anesthesia			
General anesthesia	57,619 (73.8)	54,423 (89.5)	4 (40)
Intravenous sedation anesthesia	18,100 (23.2)	4057 (6.7)	3 (30)
Regional and other anesthesia techniques	2345 (3)	2316 (3.8)	3 (30)

[a]A total of 13 patients were classed as ASA VI, who were admitted for organ transplant

Table 5 Poisson regression analysis of the risk factors in the occurrence of postanesthesia falls

Risk factor	Regression coefficient	95 % CI	*P* value
Intercept	−34.434	(−36.158, −32.711)	<0.001
Gender			
Male	Ref	Ref	NA
Female	−0.012	(−1.303, 1.280)	0.986
Age			
≦30 years old	Ref	Ref	NA
31–50 years old	23.799	(21.489, 26.108)	<0.001
51–70 years old	25.408	(23.982, 26.834)	<0.001
>70 years old	25.555	(25.555, 25.555)	NA
ASA class			
I–II	Ref	Ref	NA
III–IV	−0.132	(−1.498, 1.235)	0.850
Anesthesia technique			
General anesthesia	Ref	Ref	NA
Intravenous sedation anesthesia	2.364	(0.853, 3.875)	0.002
Regional anesthesia	2.828	(1.267, 4.390)	<0.001

Reference groups were chosen according to the subgroup with highest proportion (i.e., male group, ASA class, and general anesthesia) or the first subgroup in the analysis
CI confidence interval, *Ref* reference value, *NA* not applicable

The Hualien Buddhist Tzu Chi General Hospital is a tertiary university hospital and admits all patient populations. The in-hospital postanesthesia visit recorded the anesthetic outcomes and complications detected within 24 h after anesthesia, with an average annual conclusion rate of greater than 97 % in 2009 to 2013. Therefore, the postanesthesia visiting records in our department may provide a reliable database for the analysis of the in-hospital adverse events that happened after anesthesia in the general population. All postoperative adverse events were reported by the ward nurses and our nurse anesthetists recorded the events occurred within 24 h after anesthesia, as the pharmacologic effects of anesthetic agents are theoretically diminished and most of the patients are recovered from the neuromuscular block.

A total of ten events of postanesthesia falls were recorded from 60,796 in-hospital anesthesia procedures during the 5-year study period. The incidence proportion of falls after operation was considerably less than that reported by Church et al. (0.016 vs 1.6 %). Obviously, the observational period of the later was longer (24 h vs 30 days postoperatively) and the later recruited surgical patients who received only local anesthesia. Contrarily, postanesthesia falls developed within 24 h after anesthesia resulted in much more serious injuries that required surgical or medical interventions (30 vs 0.3 %). These serious complications included traumatic head injury, bone fracture and ICU admission, and thus lengthening the in-hospital treatment course. Head-to-head comparison of the severity of outcomes after falling between these two studies is infeasible, since the studied populations and anesthetic interventions were incommensurable. In our opinion, the residual anesthetic and neuromuscular blocking effects might have contributed to the more severe adverse clinical outcomes in patients with postanesthesia falls.

Our study outlined a few extraordinary findings in the occurrence of falls after anesthesia. More postanesthesia falls happened during at the bedside, with the presence of caregivers and after the first uneventful getting off the bed. Consistent with a most recent study (Ikutomo et al. 2015), our study also found that in-hospital falls were often reported during daytime. Patients and the accompanists could become less cautious when the patients moved about in these situations, as these are generally considered as safer scenarios during postoperative care. In addition, we also found that all events of postanesthesia falls occurred at general wards, but not in other special care units, since patients admitted to these units are more seriously ill and are mostly confined to bed after operation. Although these characteristic analyses of falls are descriptive and statistical analysis is not applicable, our study underscores that the preventive strategy for postanesthesia falls should also be comprised to all postoperative periods during the inpatient care (Ikutomo et al. 2015).

We identified four potential independent risk factors for the development of postanesthesia falls from the postanesthesia visit records, namely gender, age, ASA classification, and types of anesthesia techniques. Advanced age has been widely recognized as an independent risk factor for inpatient falls (Marschollek et al. 2012; Oliver et al. 2010). In traumatic patients, male gender is associated with high incidence of in-hospital falls (Brown et al. 2013). The ASA classification is a useful functional assessment tool for the physical status of surgical patients. Higher ASA classes predict the occurrence of falls in the postoperative periods (Church et al. 2011). These common reported factors were included in our analysis. In comparison to subpopulation groups (i.e., trauma and veteran patients) (Church et al. 2011; Brown et al. 2013), our study in the general patient population did not suggest that differences in gender and ASA classification affect the occurrence of falls within 24 h after anesthesia. In our hospital, patients with advanced ASA classes (≥III) were more often admitted to the special medical units for intensive postoperative care and thus might reduce the potential risk of falling during the first postoperative day. Nevertheless, we admit that patients with impaired physical status (high ASA classes) are conceivably more vulnerable to falling in the subsequent hospital care after operation (>24 h). Consistent with the previous reports, our investigation indicated that the incidence proportion of postanesthesia falling is significantly increased in patients with older age (mean age of 65 ± 15 years). Patients of older ages are more susceptible to falls due to multiple interacting intrinsic and extrinsic etiologies, such as comorbidity diseases, postural hypotension, muscle weakness, impaired gait, and presence of environmental hazards in hospital (Rubenstein 2006; Gschwind et al. 2011).

The core objective of this study is to determine the impact of anesthesia in the development of falls after surgical or other invasive interventions in the general population. Poisson statistical analysis clearly indicates that types of anesthesia significantly affect the occurrence of in-hospital falls within 24 h after anesthesia management. Incidence proportion of postanesthesia falls was significantly increased in patients who received neuroaxial block. Although neuroaxial blockade does not seem to impair the balance control (Suarez and Macadar 2008), the recovery of sensory and muscle power is usually unpredictable and the unassisted ambulation is longer than it is assumed (Imarengiaye et al. 2003). Furthermore, the motor and functional recoveries are variable between individual subjects following intrathecal administration of different local anesthetics (Frey et al. 1998). In clinical practice, we recommend that patient ambulation should only be allowed 8 h after regional block, and we do not routinely check the recovery profiles of patients after discharged from the recovery room. Therefore, it could be the main reason that patients might undertake unassisted ambulation without recognizing the incomplete recovery of muscle power of the lower extremities, and thus resulted in falling. We also realize that the three patients who fell after spinal anesthesia were even older (52, 76, and 92 years) than the mean age of all other falling cases (62 years). Furthermore, there was a postoperative fall patient received inhalational anesthesia via laryngeal mask for knee replacement surgery, and single injection of femoral nerve block was applied as an adjunct for perioperative pain management. Although the sample size is too small to draw any conclusive statements, our results are consistent with the previous reports that suggested that regional nerve blockade in older patients could further increase the risk of postoperative falls (Wasserstein et al. 2013). Administration of peripheral nerve block in knee operation has been reported to increase the risk of postoperative falls (Muraskin et al. 2007; Sharma et al. 2010), particularly with the application of continuous lumbar plexus blockade (Johnson et al. 2013). Therefore, any pharmacologic inhibition of nerve conduction in lower extremities following central or peripheral nerve blockade could contribute to the increased risk of postoperative falls. In addition, we detected a significant increased incidence proportion of postoperative falls in patients who received intravenous sedation anesthesia for less invasive procedures, such as endoscopic examination and simple hemorrhoidectomy. These three patients who received intravenous anesthesia were generally less seriously ill (ASA class II-III), and falls happened within 4 h after anesthesia. The reasons for post-anesthesia falls in patients received sedation anesthesia are unclear, but these fall events could probably be preventable if higher attention was applied to the post-operative period, even though the anesthesia management was less invasive.

Limitations of the study

There are several limitations in our study. This is a retrospective case-series chart-review study, and it could therefore be subjected to incomplete collection of all cases throughout the studied period. However, we admit that in-hospital falls has been an imperative monitoring parameter of health care quality assurance in our hospital. Therefore, missing of case record is most unlikely to happen. In addition, prevention of in-hospital falls has been one of the most important medical care issues in our hospital, as the "anti-falling partition board" was established by the medical and nursing staff in 2005. The occurrence of falling has thus significantly reduced after the application of fall prevention programs. Following the introduction of laryngeal mask airway, the use of regional anesthesia has reduced in our hospital due to the improved safety profile with general anesthesia. As a result, the total number of regional anesthesia in our hospital is relatively lower than other institutes. Our postanesthesia visit recorded only the identifications of the patients and did not contain patients' laboratory data and the perioperative medicine. Hence, we were not able to demonstrate the potential effects of these factors in the occurrence of in-hospital falls after anesthesia. Nevertheless, gender, age, ASA class, and anesthesia techniques are the four most indispensable patient demographical data that should be available in the record of all institutes worldwide. We address that these simple, but basic parameters, may provide useful information in the identification of the high-risk groups of postanesthesia falls.

Conclusion

The overall incidence proportion of postanesthesia falls is at least 1.6 cases per 10,000 patients over a 24-h observation period. Falls are more commonly happened during the less expected periods after operation and are increased in the elderly and patients who received regional anesthesia. This study highlights that more comprehensive clinical practice guidelines for postoperative care should be exercised to prevent the in-hospital falls.

Abbreviations

ASA: American Society of Anesthesiologists; IRB: institutional review board.

Acknowledgements

This work was supported by research funds from the Buddhist Tzu Chi General Hospital (grant numbers TCRD104-27 to C.F.L. and TCRD104-26 to T.Y.C.).

Authors' contributions

CF contributed to the study conception, study design, data analysis, and writing the article. SY, HS, and XZ carried out the data collection and clinical case analysis. JH performed the data analysis and interpretation. YC contributed to the data analysis and critical revision of the article. TY conceived the study and participated in its design and coordination. All authors read and approved the final manuscript.

Competing interests

The authors declare that they have no competing interests.

Author details

[1]Department of Anesthesiology, Buddhist Tzu Chi General Hospital and Tzu Chi University School of Medicine, No 707, Chung-Yang Road Section 3, Hualien 970, Taiwan, Republic of China. [2]Department of Medical Research, Tzu Chi General Hospital, Hualien, Taiwan. [3]Department of Health Administration, Tzu Chi University of Science and Technology, Hualien, Taiwan.

References

Amador LF, Loera JA. Preventing postoperative falls in the older adult. J Am Coll Surg. 2007;204:447–52.

Barnett S, Moonesinghe SR. Clinical risk scores to guide perioperative management. Postgrad Med J. 2011;87:535–41.

Bates DW, Pruess K, Souney P, Platt R. Serious falls in hospitalized patients: correlates and resource utilization. Am J Med. 1995;99:137–43.

Brown CV, Ali S, Fairly R, Lai BK, Arthrell J, Walker M, Tips G. Risk factors for falls among hospitalized trauma patients. Ann Surg. 2013;79:465–9.

Church S, Robinson TN, Angles EM, Tran ZV, Wallace JI. Postoperative falls in the acute hospital setting: characteristics, risk factors, and outcomes in males. Am J Surg. 2011;201:197–202.

Frey K, Holman S, Mikat-Stevens M, Vazquez J, White L, Pedicini E, Sheikh T, Kao TC, Kleinman B, Stevens RA. The recovery profile of hyperbaric spinal anesthesia with lidocaine, tetracaine, and bupivacaine. Reg Anesth Pain Med. 1998;23:159–63.

Gschwind YJ, Wolf I, Bridenbaugh SA, Kressig RW. Basis for a Swiss perspective on fall prevention in vulnerable older people. Swiss Med Wkly. 2011;141:w13305.

Haines TP, Hill AM, Hill KD, Brauer SG, Hoffmann TT, Etherton-Beer C, McPhail SM. Cost effectiveness of patient education for the prevention of falls in hospital: economic evaluation from a randomized controlled trial. BMC Med. 2013;11:135.

Hariharan S, Zbar A. Risk scoring in perioperative and surgical intensive care patients: a review. Curr Surg. 2006;63:226–36.

Hempel S, Newberry S, Wang Z, Booth M, Shanman R, Johnsen B, Shier V, Saliba D, Spector WD, Ganz DA. Hospital fall prevention: a systematic review of implementation, components, adherence, and effectiveness. J Am Geriatr Soc. 2013;61:483–94.

Ikutomo H, Nagai K, Nakagawa N, Masuhara K. Falls in patients after total hip arthroplasty in Japan. J Orthop Sci. 2015;20:663–8.

Imarengiaye CO, Song D, Prabhu AJ, Chung F. Spinal anesthesia: functional balance is impaired after clinical recovery. Anesthesiology. 2003;98:511–5.

Johnson RL, Kopp SL, Hebl JR, Erwin PJ, Mantilla CB. Falls and major orthopaedic surgery with peripheral nerve blockade: a systematic review and meta-analysis. Br J Anaesth. 2013;110:518–28.

Marschollek M, Govercin M, Rust S, Gietzell M, Schulze M, Wolf KH, Steinhagen-Thiessen E. Mining geriatric assessment data for in-patient fall prediction models and high-risk subgroups. BMC Med Inform Decis Mak. 2012;14:12–9.

Mion LC, Chandler AM, Waters TM, Dietrich MS, Kessler LA, Miller ST, Shorr RI. Is it possible to identify risks for injurious falls in hospitalized patients? Jt Comm J Qual Patient Saf. 2012;38:408–513.

Muraskin SI, Conrad B, Zheng N, Morey TE, Enneking FK. Falls associated with lower-extremity-nerve blocks: a pilot investigation of mechanisms. Reg Anesth Pain Med. 2007;32:67–72.
Oliver D, Healey F, Haines TP. Preventing falls and fall-related injuries in hospitals. Clin Geriatr Med. 2010;26:645–92.
Rubenstein LZ. Falls in older people: epidemiology, risk factors and strategies for prevention. Age Ageing. 2006;35:ii37–41.
Sharma S, Lorio R, Specht LM, Davies-Lepie S, Healy WL. Complications of femoral nerve block for total knee arthroplasty. Clin Orthop Relat Res. 2010;468:135–40.
Suarez A, Macadar O. The effect of general and spinal anesthesia on balance control in elderly patients. Int Tinnitus J. 2008;14:146–51.
Wasserstein D, Farlinger C, Brull R, Mahomed N, Gandhi R. Advanced age, obesity and continuous femoral nerve blockade are independent risk factors for inpatient falls after primary total knee arthroplasty. J Arthroplasty. 2013;28:1121–4.

3

A prospective case series evaluating use of an in-line air detection and purging system to reduce air burden during major surgery

Yussr M. Ibrahim[1], Nicole R. Marques[1], Carlos R. Garcia[1], Michael Salter[1], Christopher McQuitty[1], Michael Kinsky[1*], Mindy Juan[2] and Achiau Ludomirsky[3]

Abstract

Background: Intravascular air embolism (AE) is a preventable but potentially catastrophic complication caused by intravenous tubing, trauma, and diagnostic and surgical procedures. The potentially fatal risks of arterial AE are well-known, and emerging evidence demonstrates impact of venous AEs on inflammatory response and coagulation factors. A novel FDA-approved in-line air detection and purging system was used to detect and remove air caused by administering a rapid fluid bolus during surgery.

Methods: A prospective, randomized, case series was conducted. Subjects were observed using standard monitors, including transesophageal echocardiography (TEE) in the operating room. After general anesthesia was induced, an introducer and pulmonary artery catheter was inserted in the right internal jugular to administer fluids and monitor cardiac pressures. Six patients undergoing cardiac surgery were studied. Each patient received four randomized fluid boluses: two with the in-line air purging device, two without. For each bolus, a bulb infuser was squeezed three times (10–15 mL) over 5 s. The TEE was positioned in the mid-esophageal right atrium (RA) to quantify peak air clearance, and images were video recorded throughout each bolus. Air was quantified using optical densitometry (OD) from images demonstrating maximal air in the RA.

Results: All subjects demonstrated significantly lower air burden when the air reduction device was used ($p = 0.004$), and the average time to clear 90% of air was also lower, 3.7 ± 1.2 s vs. 5.3 ± 1.3 s ($p < 0.001$).

Conclusion: An air purging system reduced air burden from bolus administration and could consequently reduce the risk of harmful or fatal AEs during surgery.

Keywords: Air embolism, Intravenous, ClearLine IV, Anesthesia, Fluid warmers

Background

Intravascular air embolism (AE) occurs when undesired air enters the venous or arterial circulation, typically during medical procedures (Mirski et al. 2007; McCarthy et al. 2017). Once air enters the patient, symptoms range from subtle physiologic changes to potentially catastrophic events. The impact of AEs depends upon factors including the patient's physiology, size of the air mass, and the path air takes through the anatomy (Mirski et al. 2007; Orliaguet and Martin 2000; Brull and Prielipp 2017). AEs may enter the vasculature during major surgeries such as neurosurgery, or during less complex procedures including administration of medications, fluids, or blood products through intravenous tubing, intravenous catheter placement, or during diagnostic procedures (Bayliss et al. 2014). AEs may be comprised of atmospheric air or medical gases including nitrous oxide, carbon dioxide, helium, and nitrogen (Mitchell et al. 2000; McGrath et al. 1989).

When entering the venous system in healthy individuals, air is usually broken up in the capillary bed of the lungs. However, studies demonstrate that entrapment of venous air in the pulmonary microcirculation can decrease gas exchange and cause pulmonary vascular

* Correspondence: mkinsky@utmb.edu
[1]Department of Anesthesiology, The University of Texas Medical Branch, Galveston, TX, USA
Full list of author information is available at the end of the article

obstruction, potentially leading to release of vasoactive mediators. Ultimately, this may result in cellular injury and lung edema (van Hulst et al. 2003). Larger volumes of venous air can increase pulmonary artery pressure and right ventricular strain, resulting in systemic cardiovascular collapse (Muth and Shank 2000; Agarwal et al. 2009).

A paradoxical AE occurs when venous air enters arterial circulation, such as in the case of an atrial or ventricular septal defect (ASD and VSD). In cases of large venous AE, the filter capacity of the pulmonary capillary bed becomes overwhelmed and air may translocate to the arterial circulation, more often in patients with a patent foramen ovale (PFO) as well as an ASD or VSD, thereby allowing direct air passage from the venous to arterial system (Girard et al. 2003; Park et al. 2010). This phenomenon provides considerable risk since most PFOs are undiagnosed and occur in 10 to 25% of the population (Mirski et al. 2007; Brull and Prielipp 2017; Vesely 2001; Foster et al. 2003). The closer the air entry to the right heart, the lesser the volume of air required to cause fatality (McCarthy et al. 2017). Systemic inflammatory response syndrome (SIRS) can also result from AEs (Kapoor and Gutierrez 2003; Hsieh et al. 2009).

Clinicians are trained to reduce AE risk by priming intravenous tubing and use devices including Luer-lock connectors, filters, and modern infusion systems which may alarm on detection of AE. Despite this, AEs have been reported in cases of emergency, in cases of home intravenous treatment, or due to failures of pump air-in-line sensors or other device malfunctions (Laskey et al. 2002; Wilkins and Unverdorben 2012; Paul Pelletier and Fisher 2017).

The use of pressure infusion devices and fluid-warmers increases AE risk. Pressurized infusion devices rapidly deliver intravenous (IV) fluid, and air entrainment can occur from errors in manual setup. Pressurized infusion devices have limited and variable capability to detect and remove air during infusions (Schnoor et al. 2004; Zoremba et al. 2011; Woon and Talke 1999; Smith et al. 2001). As fluid is warmed, micro- and macro-bubbles dissipate from the fluid as it is heated. Air from IV tubing can be due to direct air injection or delivered into the circulation when IV fluid is heated. Specifically, this occurs when fluids are actively heated from room temperature (as often case with crystalloid fluids) or from chilled (blood and blood products). The concentration of dissolved air is based on pressure and temperature. According to Henry's law, the dissolved gas is a function of temperature, where, as temperature increases, dissolved gas/air comes out of solution in form of bubbles. Outgassing and air production when heated to 41 °C can yield 1–5 mL per liter of fluid (with colder fluids such as blood products yielding higher volumes) (Varga et al. 2016). While in-line filters help remove particulate contamination and entrapped air, they may increase flow resistance, limiting usefulness when administering rapid fluid boluses. AEs are costly events. Data from the American Society of Anesthesiologists Closed Claims Project showed 100% of claims for venous AE resulted in payment with a median of $325,000 (Brull and Prielipp 2017).

A novel device ClearLine IV™ (ClearLine MD, Woburn, MA, USA) is cleared by the FDA for automatic detection and removal of in-line air at a minimum volume of 25 μL, a quantity below that is shown to cause patient harm. This pilot study was conducted to quantify air entering a patient during bolus infusion and to test our hypothesis that ClearLine IV successfully identifies and reduces patient's air burden during major surgery.

Methods

The study protocol was approved by the Institutional Review Board (IRB), and all patients provided written informed consent prior to undergoing study procedures. Eligible patients included adults, ages 18 to 80, undergoing cardiac surgery, who were not pregnant at the time of screening. Major exclusions include malignant hypertension, esophageal disease, severe heart failure, pulmonary hypertension, and those undergoing emergency surgery. Cardiac surgery patients were chosen since they normally undergo monitoring that would permit the quantification of air necessary for the study.

The study was a case series of prospective, randomized, crossover design conducted at a single center. Enrollment occurred between November 2016 and January of 2017. Following consent, standard of care monitors and central lines were used to administer general anesthesia. After induction of anesthesia, an 8.5-Fr Cordis introducer with a pulmonary artery catheter (Edwards Lifescience, Irvine, CA, USA) was inserted in the right internal jugular to administer fluids and monitor cardiac pressures. Warmed crystalloid was delivered using HOTLINE® (HL90 Hotline Level 1, Smiths Medical, Rockland, MD, USA) with a blood filter and pressure pump (Baxter, Deerfield, IL, USA) in-line with the ClearLine IV (treatment) or via tubing, bypassing the ClearLine IV system (control) (Fig. 1).

ClearLine IV consists of a control unit and a sterile disposable component (infusion catheter). The device connects to infusion lines and uses ultrasonic sensors to detect air volumes as small as 25 μL. Once detected, the device diverts fluid flow to a waste collection bag and a second ultrasonic sensor detects when the air has been removed, at which time the controller automatically restarts the infusion flow to the patient. This device only briefly (seconds) interrupts the intravenous infusion and results in less than 10 mL fluid lost per air-removal cycle.

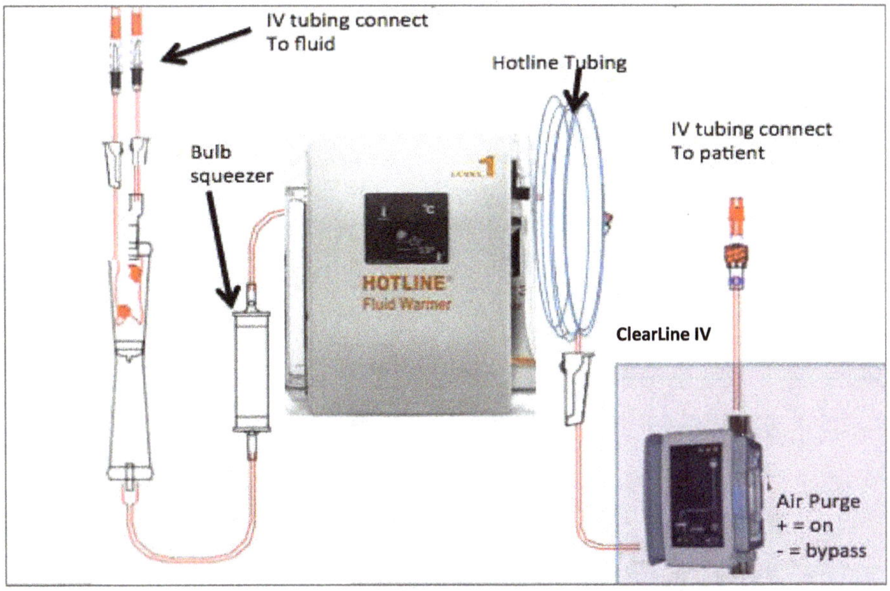

Fig. 1 Setup for IV fluid administration. Fluid administration setup with ClearLine IV. Ultrasound sensing technology detects and diverts air from the IV line to a collection bag through opening of a valve to a waste reservoir. The fluid is redirected to the patient line after the air is entrapped through another valve opening or can be bypassed (blue lines). IV: intravenous

For each bolus delivery, a pressure infuser (bulb) was squeezed three times, delivering a volume of 10 to 20 mL each time over the course of 5 s per single bolus, as is done per standard of care during cardiac procedures. Flow rates were measured by a modified scale that measured the change in mass (grams) over time (min). Each IV fluid bag was suspended from the scale and zeroed prior to bolus. We assumed that each 1 g was equivalent to 1 mL. Each bolus was followed by a 60- to 90-s pause. Each patient received four randomized boluses: two with ClearLine IV and two control boluses. Bolus order was assigned using a randomized block design to determine assignment of the first fluid bolus. Thereafter, the first and third and the second and fourth boluses were paired. Transesophageal echocardiography (TEE) (Vivid GE, Milwaukee WI) was used throughout the procedure.

When fluids are heated by warming systems, such as the Hotline, small amount of air is generated secondary to decrease in gas solubility with increasing temperature. Squeezing the bulb several times provides high infusion rates that also generate small bubbles. This is similar to rapidly injecting agitated saline to check for an inter-atrial shunt. Thus, by rapidly mixing the syringe, small air bubbles come out of solution and can be observed via TEE. The amount of air bubbles produced would be on a much larger scale by squeezing the bulb and warming the fluid.

Quantification of air burden

While TEE is the most sensitive means to determine the presence of air, to our knowledge, there is no specific ultrasound software available to quantify the amount of air in the heart. We therefore used a commercially available software from NIH (ImageJ software for MAC, NIH, Bethesda, MD, USA) to determine the maximal amount of air present in the right atrium. As this study is first to describe this methodology to assess and quantify air in the heart using this technique, we believe that this approach is novel, since ultrasound naturally has a contrast between air and fluid, which allows for visual patterns to be at least semi-quantifiable. Video sections of the right atrium (RA) and right ventricle (RV) were obtained by TEE positioned in a mid-esophageal RA view for peak air amount and clearance. TEE was chosen both because it is routinely available in the hospital and it is the most sensitive and specific indicator of intravascular air. TEE images were video recorded throughout each bolus of warmed crystalloid.

Images throughout bolus administration were reviewed, and the image at the time of maximal air in the chambers was selected and screen locked for each bolus. A control image for each patient was established where no air was present. The left atrium was used as negative control as it had similar contrast values but no air present. The images were then uploaded, the RA was outlined, and the amount of air was quantified using optical densitometry (OD) software (ImageJ software for MAC, NIH, Bethesda, MD, USA). Mean OD was determined by subtracting the peak image from the control image (Fig. 2). Mean OD values for the control versus the ClearLine IV group were determined by two independent investigators and then averaged for each subject.

Air clearance, defined as the time that 90% of air from the RA was eliminated, was also calculated.

Statistical analysis

Sample size estimate

Previous animal studies showed that the ClearLine IV could reduce air entrainment by at least 50%. Thus, we calculated that air in the right atrium without ClearLine IV to maximally cover 50% of the right atrium, ± 20% standard deviation. Our preliminary animal studies (data not shown) demonstrated that this could be reduced by half. Thus, we tested the hypothesis that ClearLine IV could reduce air entrainment to 25% with a 20% standard deviation. Based on a power of 0.80 and alpha of 0.05, $n = 6$ subjects per group would be needed to test this statistical hypothesis. Data were collected and entered in Excel for statistical analysis. Means and standard deviations for the air burden and air clearance were calculated by two independent investigators, and the final analysis included the values of both investigators. A

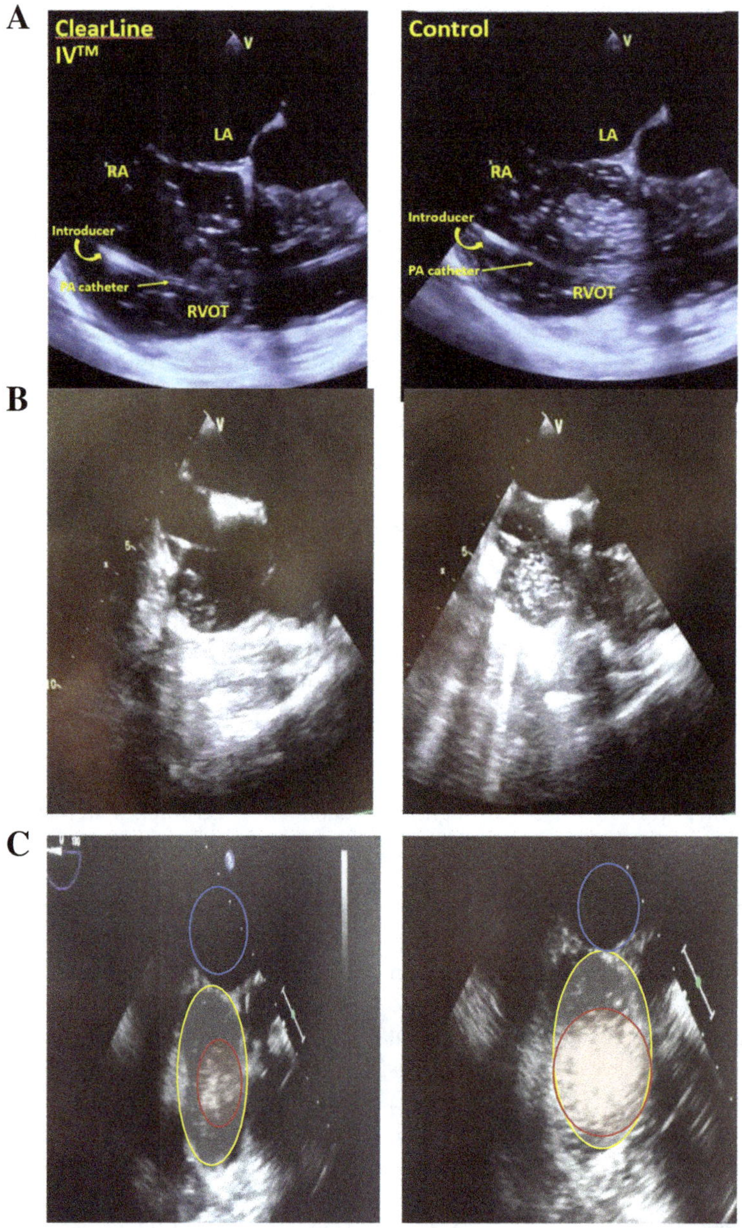

Fig. 2 Air quantification in the right atrium by optical densitometry (OD). ClearLine IV (left) versus control (right). **a**–**c** TEE images during bolus. LA: left atria, RA: right atria, RVOT: right ventricular outflow tract

paired-sample t test was conducted to compare the means of the ClearLine IV and control groups with the significance level set at $p = 0.05$.

Results

Six subjects completed the study, five males and one female (Table 1). Air quantification was conducted by two independent investigators, and the results in all cases had less than 10% error between the investigators. The flow rates of fluid boluses were similar, 145 ± 22 mL/min for ClearLine IV and 137 ± 45 mL/min for control (Table 2). Subjects demonstrated significantly less mean RA air in the ClearLine IV group (OD = 16 ± 3%) compared with those in the control group (OD = 46 ± 7%), $p = 0.004$ (Fig. 3). Air clearance time was significantly lower with the use of ClearLine IV (3.7 ± 1.2 s) compared to control (5.3 ± 1.3 s), $p < 0.001$.

Discussion

Air embolism is an uncommon but potentially life-threatening event for which prompt diagnosis and treatment can lead to a better patient outcome. Air embolism formation requires a connection and pressure gradient between the blood vessel and the gas. The air bubbles have the deteriorating effect as they can migrate to different vital organs, thus negatively affecting patient morbidity and mortality. Most air emboli in the vascular system are iatrogenic in nature (Mirski et al. 2007). Venous air emboli may occur during pressured venous infusion and/or catheter manipulation such as during insertion of intravascular catheters, including peripheral and central venous cannula and diagnostic and therapeutic catheters. Air embolism in the venous circulation usually travels into the right atrium and ventricle and then reaches the pulmonary circulation. Since a large percentage of the population carries the diagnosis of patent foramen ovale (PFO), a risk of paradoxical embolus is present when the air bubble travels across the PFO into the systemic circulation, hence reaching vital organs like the brain and kidneys. Arterial air embolism most often occurs during significant invasive procedures. These include bronchoscopy, craniotomies, esophagogastroscopy, and lung and liver biopsies.

The literature reports an increased incidence of cases of air emboli during cardiac surgeries that require the patient to be on the heart-lung machine, extracorporeal membranous oxygenation (ECMO), and/or left-sided assist devices (LVAD). In the case of arterial air embolism, the air may flow in a retrograde way via different arteries and reach the cerebral circulation. If the air reaches the left ventricle, there is a possibility that the air will enter the coronary arteries and cause significant cardiac ischemia and arrhythmia.

During the last two decades, a breakthrough has been achieved in the treatment of ischemic and congenital heart disease via a transcatheter approach. These procedures are high-risk and invasive in nature. Currently, we can perform balloon dilation of small vessel and stenotic valves among other procedures. The technology also provides the interventionists with tools to perform atrial and ventricular septal defect closure as well as valve repair and replacement via a catheter approach. The duration of these complex and innovative procedures is long and requires multiple arterial and venous axes. Continuous flow is necessary to keep these lines, arterial and venous, patent and ready for catheter manipulations. Different maintenance solutions including blood products and both cardiac and anesthetic medication are administered to the patient via these lines. These manipulations significantly increase the risk of air embolism in this population of patients.

A large air embolism may cause catastrophic events and lead to death regardless if it is in the systemic or pulmonary circulations. In the venous system, large amounts of air (300–500 mL) may lead to RV failure, cardiogenic shock, and death. In contrast, small amounts of air in the arterial circulation can be fatal and lead to coma, seizures, myocardial ischemia and infarction, arrhythmia, and heart failure (Toung et al. 2001).

It is known that even small amounts of air emboli have negative effects on different tissues. A surge of inflammatory response occurs as a marker for physiological tissue impairment. There is also non-obvious damage caused by bubbles in the microcirculation, which include tissue ischemia, micro-thrombosis, endothelial damage, and cytokine release.

Varga and colleagues introduced the concept of "The Partially Invisible Phenomenon" which was noticed also by other investigators (Varga et al. 2016). This phenomenon describes the potential harm caused by outgassing from intravenous fluid or cold blood products during warming to normal body temperature. The dissolved gas is invisible and can be administered unintentionally and undetectably. Since many institutes are using warmers as a standard of care in their patients' circuits, it is crucial that we pay serious attention to potential air embolism symptoms. It requires close monitoring of cardiac and brain activity (Barak and Katz 2005).

Table 1 Baseline demographics

	Gender	Age	Race/ethnicity
Subject 1	Male	72	White/non-Hispanic
Subject 2	Male	61	White/non-Hispanic
Subject 3	Male	60	Black/non-Hispanic
Subject 4	Male	65	White/non-Hispanic
Subject 5	Male	49	White/Hispanic
Subject 6	Female	73	White/non-Hispanic

Table 2 Air quantification by optical densitometry (OD)

	ClearLine IV mean ± SD	Control mean ± SD	*p* value
Fluid flow rates (mL/min)	145 ± 22	137 ± 45	NS
Mean RA air by OD (%)	16 ± 3	46 ± 7	$p = 0.004$
Air clearance time (s)	3.7 ± 1.2	5.3 ± 1.3	$p < 0.001$

The objective of this study was to quantify air entering a patient during bolus infusion during surgery and to test whether ClearLine IV reduced patient's air burden. Several factors related to fluid warming and infusion place patients undergoing major surgery at risk of AE. Fluid warming and pressurized infusion devices are common in the operating room setting, and studies have shown that these devices increase AE risk (Orliaguet and Martin 2000; Zoremba et al. 2011). Further, fluid flow rates create variability in air introduction, as the volume of air introduced increases as the infusion flow rate decreases. Other factors may unpredictably impact the air volume introduced, as gas bubbles are dynamic, and, as they flow and come into contact with other emboli, may combine to form larger emboli more likely to cause patient harm (Van Liew and Burkard 1995). Taken together, these findings suggest that any quantity of air should be removed, if possible, to mitigate risk. In-line filters, while widely accepted for air and particle removal, are unable to remove all air from circulation and increase resistance in the line, making their utility challenging, particularly in the setting of bolus infusion (Herbst and Najm 2012). While some fluid warming devices can detect air, the air elimination capability of these systems demonstrates variable results, particularly in the setting of pressurized infusions (Pelletier and Fisher 2017; Schnoor et al. 2004; Zoremba et al. 2011a; Woon and Talke 1999; Smith et al. 2001). ClearLine IV has been shown to successfully detect air using an ultrasound sensor, as small as 25 μl, and thereby eliminate air from entering into IV tubing. While ClearLine IV can eliminate large volumes of air (> 50 mL), flow rate is the limiting factor. Specifically, the ClearLine IV sensor triggers a diverter "switch" enabling air to be bypassed. ClearLine IV can accommodate and remove air semi-continuously as long as the flow rate does not exceed 400 mL/min (product safety studies). Commercialized IV fluid pumps on the market rarely deliver fluid exceeding this rate. Few infusion pumps exceed 100 mL/min. Prior to this clinical study, we tested the Clearline IV in our lab. Using a similar setup (bulb-squeezer pressure pump connected to Hotline) shown in "Methods", a Doppler flow probe (in-line, Transonic flow meter, Ithaca, NY, USA) was placed on the IV tubing connected to an 8.5-Fr Cordis line. We demonstrated that the maximum flow rate during a rapid bolus using the Hotline with a bulb squeezer did not exceed 250 mL/min. We appreciate that devices for large-volume resuscitation, e.g., Level 1 (under high driving pressure) or Belmont rapid infuser, can deliver fluids at 500 mL/min. Both of these commercialized products have a separate air trap device. In these cases, using the Belmont or Level 1, the

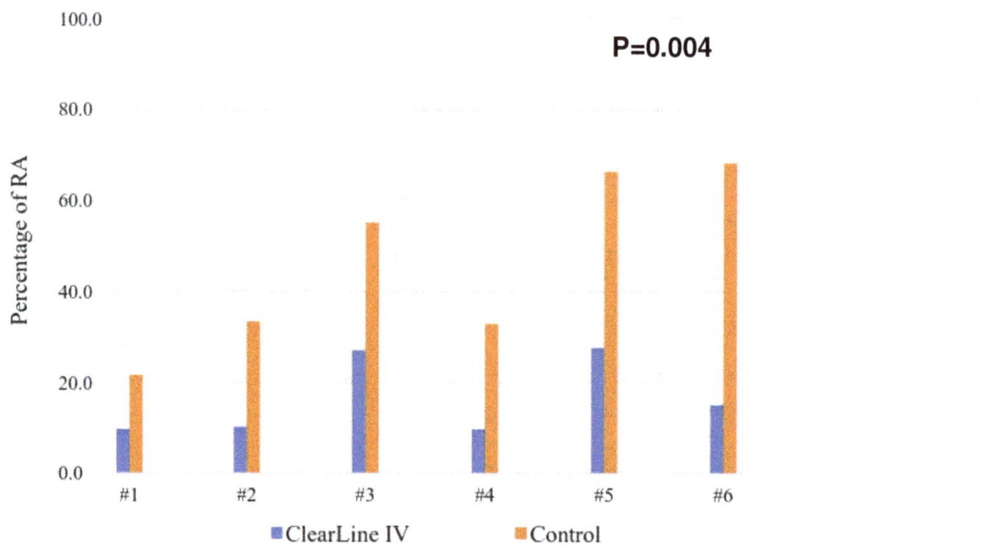

Fig. 3 Air quantification as measured in the right atrium (RA) by TEE images and optical densitometry (OD). Less air was quantified in the RA following boluses administered in-line with the ClearLine IV system. TEE: transesophageal echocardiography

flow rate would exceed the capability of the ClearLine IV device.

Therefore, identification of additional technological options to mitigate the residual risk of AE is clinically important and motivated us to conduct this investigation of the ClearLine IV system.

The results of our investigation confirm that during major surgery, particularly in the setting of fluid warming devices and pressure and bolus infusions, quantifiable AEs are introduced into the patient's vasculature. While left-sided air is common during cardiac surgery and enters the cerebral circulation and other systemic organs, the potential presence of a PFO, ASD, or VSD and the risk of right-sided AEs offer additional clinical risk. Further, increasing evidence suggests that AEs of any size can result in patient harm. In fact, neuropsychological injury arising from small volumes of air following cardiopulmonary bypass remains one of the most serious and costly complications of the procedure. These microemboli arise from surgical and manual manipulation of the heart and arteries and the components of the extracorporeal circuit (Lou et al. 2011).

While none of the subjects in this study experienced a detectable adverse experience from the air introduced, patients who are compromised or have a PFO/ASD/VSD could be at higher risk for negative impact of AE. Special consideration can be taken for patients with a known PFO to prevent paradoxical embolization, although given the high rate of undiagnosed PFO and high cost of AE, the ClearLine IV system may provide an important role in all surgical patients to avoid this potential risk.

Limitations

The sample size for this study was small ($n = 6$). The study was not designed to impact the outcome but rather was performed to determine if the ClearLine IV system could significantly reduce the delivery of intravenous air into the right heart. While the series was randomized, the investigators were not blinded when they quantified the air in the RA images, since audiovisual files were created to distinguish the timing of sequential fluid boluses. The investigators of this study were not aware of any commercially available software to objectively quantify air in the RA. While the OD (optical densitometry) methodology is not officially validated for determining intra-atrial air, the use of the ImageJ software provided a well-known method for calculating OD. Further, the fact that two investigators scored all images independently and measures were within 10% of each other reduces the risk of error or bias introduced in this process. We also recognize that we are using two-dimensional measurements, and "air", which is not lucid via ultrasound, will be reduced in the far field (away from the probe). Thus, air in the far field would not be as reflective. However, we suggest that this limitation would be present in both assessments with and without the ClearLine IV group. Although this study did not measure the effects of asymptomatic air emboli (e.g., inflammatory response to micro-air emboli without evidence of hemodynamic collapse), it is possible that this factor would be attenuated given the threefold reduction in overall air entrainment with the ClearLine IV system.

Conclusion

Our study found that use of ClearLine IV in-line with the circuit significantly reduced the quantity of RA air when delivering a warmed solution at a fast rate without changing the rate of bolus infusion or creating resistance in the circuit. Subsequently, the clearance time for air was also significantly faster in the ClearLine IV circuit. This device could thereby reduce risk of harmful and potentially fatal AEs. While the total volume of air removed was relatively small in these cases (3–7 mL), given the nature of rapid bolus, error could result in administration of greater volumes of air during these procedures and even small amounts of air could result in harm. The results of this study demonstrate the utility of the ClearLine IV system to reduce the amount of air introduced into the patient when delivering a warm solution at a fast rate during major surgery. Further studies are warranted to assess efficacy in preventing harmful sequelae of air embolism such as coagulation changes, systemic inflammatory response syndrome (SIRS), pulmonary edema, and ischemia.

Abbreviations

AE: Air embolism; ECMO: Extracorporeal membranous oxygenation; IRB: Institutional Review Board; LVAD: Left-sided assist devices; OD: Optical densitometry; PFO: Patent foramen ovale; RA: Right atrium; RV: Right ventricle; TEE: Transesophageal echocardiography

Acknowledgements

The authors wish to acknowledge Bethany Muhlebach for editorial support.

Funding

This study was supported by a research grant from ClearLine MD, Woburn, MA, USA.

Achiau Ludomirsky MD is Chairman of the Clinical Advisory Board for ClearLine MD.

Authors' contributions

YI analyzed and interpreted patient data regarding the amount of air that entered the right atrium in the control and non-control boluses and how much air was removed from each of the surgeries. YI played a role in writing the abstract and manuscript. NM analyzed and interpreted patient data regarding the amount of air that entered the right atrium in the control and non-control boluses and how much air was removed from each of the surgeries. NM was also present intraoperatively during each data collection. NM played a role in writing the abstract and manuscript. CG was present intraoperatively during each data collection. CG was involved in some portions of data analysis.

MJ was present intraoperatively during each data collection. MS was present intraoperatively during each data collection. MS was involved in data extraction. CM was present intraoperatively during each data collection. MK was present intraoperatively during each data collection. MK was involved in data extraction. MK analyzed and interpreted patient data regarding the amount of air that entered the right atrium in the control and non-control boluses and how much air was removed from each of the surgeries. All authors read and approved the final manuscript.

Competing interests

AL is the Chairman of the Clinical Advisory Board for ClearLine MD. The remaining authors declare that they have no competing interests.

Author details

[1]Department of Anesthesiology, The University of Texas Medical Branch, Galveston, TX, USA. [2]Department of Anesthesiology, Kadlec Regional Medical Center, Pasco, WA, USA. [3]Department of Pediatrics, NYU Langone Health, School of Medicine , New York, NY, USA.

References

Agarwal SS, Kumar L, Chavali KH, Mestri SC. Fatal venous air embolism following intravenous infusion. J Forensic Sci. 2009;54(3):682–4.

Barak M, Katz Y. Microbubbles. Chest. 2005;128:2918–32.

Bayliss Y, Balogh A, Burrowes P, Brunet G, Jensen K. A quality review of the occurrence of a non-fatal venous air embolism event following CT contrast enhanced administration for the purpose of radiation therapy planning. J Radiother Pract. 2014;13(1):29–34.

Brull SJ, Prielipp RC. Vascular air embolism: a silent hazard to patient safety. J Crit Care. 2017;42:255–63.

Foster PP, Boriek AM, Butler BD, Gernhardt ML, Bové AA. Patent foramen ovale and paradoxical systemic embolism: a bibliographic review. Aviat Space Environ Med. 2003;74(6 Pt 2):B1–B64.

Girard F, Ruel M, McKenty S, Boudreault D, Chouinard P, Todorov A, Molina-Negro P, Bouvier G. Incidences of venous air embolism and patent foramen ovale among patients undergoing selective peripheral denervation in the sitting position. Neurosurgery. 2003;53(2):316–9 discussion 9-20.

Herbst DP, Najm HK. Development of a new arterial-line filter design using computational fluid dynamics analysis. J Extra Corpor Technol. 2012;44(3): 139–44.

Hsieh TK, Hsieh JP, Lin MC, Ho ST, Hsing CH, Wang JJ, Chu CC. Fatal venous air embolism during emergence from anesthesia. Acta Anaesthesiol Taiwanica. 2009;47(3):138–42.

Kapoor T, Gutierrez G. Air embolism as a cause of the systemic inflammatory response syndrome: a case report. Crit Care. 2003;7(5):R98–r100.

Laskey AL, Dyer C, Tobias JD. Venous air embolism during home infusion therapy. Pediatrics. 2002;109(1):E15.

Lou S, Ji B, Liu J, Yu K, Long C. Generation, detection and prevention of gaseous microemboli during cardiopulmonary bypass procedure. Int J Artif Organs. 2011;34(11):1039–51.

McCarthy CJ, Behravesh S, Naidu SG, Oklu R. Air embolism: diagnosis, clinical management and outcomes. Diagnostics. 2017;7(1):5.

McGrath BJ, Zimmerman JE, Williams JF, Parmet J. Carbon dioxide embolism treated with hyperbaric oxygen. Can J Anaesth. 1989;36:586–9.

Mirski MA, Lele AV, Fitzsimmons L, Toung TJ. Diagnosis and treatment of vascular air embolism. Anesthesiology. 2007;106:164–77.

Mitchell SJ, Benson M, Vadlamudi L, Miller P. Cerebral arterial gas embolism by helium: an unusual case successfully treated with hyperbaric oxygen and lidocaine. Ann Emerg Med. 2000;35:300–3.

Muth CM, Shank ES. Gas embolism. N Engl J Med. 2000;342(7):476–82.

Orliaguet GA, Martin J. Management of venous air embolism. Cahiers d'anesthesiologie. 2000;48(4):251–60.

Park YH, Kim HJ, Kim JT, Kim HS, Kim CS, Kim SD. Prolonged paradoxical air embolism during intraoperative intestinal endoscopy confirmed by transesophageal echocardiography - a case report. Korean J Anesthesiol. 2010;58(6):560–4.

Paul Pelletier N, Fisher A. Infusion pump in UH60L/M flight in Afghanistan: why failures occur. Air Med J. 2017;36(5):248–57.

Schnoor J, Macko S, Weber I, Rossaint R. The air elimination capabilities of pressure infusion devices and fluid-warmers. Anaesthesia. 2004;59(8):817–21.

Smith CE, Kabbara A, Kramer RP, Gill I. Evaluation of a new IV fluid and blood warming system to prevent air embolism. Trauma Care. 2001;11:78–82.

Toung TJ, Rossberg MI, Hutchins GM. Volume of air in lethal venous air embolism. Anesthesiology. 2001;94:360–1.

van Hulst RA, Klein J, Lachmann B. Gas embolism: pathophysiology and treatment. Clin Physiol Funct Imaging. 2003;23(5):237–46.

Van Liew HD, Burkard ME. Bubbles in circulating blood: stabilization and simulations of cyclic changes of size and content. J Appl Physiol (1985). 1995; 79(4):1379–85.

Varga C, Lutia I, Gravensterein N. Intravenous air: the partially invisible phenomenon. Anesth Analg. 2016;123(5):1149–55.

Vesely TM. Air embolism during insertion of central venous catheters. J Vasc Interv Radiol. 2001;12(11):1291–5.

Wilkins RG, Unverdorben M. Accidental intravenous infusion of air: a concise review. J Infus Nurs. 2012;35(6):404–8.

Woon S, Talke P. Amount of air infused to patient increases as fluid flow rates decrease when using the Hotline HL-90 fluid warmer. J Clin Monit Comput. 1999;15(3–4):149–52.

Zoremba N, Gruenewald C, Zoremba M, Rossaint R, Schaelte G. Air elimination capability in rapid infusion systems. Anaesthesia. 2011;66(11):1031–4.

Validity of the Postoperative Morbidity Survey after abdominal aortic aneurysm repair

Ben A. Goodman[1], Alan M. Batterham[2], Elke Kothmann[3], Louise Cawthorn[3], David Yates[4], Helen Melsom[5], Karen Kerr[6] and Gerard R. Danjoux[2,3*]

Abstract

Background: Currently, there is no standardised tool used to capture morbidity following abdominal aortic aneurysm (AAA) repair. The aim of this prospective observational study was to validate the Postoperative Morbidity Survey (POMS) according to its two guiding principles: to only capture morbidity substantial enough to delay discharge from hospital and to be a rapid, simple screening tool.

Methods: A total of 64 adult patients undergoing elective infrarenal AAA repair participated in the study. Following surgery, the POMS was recorded daily, by trained research staff with the clinical teams blinded, until hospital discharge or death. We modelled the data using Cox regression, accounting for the competing risk of death, with POMS as a binary time-dependent (repeated measures) internal covariate. For each day for each patient, 'discharged' (yes/no) was the event, with the elapsed number of days post-surgery as the time variable. We derived the hazard ratio for any POMS morbidity (score 1–9) vs. no morbidity (zero), adjusted for type of repair (endovascular versus open), age and aneurysm size.

Results: The hazard ratio for alive discharge with any POMS-recorded morbidity versus no morbidity was 0.130 (95 % confidence interval 0.070 to 0.243). The median time-to-discharge was 13 days after recording any POMS morbidity vs. 2 days after scoring zero for POMS morbidity. Compliance with POMS completion was 99.5 %.

Conclusions: The POMS is a valid tool for capturing short-term postoperative morbidity following elective infrarenal AAA repair that is substantial enough to delay discharge from hospital. Daily POMS measurement is recommended to fully capture morbidity and allow robust analysis. The survey could be a valuable outcome measure for use in quality improvement programmes and future research.

Keywords: Aneurysm, AAA, Postoperative, Morbidity, POMS, Complications, Outcome

* Correspondence: Gerard.Danjoux@stees.nhs.uk
The results of the study were presented in part to the Anaesthetic Research Society Meeting, London, UK, October 2013, and the Preoperative Association National Conference, York, UK, Nov 2013; published in abstract form as Br J Anaesth 2014;112(1):181P-199P
A secondary analysis of the study was submitted as a dissertation in partial fulfilment of the requirements of Teesside University for the degree of MSc Evidence Based Medicine (Anaesthetics) in May 2014 by Dr Ben A. Goodman. All relevant regulations of the Teesside University were followed. The dissertation has not been made publically available, thereby avoiding redundant or dual publication.
[2]Health and Social Care Institute, Teesside University, Middlesbrough, UK
[3]Department of Academic Anaesthesia, James Cook University Hospital, Marton Road, Middlesbrough TS4 3BW, UK
Full list of author information is available at the end of the article

Background

The Abdominal Aortic Aneurysm (AAA) Quality Improvement Programme (AAAQIP) was introduced in 2009 with the explicit remit of halving national mortality following elective repair by 2014. Latest published outcomes show the dramatic effect the AAAQIP has had, with mortality figures superior to those initially targeted at 2.4 % (open and endovascular outcomes combined) (Potgieter et al. 2012). As care improves for patients undergoing surgery, mortality becomes less common and therefore becomes a less sensitive measure of differences in the quality of care (Patila et al. 2006). Morbidity following AAA repair is significantly higher than mortality, with an estimated prevalence of 28 % following open repair and 12 % following EVAR (Giles et al. 2010). Despite this, morbidity is not robustly captured in the AAAQIP outcome dataset. Introducing standardised morbidity reporting would represent a logical next step to ensuring transparency of outcomes, whilst providing a more sensitive measure for differences in quality of care.

Capturing postoperative complications is highly relevant given their strong association with adverse outcomes for both patient and institution including prolonged hospital stay, poor functional ability on hospital discharge, reduced life-expectancy, reduced quality of life and increased hospital resource utilisation (Khuri et al. 2005; Head et al. 2008). Despite this, there is no standardised tool used to reliably capture morbidity following AAA repair. Beyond being able to identify complications postoperatively, a robust recording system would also facilitate quality assurance of hospital care and determine the effects of new surgical interventions.

The Postoperative Morbidity Survey (POMS) is a nine-domain tool that prospectively describes in-hospital morbidity following major surgery (Bennett-Guerrero et al. 1999). The POMS is able to detect a range of complication severities—from minor to life threatening—and classify morbidity by organ system, thereby representing a particularly useful scoring system. The original research from which the POMS tool was derived consisted of a heterogeneous population of surgical patients, including a minor cohort undergoing vascular surgery. Subsequent studies demonstrate the POMS has good inter-rater reliability, high patient satisfaction, accurately describe all postoperative complications (Grocott et al. 2007; Davies et al. 2013) and is associated with length of stay (LOS) (Grocott et al. 2007; Davies et al. 2013; Wakeling et al. 2005; Ackland et al. 2007; Ackland et al. 2010; Snowden et al. 2010; Ackland et al. 2011; Sanders et al. 2011; Ausania et al. 2012; Jones et al. 2013; Moonesinghe et al. 2014; West et al. 2014; Lee et al. 2014).

To date, the POMS has not been specifically evaluated in vascular surgery patients. Moreover, the POMS has not been validated against the primary guiding principle for its design—that it should capture morbidity substantial enough to delay discharge from hospital (Bennett-Guerrero et al. 1999). Rather, previous studies have used POMS scores on an arbitrary day post-surgery, for example, day 3 or 5 (Grocott et al. 2007; Davies et al. 2013). The aim of the present study therefore was to validate the POMS following elective AAA repair, both open and endovascular (EVAR), using repeated daily measurement in each patient up to the point of discharge or competing event (death). Consistent with the key guiding principle of the POMS, the primary objective was to estimate the instantaneous relative risk of being discharged from hospital, at any time-point, with any POMS-recorded morbidity (POMS score 1–9) versus no morbidity. A secondary objective was to assess the POMS against the second guiding principle in its development; that it should be a simple and rapid patient-screening tool.

Methods

This study was a four-centre, prospective observational cohort study that recruited patients from the James Cook University Hospital, Middlesbrough; York Hospital; University Hospital of North Durham and the Northern General Hospital, Sheffield, between July 2012 and March 2013. All patients ≥18 years of age and with capacity to give informed consent, undergoing elective infrarenal AAA repair, were eligible for inclusion. Exclusion criteria were the following: inability to provide informed consent, surgery for suprarenal thoracic or non-elective aneurysms and non-operative management.

A study investigator approached consecutive patients with an information sheet at the preoperative assessment or vascular surgical clinics, and written informed consent was obtained on admission to hospital for the surgical procedure. The study was approved by the West Midlands—Coventry & Warwickshire Research Ethics Committee (reference 12/WM/0114) and locally in recruiting centres (South Tees Hospitals Research and Development Department, York Foundation Trust Research and Development Unit, County Durham and Darlington Centre for Clinical Research and Innovation and the Sheffield Teaching Hospitals Clinical Research Office).

Study procedure

Patients underwent preoperative assessment and multidisciplinary team discussion based on the AAAQIP care pathway as part of their usual care. Baseline data were collected from preoperative assessment prior to open or endovascular AAA repair. Anaesthetic and surgical techniques were used at the discretion of attending clinicians.

Following surgery, the POMS (Table 1) was recorded daily, by trained research staff, until hospital discharge or death. A modification was made a priori, to reflect changes in clinical practice away from intravenous opioid analgesics towards oral formulations (Pergolizzi et al. 2012). The medical notes were reviewed on a daily basis with any postoperative morbidity not identified by the POMS recorded as free text. Postoperative patient management was otherwise performed per routine clinical practice at the discretion of the attending clinical teams, who were blinded to the POMS data. If patients remained in hospital with no morbidity, the reason for continued admission was recorded as free text. Critical care and overall hospital length of stay were recorded in addition to in-hospital mortality.

Sample size and statistical analysis

Sample size and power estimations were conducted using R® software (Qiu et al. 2012). We predicted that at least 60 patients could be recruited over 9 months. This sample size provides 85 % power to detect a clinically relevant hazard ratio of ~0.4 reflecting a substantially lower instantaneous relative risk of being discharged at any time with any POMS-recorded morbidity versus no morbidity (with $2P = 0.05$, an expected discharge rate of 95 %, a predicted proportion of the sample with POMS morbidity at discharge of 25 % and a correlation coefficient of 0.1 between the primary exposure (POMS) and the other covariates in the model (see below).)

We analysed the data using a simple multistate Cox regression model to derive the cause-specific association between morbidity and hospital discharge (alive), accounting for the competing risk of in-hospital death (Beyersmann et al. 2012). For each day for each patient, 'discharged' (yes/no) was the event, with the elapsed number of days post-surgery as the time variable. The POMS score (yes = 1–9, no = zero) was a binary time-dependent internal covariate. Analysis was conducted using Stata® software (StataCorp. 2013. *Stata Statistical Software: Release 13*. College Station, TX: StataCorp LP). The hazard ratio (95 % confidence interval) for the effect of any POMS morbidity vs. no morbidity was estimated, controlling for type of repair (open vs. EVAR), patient age and size of aneurysm. These three variables were selected, a priori, as each may be predicted to affect length of stay independent of POMS morbidity (Schouten et al. 2006; Lee et al. 2004). Sex was not included as a covariate as the sample was 95 % male. The hazard ratio reflects the instantaneous relative risk of alive discharge for a state of morbidity vs. no morbidity.

Table 1 The Postoperative Morbidity Survey (Bennett-Guerrero et al. 1999)

Morbidity type	Criteria	Source of data
Pulmonary	New requirement for supplemental oxygen or other respiratory support	Patient observation Treatment chart
Infectious	Currently on antibiotics or temperature >38 °C in the last 24 h	Treatment chart Observation chart
Renal	Presence of oliguria (500 mL 24 h^{-1}), increased serum creatinine (>30 % from preoperative level) or urinary catheter in place	Patient observation Fluid balance chart Biochemistry result
Gastrointestinal	Unable to tolerate an enteral diet for any reason, including nausea, vomiting, and abdominal distension *or use of anti-emetic*[a]	Patient questioning Fluid balance chart Treatment chart
Cardiovascular	Diagnostic tests or therapy within the last 24 h for any of the following: new myocardial infarction or ischaemia, hypotension (requiring pharmacological therapy or fluid therapy >200 mL h^{-1}), atrial or ventricular arrhythmias, cardiogenic pulmonary oedema or thrombotic event (requiring anticoagulation)	Treatment chart Note review
Neurological	Presence of new focal deficit, confusion, delirium or coma	Note review Patient questioning
Wound	Wound dehiscence requiring surgical exploration or drainage of pus from the operation wound with or without isolation of organisms	Note review Pathology result
Haematological	Requirement for any of the following within the last 24 h: packed erythrocytes, platelets, fresh-frozen plasma or cryoprecipitate	Treatment chart Fluid balance chart
Pain	New postoperative pain significant enough to require *strong*[b] opioids or regional analgesia	Treatment chart Patient questioning

[a]Change made by Grocott et al. 2007
[b]Change for the present study (previously *parenteral*)

One patient was discharged 8 days post-surgery but due to administrative error had no POMS scores recorded after day 5. To include this patient's event data in the analysis, we carried forward the day 5 morbidity (in the gastrointestinal domain) for days 6–8—a conservative approach in this context.

With respect to the validity of POMS as conceptualised in the current study, there are two types of 'error' versus the reference method of the discharge decision by the vascular team. First, a patient might attain a zero score for POMS on a particular day but not be discharged within 24 h of that time-point. Second, a patient might be discharged despite having recorded POMS morbidity. We present a summary of both of these categories in the 'Results' section.

We also conducted a sensitivity analysis to examine the effect that patients who were not discharged within 24 h of achieving a zero score had on the validity of the POMS (degree of attenuation of the observed hazard ratio). To conduct this analysis, we first manually edited the data to reflect a scenario in which all patients who reached a zero for POMS had been discharged immediately (i.e. within 24 h).

Results

Participant flow

Out of the 104 potential participants screened for inclusion, 81 met the inclusion criteria and were approached by an investigator, of which 64 were recruited into the study. Reasons for non-enrolment were non-operative management ($n = 8$), surgery performed outside recruitment window ($n = 5$), refusal ($n = 3$) and cognitive dysfunction precluding informed consent ($n = 1$). All 64 patients completed follow-up and were included in the analysis.

Sample characteristics

Patient and perioperative characteristics are described in Table 2. Prevalence of daily presence of POMS morbidity and the count of the number of domains affected are presented in Table 3. Data are presented up to day 6, when approximately 50 % of the overall sample had been discharged. One patient (1.6 % of the total sample) died on the ninth postoperative day after an open AAA repair from multi-organ failure. One patient had postoperative limb ischaemia suspected clinically, resulting in further investigation, but did not meet any of the existing POMS domain criteria.

Validity of the POMS

Compliance with POMS completion was 99.5 %, with just three missing days for one patient from a total of 608 possible observations (see 'Methods'). The hazard ratio for discharge with any POMS-recorded morbidity versus no morbidity was 0.130 (95 % confidence interval 0.070 to 0.243). The median time-to-discharge was 13 days after recording any POMS morbidity vs. 2 days after scoring zero for POMS morbidity.

Twenty-nine patients remained in hospital beyond 24 h of first attaining a zero score for POMS. For 10 of these patients, nothing was documented in the patient notes that might shed light on reasons for any delay. For the other 19 patients, the notes suggested that 4 were awaiting the results of diagnostic tests, 7 had evidence of social/non-medical reasons that delayed discharge, 3 remained in hospital for medical reasons, and 5 developed morbidity very shortly after first reaching zero POMS morbidity: 2 with an infective complication, 2 with pain, and 1 with atrial fibrillation. The sensitivity analysis assuming that all of these 29 patients had been discharged when they first reached a zero score for POMS revealed a hazard ratio for morbidity vs. no morbidity of 0.058 (0.030 to 0.114).

Nineteen patients were discharged with a POMS score of >0 (morbidity in one or more POMS domains). The majority of these ($n = 17$) had recorded morbidity in a single POMS domain: 10 for Infectious, 4 for Pain, and one each for Gastrointestinal, Cardiovascular and Pulmonary. Two patients had recorded morbidity in two POMS domains—Cardiovascular plus Pain and Infectious plus Pain.

Discussion

Validity

This is the first study to validate the POMS specifically in patients undergoing abdominal aortic aneurysm repair. The observed hazard ratio reveals that the chances of being discharged by usual clinical decision-making at any time-point with any POMS-recorded morbidity are approximately 1/8 those of being discharged in the absence of POMS morbidity—a very large effect size. There was also a very large difference for the median time-to-discharge in the morbidity vs. no morbidity states. Taken together, these findings provide strong evidence for the validity of the POMS against its primary guiding principle—to only capture morbidity that is of a type and severity to delay discharge from hospital. Following abdominal aortic aneurysm repair the POMS therefore has good, albeit not perfect, validity.

The factor primarily responsible for the non-perfect validity of the POMS in this context is the 19 patients who were discharged with a POMS score >0. The majority of these patients had POMS-recorded morbidity in a single domain—most frequently 'Infectious', followed by 'Pain'. If these 19 patients had instead not been discharged (censored data, i.e. 'event' did not occur) then the hazard ratio for morbidity vs. no morbidity would have been essentially zero, as the POMS morbidity covariate at the point of discharge would have been

Table 2 Patient and perioperative characteristics

Variable	*n*	Total ($n = 64$)	EVAR ($n = 31$)	Open ($n = 33$)
Age (years)	64	72.7 (7.9)	75.6 (6.2)	70.0 (8.5)
Male:female	64	61:3	29:2	32:1
Body mass index (kg m^{-2})	62	28.2 (5.0)	28.0 (4.6)	28.4 (5.4)
ASA-PS	64			
2		11	1	10
3		47	26	21
4		6	4	2
Revised cardiac risk index (Lee et al. 1999)	64			
1		26	12	14
2		30	16	14
3		8	3	5
Estimated glomerular filtration rate (Levey et al. 1999) (ml min^{-1})	64	76.7 (21.5)	75.9 (22.8)	77.6 (20.6)
Size of AAA (cm)	64	6.7 (1.3)	6.4 (1.2)	7.1 (1.4)
Duration of procedure (h)	57	3.2 [2.2–5.4]	2.5 [2.0–3.6]	4.0 [3.0–6.3]
Aortic cross-clamp time (h)	28	1.1 [0.8–1.8]	n/a	1.1 [0.9–1.8]
Estimated blood loss (L)	44	1.2 [0.5–3.8]	0.5 [0.3–0.6]	2 [1.2–4.6]
Type of anaesthetic	64			
General		45	12	33
Spinal		4	4	0
Epidural		32	2	30
Combined spinal-epidural		14	14	0
In-hospital mortality	64	1	0	1
Postoperative LOS (days)	64	6 [4–11]	4 [3–6]	9 [6–13]
Critical care LOS (days)	64	2 [1–4]	1 [1–2]	4 [2–6]

Data are mean (SD), median [interquartile range] or number
ASA-PS American Society of Anesthesiologists Physical Status, *LOS* length of stay, *EVAR* endovascular aneurysm repair

constant across the sample. The sensitivity analysis revealed that the 29 patients who were not discharged within 24 h of first reaching a POMS score of zero attenuated the observed hazard ratio by >50 % (0.130 vs. 0.058). This implies that if all 29 had in fact been discharged within 24 h of first reaching zero, the chances of being discharged with a POMS score >0 compared to a POMS score =0 would decrease significantly from 1/8 (the value we observed) to 1/17. This difference can be explained by imperfections in the healthcare system (delayed recognition of recovery from perioperative morbidity) or by the presence of factors preventing discharge that were not identified by either the POMS or the patient notes—see below for a critique of the POMS.

Table 3 Prevalence of any POMS-recorded morbidity (yes/no) and POMS count for those patients remaining in hospital at that time-point

	EVAR ($n = 31$)		Open ($n = 33$)		All ($n = 64$)	
Day	Prevalence	Count	Prevalence	Count	Prevalence	Count
1	100 %	3 (2–3)	100 %	5 (4–6)	100 %	4 (3–5)
2	74 %	1 (0–3)	100 %	4 (4–5)	88 %	3.5 (1–4)
3	39 %	0.5 (0–2)	100 %	4 (2–5)	70 %	2 (1–4)
4	29 %	0 (0–2)	85 %	3 (1–5)	58 %	2 (0–4)
5	26 %	1 (0–1)	76 %	2.5 (1–4.75)	52 %	1 (0–4)
6	19 %	1 (0.25–1)	70 %	2 (0.5–5)	45 %	1 (0.5–4)

Data are % of total *n*, median (interquartile range)
EVAR endovascular aneurysm repair

With respect to delayed discharge, hospital length of stay is affected by social and organisational factors unrelated to the patients' physiological recovery from surgery (Bennett-Guerrero et al. 1999; Grocott et al. 2007). Grocott et al. reported that 161 out of 200 patients (81 %) remained in hospital with no identifiable morbidity following major surgery (Grocott et al. 2007). In contrast, the current study found fewer than half of the patients stayed in hospital beyond the day on which POMS first identified zero morbidity. This disparity could be due to differences between the study samples, differing discharge practices between institutions (de Jong et al. 2006) or the emphasis on throughput and efficiency in the NHS in recent years (Paton et al. 2014), resulting in more prompt discharge once postoperative morbidity has resolved.

Potential use

Our strategy of collecting daily POMS count facilitates objective 'morbidity tracking' and discharge planning for individual patients in the postoperative period. Considering the former, progressive improvements in POMS count can be used as an indicator of patient recovery leading towards appropriately targeted discharge planning once no morbidity is recorded. Conversely, an upward trend in POMS count should trigger appropriate senior level review and reconsideration of 'fitness for discharge'. In this respect, we propose POMS to be an adjunct, rather than replacement, for other regularly recorded physiological scoring systems, e.g. National Early Warning Score (NEWS) (Royal College of Physicians of London 2012). The organ-specific structure of the POMS may guide clinicians making diagnostic and treatment decisions in the postoperative period, over and above the non-specific information from NEWS. Using two complementary systems enables early identification of postoperative complications, when patients can be more easily rescued. This could be achieved without undue time-burden on attending healthcare professionals as we expand on below.

The concept of enhanced discharge decision-making is particularly pertinent when considering the aforementioned pressures to increase efficiency and decrease hospital length of stay. This situation creates a significant risk of discharging patients before they are truly ready, resulting in increased readmissions (Kaboli et al. 2012) and resultant financial penalties for NHS trusts (Department of Health 2013). The objective nature of POMS provides a safeguard against this particularly with daily tracking. Standardising the level of recovery at which patients are discharged through use of the POMS could therefore prevent both premature and late discharge. In addition, the objective nature enables nurse initiated discharge and reduction in burden on senior medical staff.

Contrary to widespread belief, we believe that it is indeed permissible to sum POMS domains into a total score. The misconception is based on the low–moderate internal consistency reported for the nine POMS domains, which has led researchers into believing that the items may not be summed into a unidimensional scale (Grocott et al. 2007; Davies et al. 2013; Moonesinghe et al. 2014). However, the POMS is clearly composed of so-called 'causal indicators' rather than 'effect indicators' (Streiner 2003). With *scales* composed of effect indicators, the items are manifestations of an underlying construct. For example, in a scale consisting of multiple items to measure the construct of depression, scores for all items would be expected to increase or decrease together if depression got worse or better, respectively. For such scales, therefore, unidimensionality (evaluated via confirmatory factor analysis) and high internal consistency are indeed important. However, for *indexes* composed of causal indicators, where the items taken together define the construct—in this case postoperative morbidity—internal consistency is not relevant. Indeed, the low–moderate correlation between the POMS domains is a direct consequence of its design, focusing on multiple physiological systems. In short, these domains are sometimes largely independent (e.g. 'Pain' and 'Renal') and other times correlated (e.g. 'Wound' and 'Infectious'). This differentiation between a scale and an index is critical; with due caution, the nine domains of the POMS may be summed into an index to reflect the magnitude of postoperative morbidity. This index should be validated in larger studies prior to further use.

Critique of the POMS

A guiding principle in the development of the POMS was that data collection should be low-burden. Feedback from the research team confirmed this to be true and compliance with POMS completion was excellent in the current study. Indeed, the simplicity of the POMS is one of its core strengths. It has previously been shown to have good reliability even when used by researchers previously unfamiliar with its use (Davies et al. 2013). With definitions that are understandable and simple to answer by the clinical team caring for patients, it could easily be incorporated into routine postoperative monitoring. We chose to keep the existing structure of POMS to enable this goal. In comparison, the recently developed and validated cardiac-POMS (Sanders et al. 2012) changed and added definitions to develop a 13-domain survey suited to patients recovering from cardiac surgery. However, our data do suggest one change to the POMS to make it suitable for patients undergoing vascular surgery: the addition of *limb ischaemia* to the cardiovascular domain definition.

The POMS may not capture all relevant reasons why patients remain in hospital following surgery. General deconditioning and reduced mobility can require a period of rehabilitation, delaying hospital discharge without falling into one of the POMS domains. In the study by Grocott et al. (Grocott et al. 2007), 41 out of 200 patients remained in hospital on day 8 due to postoperative mobility problems. No formal assessment of reduced mobility was used in that study or in ours. Had one been used, it may have revealed some of the unexplained delayed discharges. The newly developed cardiac-POMS added a separate domain for assisted ambulation (Sanders et al. 2012). Impaired mobility can arguably be considered as postoperative morbidity that is currently unrecognised by the POMS and could be addressed in future research with a similar modification. However, any such change would have to be carefully evaluated, as adding further domains would increase the complexity of the tool, making it more burdensome to use.

Several alternative instruments have been developed to measure morbidity following surgery, although many have not gained widespread popularity (Clavien et al. 1992; Pomposelli et al. 1997; Gawande et al. 1999; Pillai et al. 1999; Dindo et al. 2004; Slankamenac et al. 2013; Strasberg et al. 2009). The Clavien-Dindo classification of postoperative complications (Dindo et al. 2004) is perhaps the most commonly used alternative system. It retrospectively classifies complications by type of treatment required to manage them. Some of the problems encountered with the system include as follows difficulties in categorising some cases (Clavien et al. 2009), differing morbidity may be classified similarly and the same complication may be classified differently depending on the treatment given (Rassweiler et al. 2012)—although this criticism can also be levelled at the POMS. It is unclear whether the original description and validation study of the Clavien-Dindo classification (Dindo et al. 2004) or its subsequent analysis (Clavien et al. 2009) specifically assessed its use in vascular surgery. Although it has subsequently been used in several publications in the vascular literature (Pol et al. 2011; Desai et al. 2011; Arya et al. 2015; Visser et al. 2014; Patel et al. 2015; Gunawansa et al. 2011), it was not used by the AAAQIP (AAAQIP 2011). The National Surgical Quality Improvement Program has been widely adopted in the USA, but the definitions of the postoperative complications are not publically available (https://www.facs.org/quality-programs/acs-nsqip). A high-profile pilot scheme is soon to be launched across the UK in a combined venture between the Health Services Research Centre and National Institute of Academic Anaesthesia. The Perioperative Quality Improvement Programme aims to capture postoperative complications, mortality and patient reported outcome in a structured fashion utilising using a range of validated instruments (Moonesinghe and Grocott 2015). This venture should provide further much needed clarity around the optimal strategy for recording postoperative complications.

Strengths and limitations

The key strength of the current study is that it is the first to validate the POMS according to its primary guiding design principle—to only capture morbidity substantial enough to delay discharge from hospital. This required careful blinding of the clinical teams to the POMS scores and daily POMS recording up until the point of discharge or competing event (a range of over 3 months). A limitation is the relatively small sample. However, this sample size, together with multiple measures per patient, afforded adequate precision to estimate the effect of any morbidity versus no morbidity. Our design is statistically very efficient, as the expected event rate (discharge) is very high (>95 %) which results in a smaller sample size requirement versus studies in which the outcome occurs less frequently. Moreover, our sample is representative of this patient population, with age and length of stay for EVAR and open repair patients equivalent to national data (Potgieter et al. 2012). Furthermore, the multi-centre design of our study adds to its external validity. The institutions include those traditionally described as both teaching hospitals and district general hospitals, reflecting current practice in the UK.

Another limitation is the lack of observation following hospital discharge. Nineteen patients were discharged with POMS morbidity recorded. Given the experience of previous researchers, where patients remained in hospital with no postoperative morbidity (Grocott et al. 2007), we did not consider the alternative situation when planning the study. It may have been informative to have followed these participants after hospital discharge to see whether they had an increased rate of re-admission or use of primary care.

From a wider-reaching perspective, robust postoperative morbidity capture is highly relevant. The development of early postoperative complications is of greater prognostic significance than preoperative comorbidity in determining long-term survival (Khuri et al. 2005). In this setting, although the POMS describes only in-hospital morbidity, a recent study demonstrated its association with increased mortality for up to 2 years following surgery (Moonesinghe et al. 2014). In addition, objective postoperative morbidity data would add to the existing mortality and length of stay information used to benchmark institutions comparatively. Furthermore, daily POMS recording as part of perioperative care pathways might highlight areas for improvement and be used to audit any resultant change in practice. The POMS could therefore act as an informative tool both locally and nationally to drive quality improvement and institution benchmarking.

Conclusions

This study has demonstrated the POMS to be a valid tool to measure short-term postoperative morbidity in patients undergoing elective infrarenal AAA repair. The data suggest a minor modification to ensure complete capture of morbidity. Daily POMS measurement is recommended to fully capture morbidity and allow robust analysis. The survey could be a valuable outcome measure for use in quality improvement programmes and future research, or as an adjunct to clinical decision-making in the postoperative period.

Abbreviations

AAA: abdominal aortic aneurysm; AAAQIP: National Abdominal Aortic Aneurysm Quality Improvement Programme; EVAR: endovascular aneurysm repair; LOS: length of stay; NHS: National Health Service; POMS: Postoperative Morbidity Survey.

Competing interests

The authors declare that they have no competing interests.

Authors' contributions

BG designed the study, collected data, analysed the data and drafted the manuscript. AB designed the study, analysed the data and drafted the manuscript. EK, LC, DY, HM, KK and GD designed the study, collected data and drafted the manuscript. All authors read and approved the final manuscript.

Acknowledgements

This research was funded by a small grand award from South Tees Hospitals NHS Trust and local departmental funds in each recruiting centre.

Author details

[1]Department of Perioperative Care, Royal Victoria Infirmary, Newcastle upon Tyne, UK. [2]Health and Social Care Institute, Teesside University, Middlesbrough, UK. [3]Department of Academic Anaesthesia, James Cook University Hospital, Marton Road, Middlesbrough TS4 3BW, UK. [4]Department of Anaesthesia, York Hospital, York, UK. [5]Department of Anaesthesia, University Hospital of North Durham, Durham, UK. [6]Department of Anaesthesia, Northern General Hospital, Sheffield, UK.

References

AAAQIP. National Abdominal Aortic Aneurysm Quality Improvement Programme Interim report. 2011.

Ackland GL, Scollay JM, Parks RW, De Beaux I, Mythen MG. Pre-operative high sensitivity C-reactive protein and postoperative outcome in patients undergoing elective orthopaedic surgery. Anaesthesia. 2007;62:888–94.

Ackland GL, Harris S, Ziabari Y, Grocott M, Mythen M. Revised cardiac risk index and postoperative morbidity after elective orthopaedic surgery: a prospective cohort study. Br J Anaesth. 2010;105:744–52.

Ackland GL, Moran N, Cone S, Grocott MPW, Mythen MG. Chronic kidney disease and postoperative morbidity after elective orthopedic surgery. Anesth Analg. 2011;112:1375–81.

Arya S, Kim SI, Duwayri Y, Brewster LP, Veeraswamy R, Salam A, et al. Frailty increases the risk of 30-day mortality, morbidity, and failure to rescue after elective abdominal aortic aneurysm repair independent of age and comorbidities. J Vasc Surg. 2015;61:324–31.

Ausania F, Snowden CP, Prentis JM, Holmes LR, Jaques BC, White SA, et al. Effects of low cardiopulmonary reserve on pancreatic leak following pancreaticoduodenectomy. Br J Surg. 2012;99:1290–4.

Bennett-Guerrero E, Welsby I, Dunn TJ, Young LR, Wahl TA, Diers TL, et al. The use of a postoperative morbidity survey to evaluate patients with prolonged hospitalization after routine, moderate-risk, elective surgery. Anesth Analg. 1999;89:514–9.

Beyersmann J, Schumacher M, Allignol A. Time-dependent covariates and multistate models. In: Competing Risks and Multistate Models with R. New York: Springer; 2012. p. 211–26. [Use R!].

Clavien PA, Sanabria JR, Strasberg SM. Proposed classification of complications of surgery with examples of utility in cholecystectomy. Surgery. 1992;111:518–26.

Clavien PA, Barkun J, de Oliveira ML, Vauthey JN, Dindo D, Schulick RD, et al. The Clavien-Dindo classification of surgical complications: five-year experience. Ann Surg. 2009;250:187–96.

Davies SJ, Francis J, Dilley J, Wilson RJT, Howell SJ, Allgar V. Measuring outcomes after major abdominal surgery during hospitalization: reliability and validity of the Postoperative Morbidity Survey. Perioper Med. 2013;2:1.

de Jong JD, Westert GP, Lagoe R, Groenewegen PP. Variation in hospital length of stay: do physicians adapt their length of stay decisions to what is usual in the hospital where they work? Health Serv Res. 2006;41:374–94.

Department of Health. Payment by Results Guidance for 2013–14. 2013.

Desai M, Gurusamy KS, Ghanbari H, Hamilton G, Seifalian AM. Remote ischaemic preconditioning versus no remote ischaemic preconditioning for vascular and endovascular surgical procedures. In: Cochrane Database of Systematic Reviews. John Wiley & Sons, Ltd; 2011.

Dindo D, Demartines N, Clavien P-A. Classification of surgical complications. Ann Surg. 2004;240:205–13.

Gawande AA, Thomas EJ, Zinner MJ, Brennan TA. The incidence and nature of surgical adverse events in Colorado and Utah in 1992. Surgery. 1999;126:66–75.

Giles KA, Wyers MC, Pomposelli FB, Hamdan AD, Avery Ching Y, Schermerhorn ML. The impact of body mass index on perioperative outcomes of open and endovascular abdominal aortic aneurysm repair from the National Surgical Quality Improvement Program, 2005–2007. J Vasc Surg. 2010;52:1471–7.

Grocott MPW, Browne JP, Van der Meulen J, Matejowsky C, Mutch M, Hamilton MA, et al. The Postoperative Morbidity Survey was validated and used to describe morbidity after major surgery. J Clin Epidemiol. 2007;60:919–28.

Gunawansa N, Goonerathne T, Cassim R, Wijeyaratne M. Open repair of infra renal abdominal aortic aneurysms: a single center experience from the developing world. Ann Vasc Dis. 2011;4:313–8.

Head J, Ferrie JE, Alexanderson K, Westerlund H, Vahtera J, Kivimäki M. Diagnosis-specific sickness absence as a predictor of mortality: the Whitehall II prospective cohort study. BMJ. 2008;337:a1469.

Jones C, Kelliher L, Dickinson M, Riga A, Worthington T, Scott MJ, et al. Randomized clinical trial on enhanced recovery versus standard care following open liver resection. Br J Surg. 2013;100:1015–24.

Kaboli PJ, Go JT, Hockenberry J, Glasgow JM, Johnson SR, Rosenthal GE, et al. Associations between reduced hospital length of stay and 30-day readmission rate and mortality: 14-year experience in 129 Veterans Affairs Hospitals. Ann Intern Med. 2012;157:837–45.

Khuri SF, Henderson WG, DePalma RG, Mosca C, Healey NA, Kumbhani DJ. Determinants of long-term survival after major surgery and the adverse effect of postoperative complications. Ann Surg. 2005;242:326–41. discussion 341–343.

Lee TH, Marcantonio ER, Mangione CM, Thomas EJ, Polanczyk CA, Cook EF, et al. Derivation and prospective validation of a simple index for prediction of cardiac risk of major noncardiac surgery. Circulation. 1999;100:1043–9.

Lee WA, Carter JW, Upchurch G, Seeger JM, Huber TS. Perioperative outcomes after open and endovascular repair of intact abdominal aortic aneurysms in the United States during 2001. J Vasc Surg. 2004;39:491–6.

Lee A, Chiu CH, Cho MWA, Gomersall CD, Lee KF, Cheung YS, et al. Factors associated with failure of enhanced recovery protocol in patients undergoing major hepatobiliary and pancreatic surgery: a retrospective cohort study. BMJ Open. 2014;4, e005330.

Levey AS, Bosch JP, Lewis JB, Greene T, Rogers N, Roth D. A more accurate method to estimate glomerular filtration rate from serum creatinine: a new prediction equation. Ann Intern Med. 1999;130:461–70.

Moonesinghe R, Grocott M. Towards a national Perioperative Quality Improvement Programme (PQIP). Bull R Coll Anaesth. 2015;91:12–3.

Moonesinghe SR, Harris S, Mythen MG, Rowan KM, Haddad FS, Emberton M, et al. Survival after postoperative morbidity: a longitudinal observational cohort study. Br J Anaesth. 2014;113(6):977–84.

National Surgical Quality Improvement Program. [https://www.facs.org/quality-programs/acs-nsqip].

Patel SD, Constantinou J, Simring D, Ramirez M, Agu O, Hamilton H, et al. Results of complex aortic stent grafting of abdominal aortic aneurysms

stratified according to the proximal landing zone using the Society for Vascular Surgery classification. J Vasc Surg. 2015;62:319–25.e2.
Patila T, Kukkonen S, Vento A, Pettila V, Suojaranta-Ylinen R. Relation of the sequential organ failure assessment score to morbidity and mortality after cardiac surgery. Ann Thorac Surg. 2006;82:2072–8.
Paton F, Chambers D, Wilson P, Eastwood A, Craig D, Fox D, et al. Initiatives to reduce length of stay in acute hospital settings: a rapid synthesis of evidence relating to enhanced recovery programmes. Health Serv Deliv Res. 2014;2(21).
Pergolizzi JV, Raffa RB, Tallarida R, Taylor R, Labhsetwar SA. Continuous multimechanistic postoperative analgesia: a rationale for transitioning from intravenous acetaminophen and opioids to oral formulations. Pain Pract. 2012;12:159–73.
Pillai SB, van Rij AM, Williams S, Thomson IA, Putterill MJ, Greig S. Complexity- and risk-adjusted model for measuring surgical outcome. Br J Surg. 1999;86:1567–72.
Pol RA, van Leeuwen BL, Visser L, Izaks GJ, van den Dungen JJ, Tielliu IFJ, et al. Standardised frailty indicator as predictor for postoperative delirium after vascular surgery: a prospective cohort study. Eur J Vasc Endovasc Surg. 2011;42:824–30.
Pomposelli JJ, Gupta SK, Zacharoulis DC, Landa R, Miller A, Nanda R. Surgical complication outcome (SCOUT) score: a new method to evaluate quality of care in vascular surgery. J Vasc Surg. 1997;25:1007–14. discussion 1014–1015.
Potgieter R, Hindley H, Mitchell D, McCleary J. Delivering a National Quality Improvement Programme for Patients with Abdominal Aortic Aneurysms. The Vascular Society of Great Britain and Ireland; 2012.
Qiu W, Chavarro J, Lazarus R, Rosner B, Ma J. powerSurvEpi: Power and Sample Size Calculation for Survival Analysis of Epidemiological Studies. 2012.
Rassweiler JJ, Rassweiler M-C, Michel M-S. Classification of complications: is the Clavien-Dindo classification the gold standard? Eur Urol. 2012;62:256–8. discussion 259–260.
Royal College of Physicians of London. National Early Warning Score (NEWS): Standardising the Assessment of Acute-Illness Severity in the NHS. London: Royal College of Physicians; 2012.
Sanders J, Patel S, Cooper J, Berryman J, Farrar D, Mythen M, et al. Red blood cell storage is associated with length of stay and renal complications after cardiac surgery. Transfusion (Paris). 2011;51:2286–94.
Sanders J, Keogh BE, Van der Meulen J, Browne JP, Treasure T, Mythen MG, et al. The development of a postoperative morbidity score to assess total morbidity burden after cardiac surgery. J Clin Epidemiol. 2012;65:423–33.
Schouten O, Kok NFM, Hoedt MTC, van Laanen JH, Poldermans D. The influence of aneurysm size on perioperative cardiac outcome in elective open infrarenal aortic aneurysm repair. J Vasc Surg. 2006;44:435–41.
Slankamenac K, Graf R, Barkun J, Puhan MA, Clavien P-A. The comprehensive complication index. Ann Surg. 2013;258:1–7.
Snowden CP, Prentis JM, Anderson HL, Roberts DR, Randles D, Renton M, et al. Submaximal cardiopulmonary exercise testing predicts complications and hospital length of stay in patients undergoing major elective surgery. Ann Surg. 2010;251:535–41.
Strasberg SM, Linehan DC, Hawkins WG. The accordion severity grading system of surgical complications. Ann Surg. 2009;250:177–86.
Streiner DL. Being inconsistent about consistency: when coefficient alpha does and doesn't matter. J Pers Assess. 2003;80:217–22.
Visser L, Pol RA, Tielliu IFJ, van den Dungen JJAM, Zeebregts CJ. A limited and customized follow-up seems justified after endovascular abdominal aneurysm repair in octogenarians. J Vasc Surg. 2014;59:1232–40.
Wakeling HG, McFall MR, Jenkins CS, Woods WGA, Miles WFA, Barclay GR, et al. Intraoperative oesophageal Doppler guided fluid management shortens postoperative hospital stay after major bowel surgery. Br J Anaesth. 2005;95:634–42.
West MA, Lythgoe D, Barben CP, Noble L, Kemp GJ, Jack S, et al. Cardiopulmonary exercise variables are associated with postoperative morbidity after major colonic surgery: a prospective blinded observational study. Br J Anaesth. 2014;112:665–71.

Anticipated regret in shared decision-making: a randomized experimental study

Rebecca M. Speck[1,2], Mark D. Neuman[3], Kimberly S. Resnick[4], Barbara A. Mellers[5] and Lee A. Fleisher[6*]

Abstract

Background: Explicit consideration of anticipated regret is not part of the standard shared decision-making protocols. This pilot study aimed to compare decisions about a hypothetical surgery for breast cancer and examined whether regret is a consideration in treatment decisions.

Methods: In this randomized experimental study, 184 healthy female volunteers were randomized to receive a standard decision aid (control) or one with information on post-surgical regret (experimental). The main outcome measures were the proportion of subjects choosing lumpectomy vs. mastectomy and the proportion reporting that regret played a role in the decision made. We hypothesized that a greater proportion of the experimental group (regret-incorporated decision aid) would make a surgical treatment preference that favored the less regret-inducing option and that they would be more likely to consider regret in their decision-making process as compared to the control group.

Results: A significantly greater proportion of the experimental group subjects reported regret played a role in their decision-making process compared to the control counterparts (78 vs. 65 %; $p = 0.039$). Recipients of the regret-incorporated experimental decision aid had a threefold increased odds of choosing the less regret-inducing surgery (OR = 2.97; 95 % CI = 1.25, 7.09; p value = 0.014).

Conclusions: In this hypothetical context, the incorporation of regret in a decision aid for preference-sensitive surgery impacted decision-making. This finding suggests that keying in on anticipated regret may be an important element of shared decision-making strategies. Our results make a strong argument for applying this design and pursuing further research in a surgical patient population.

Keywords: Breast cancer, Anticipated regret, Decision-making, Surgery

Background

In recent years, the US health-care system has been redefining itself as one that strives to be patient-centered. Central to this idea is the belief that patients ought to be actively engaged in their health care (Barry & Edgman-Levitan 2012). One approach to accomplishing this goal is the use of "shared decision-making," in which physician and patient share information in an attempt to improve the extent to which patients select treatments that match their underlying preferences (Wennberg et al. 2002). It is thought that shared decision-making can improve care and reduce costs and is encouraged and supported by the Affordable Care Act (ACA) (Oshima & Emanuel 2013).

Shared decision-making may be particularly important in clinical situations in which there is clinical equipoise, i.e., there is no best treatment paradigm. In these "preference-sensitive" conditions, the treatment choice depends on the unique values of the patient (Wennberg 2002). Although the use of decision aids has been shown to increase patient activation, improve knowledge, and aid in the realistic perception of outcome, the size of the effect varies across studies (Wennberg et al. 2010; Stacey et al. 2011). Furthermore, randomized control trials

* Correspondence: lee.fleisher@uphs.upenn.edu
[6]Department of Anesthesiology and Critical Care, Center for Pharmacoepidemiology Research and Training, Leonard Davis Institute, University of Pennsylvania, 3400 Spruce Street, Dulles 6, Philadelphia, PA 19104, USA
Full list of author information is available at the end of the article

comparing the impact of decision aids with "no intervention," "usual care," or "alternate intervention" have found current decision aids to be no better than comparisons in improving satisfaction with decision-making, anxiety, health outcomes, or decisional regret (O'Connor et al. 2009; Goel et al. 2001).

In the current model of shared decision-making, patients are asked to make surgical decisions in which the risks of different outcomes are discussed and presented numerically. However, multiple studies have documented the public's lack of the numerical skills essential to making informed medical decisions (Reyna et al. 2009). In the area of surgical treatment of breast cancer, external forces such as celebrity treatment choice rather than evidence can influence the desire for more aggressive treatment. Nancy Reagan's choice of mastectomy over lumpectomy in the late 1980s (Lewin 1988; Nattinger et al. 1998) and more recently Angelina Jolie's decision to have a prophylactic double mastectomy are two examples (Kamenova et al. 2014).

Recent psychological research has highlighted the role of anticipated regret—the fear of "buyer's remorse"—as an important influence on individual choices across a range of domains, including health care (Zeelenberg 1999; Simonson 1992; Nelissen et al. 2011). While largely absent from past research on the design of decision aids, insights from research on anticipated regret may hold promise as a potential means of improving decision-making strategies.

In this study, we aimed to investigate whether surgical treatment choices for breast cancer would differ based on the decision aid the subjects were given. We hypothesized that subjects given an experimental decision aid which incorporated information about regret would be more likely to make a surgical treatment preference that was less regret-inducing and that they would be more likely to consider regret in their decision-making process as compared to subjects in the control group.

Methods

We conducted a randomized experimental pilot study at the University of Pennsylvania among healthy female volunteers receiving decision aids for the surgical treatment of early-stage breast cancer. Early-stage breast cancer was chosen because although it has more than one treatment option available, there is little medical evidence to suggest one treatment option is superior to another. Consequently, the ultimate treatment choice is informed by patient preference and greatly influenced by shared decision-making strategies. Furthermore, early-stage breast cancer can be treated with increasingly invasive procedures, the more invasive of which has been associated with high rates of regret after surgery.

We incorporated information about the rate at which regret occurs after surgery into standard decision aids for breast cancer and assigned volunteers to receive the standard or regret-incorporated versions.

Study participants and materials

The study received International Review Board approval through the University of Pennsylvania. A waiver for written informed consent was approved. Study subjects were healthy female volunteers, recruited through campus advertising, and offered a participant compensation of US$5. Subject recruitment and participation occurred in April 2013. There were no specific inclusion or exclusion criteria.

Study participants received decision aids on surgery for early-stage breast cancer (Additional files 1 and 2). We created two versions of the decision aid: one based on standard information and one that incorporated additional information on the rates of regret after surgical treatment. To develop the standard version, we relied on existing decision aids developed by the Informed Medical Decisions Foundation and selected those with the highest scores for the content, development process, and effectiveness criteria proposed by the International Patient Decision Aids Standards (IPDAS) collaboration. For the experimental version, we incorporated additional information on the rates of regret after surgical treatment found in the literature (Fernandes-Taylor & Bloom 2011; Lantz et al. 2005). In a study of 449 women 5 years post surgery for breast cancer, Fernandes-Taylor and Bloom (Fernandes-Taylor & Bloom 2011) found the post-surgical regret rate for mastectomy was 24.1 %. Lantz and colleagues (Lantz et al. 2005) reported a post-surgical regret rate of 11.4 % among a sample of 1633 women that underwent mastectomy as opposed to lumpectomy.

Data collection and analysis

All data collection occurred in the Wharton Behavioral Lab (WBL) on the University of Pennsylvania campus. The WBL was initially funded by the Wharton School in Spring 2005. The primary goal of the WBL is to enhance the research productivity of Wharton-affiliated faculty by minimizing the operational costs, both time and money, of conducting research. Each WBL session lasts 30 to 60 min. During a session, study subjects may complete questionnaires, participate in online experiments, or interact in groups.

For the present study, standard and regret rate-incorporated decision aids for breast cancer were distributed to participants at random. All participants were asked to complete an investigator-designed computer-based survey about their treatment preferences for breast cancer surgery, as presented in the decision aid. Participants were asked to choose between lumpectomy and mastectomy and were then questioned about the role that anticipated regret played in this decision-making process and which sections or statements in the decision aid most influenced their choice for treatment.

Demographic data was collected via an online survey platform that captured age, gender, and university affiliation. Descriptive statistics were calculated for demographic data, and the anticipated regret outcomes were compared between the experimental and control groups using the chi-square test. Frequency counts were performed for each line of each decision aid and analyzed. Referenced lines from the decision aids that used the same words with different sentence structure were collapsed and counted together.

Results

There were 189 subjects enrolled in this study. From this sample, the data collected from five of the participants were discarded due to procedural error in data collection. Of the 184 females receiving the breast cancer decision aid, 96 received the control standard version and 88 received the experimental anticipated regret-incorporated version.

Descriptive statistics of 182 study participants are available; two participants did not complete the demographic questions (Table 1). Participants were 22.0 years old on average and included undergraduates (86 %), graduate students (9 %), university staff (3 %), and others (2 %). The majority were unemployed (53.3 %), while over a third worked part-time (39.6 %) and 7.1 % worked full-time. There was a statistically significant difference between the experimental and control groups in terms of citizenship.

Quantitative data

The first outcome of interest was the difference in surgical treatment preference by the decision aid type (experimental vs. control). In the control group, which received the standard version of the decision aid, 74 out of 96 (77 %) subjects chose lumpectomy over mastectomy, whereas in the experimental group that received the regret-incorporated decision aid, 80 out of 88 (91 %) subjects chose lumpectomy over mastectomy ($p = 0.011$). Subjects in the experimental group had a threefold increased odds of choosing the less regret-inducing surgery (OR = 2.97; 95 % CI = 1.25, 7.09; p value = 0.014; Table 2).

Our other outcome of interest was whether there was a difference in consideration of regret during the decision-making process between those who received the experimental vs. the standard version of the decision aid. In the experimental group, 69 out of 88 (78 %)

Table 1 Demographics of study subjects

	All subjects (*N* = 182) Mean (SD) or *N* (%)	Experimental (*N* = 88)	Control (*N* = 94)	*p* value
Age in years	22.0 (6.6)	21.8 (5.9)	22.1 (7.2)	0.76
Employment status				
Full-time	13 (7.1)	4 (4.5)	9 (9.6)	0.43
Part-time	72 (39.6)	35 (39.8)	37 (39.3)	
Unemployed	97 (53.3)	49 (55.7)	48 (51.1)	
Academic affiliation				
Undergraduate	153 (84.1)	72 (81.8)	81 (86.2)	0.70
Graduate	21 (11.5)	13 (14.8)	8 (8.5)	
Staff	8 (4.4)	3 (3.4)	5 (5.3)	
Ethnicity				
White	54 (29.7)	24 (27.3)	30 (31.9)	0.70
Black	32 (17.6)	13 (14.8)	19 (20.2)	
Asian/Pacific Islander	68 (37.3)	35 (39.8)	33 (35.1)	
Hispanic	12 (6.6)	7 (8.0)	5 (5.3)	
Declined to state	16 (8.8)	9 (10.2)	7 (7.5)	
Citizenship				
American citizen	155 (85.1)	69 (78.4)	86 (91.5)	0.02
Green card	20 (11.0)	13 (14.8)	7 (7.4)	
No green card	2 (1.1)	1 (1.1)	1 (1.1)	
Declined to state	5 (2.8)	5 (5.7)	0	

Table 2 Preferred surgical treatment and role of regret by decision aid received

	Experimental ($N = 88$)	Control ($N = 96$)	p value
Treatment choice?			
Lumpectomy (vs. mastectomy)	80 (91 %)	74 (77 %)	0.011
Did regret play a role in your decision-making process?			
Yes (vs. no)	69 (78 %)	62 (65 %)	0.039
Odds of choosing lumpectomy (vs. mastectomy)			
	OR	95 % CI	p value
Experimental group	2.97	1.24–7.09	0.014
Odds that regret was considered in decision			
	OR	95 % CI	p value
Experimental group	1.99	1.03–3.84	0.04

reported that regret was considered during the decision-making process, compared to 62 out of 96 (65 %) in the control group ($p = 0.039$). Subjects in the experimental group had a twofold increased odds (OR = 1.99; 95 % CI = 1.03, 3.84; p value = 0.04) of considering regret during the decision-making process as compared to subjects in the control group.

Qualitative data

In order to analyze the responses to the survey question of "what part(s) of the brochure played a role in the decision you made for your treatment choice," we performed frequency counts for the various sentences reported. The top five most frequent sentences for each decision aid (experimental vs. control) are presented in Table 3. Whereas many of the top five sentences reported by the control group were also among the top five most often reported by the experimental group, there was a difference in the order of importance: sentences referencing regret displaced other sentences from the control condition. This pattern demonstrated that when participants are presented with information about regret rates, this information becomes an important factor in their decision-making process.

Discussion

In this randomized experimental study, we demonstrated that incorporating information about post-surgical regret into decision aids for breast cancer was associated with preferences toward a less regret-inducing surgical treatment option and a higher probability of considering regret during the decision-making process. These findings suggest that there is the potential that activating subjects to think pre-operatively about the states they may ruminate on post-operatively could inform the decision-making process. The concept that anticipated regret can be used to optimize decision-making behavior has been given credibility by recent neurobiological studies and neuroimaging data that have found a neural basis for the emotion of regret (Camille et al. 2004; Coricelli et al. 2005). Functional magnetic resonance imaging (fMRI) data have confirmed that the emotion of regret is subserved by specific cerebral regions and have localized processing to the orbitofrontal cortex (Chandrasekhar et al. 2008). The same pattern of activity expressed during the experience of regret has been demonstrated to be expressed in the moments preceding decision-making, suggesting that experienced regret and anticipated regret are mediated by the same neural circuitry (Coricelli et al. 2005). Furthermore, these same brain structures become active when learning of another individual's regretful outcome, suggesting that one is able to incorporate this type of information into the decision-making process as it reactivates the same neural regret network (Canessa et al. 2011). Taken together, these neuroimaging studies provide a neurobiological basis for the design of our experiment and place regret at the intersection of emotion and cognition and document its role in decision behavior.

Currently, the rates of post-surgical regret and associated morbidities represent an objective body of information that has been previously overlooked or, at best, only sporadically employed by individual physicians. The observation that patients continue to have post-surgical regret rates as high as 47 % in areas of preference-sensitive medicine suggests that there is room for improvement in the way in which we currently help patients to navigate the decision-making process (Sheehan et al. 2007). Incorporating anticipated regret into the process may be one way of achieving this outcome. Further, it holds promise for combatting one of the themes most often expressed by patients experiencing regret: dissatisfaction with information provided regarding treatment alternatives and adverse side effects, which can cause patients to later say "if only I had known…." Therefore, the patient may more appropriately choose wisely from the perspective of satisfaction after the intervention.

Table 3 Qualitative data: top five most frequent responses by decision aid

Control group standard decision aid		Experimental group regret-incorporated decision aid	
Frequency	Response	Frequency	Response
18 (19 %)	With mastectomy, after 10 years, about 8 out of 100 women will have local recurrence. With lumpectomy and radiation, after 10 years, about 10 out of 100 women will have local recurrence	19 (22 %)	With mastectomy, after 10 years, about 8 out of 100 women who have will have local recurrence. With lumpectomy and radiation, after 10 years, about 10 out of 100 women would have a local recurrence
16 (17 %)	Mastectomy removes the entire breast	18 (20 %)	If a woman undergoes mastectomy and is unable to cope with the loss of her breast… she may regret her decision to treat a cancer that could also have been cured with breast-conserving therapy. This regret may be especially pertinent if she learns that a similar woman with a similar cancer chose lumpectomy with radiation and continued to live cancer-free without the same sacrifice to her appearance
10 (10 %)	The chance of local recurrence is low after mastectomy and slightly higher after lumpectomy with radiation	17 (19 %)	Lumpectomy saves the breast
9 (9 %)	You will live the same length of time whether you choose mastectomy or lumpectomy with radiation	14 (16 %)	24.1 % of women choosing mastectomy have regretted their decision afterwards
9 (9 %)	Cancer that comes back in the breast after lumpectomy can usually be successfully treated with mastectomy	14 (16 %)	You will live the same length of time whether you choose mastectomy or lumpectomy

In our experimental, hypothetical, surgical decision-making situation, receipt of the decision aid that keyed in on anticipated regret was associated with the surgical treatment option demonstrated to be less likely to induce regret. The difference in preference between the experimental and control groups is important given that studies have suggested an association between post-surgical regret and poorer health-related quality of life (Hu et al. 2003). Of note, post-surgical regret does not appear to be dependent on having a bad outcome, as it has been shown to occur in patients that are equivalent in clinical outcome measures (Schroeck et al. 2008). If anticipated regret can help patients minimize the likelihood of post-surgical regret, then it may also spare them the decrease in quality of life with which it is associated.

Despite the implications of this study, there are several limitations. Our results are limited by the hypothetical nature for the population in which the study was tested. Specifically, the study subjects were not personally facing the need to make a decision about breast cancer surgery. Further, the average age of participants in this study was younger than the age at which breast cancers are most often diagnosed (Hayat et al. 2007). Finally, our study cohort was comprised of individuals with an education beyond high school. Over 10 % were in a graduate degree program, the remainder is in an undergraduate degree program or on staff at the institution. Therefore, although this design was useful in demonstrating feasibility, the results are not immediately generalizable to the intended surgical patient population with early-stage breast cancer, a population with a more diverse educational level.

Despite these limitations, the results of this pilot study make a strong argument for applying this design to a larger, relevant surgical patient population to further investigate the role of anticipated regret in shared medical decision-making. Specifically, this study design should be repeated in cancer patients at the time of diagnosis of early-stage breast cancer. After randomization to receive the standard or regret-incorporated versions of the decision aid, patients should be followed through their decision-making process, treatment course, and post-decisional state. Important results will include the surgical treatment selected as well as the rates of post-decisional regret. We believe that a decision process which incorporates anticipated regret could be accomplished in the surgeon's office through collaboration between the surgeon, anesthesiologist and primary caregiver as part of the consent process.

The incorporation of shared decision-making strategies into health care is becoming increasingly important with the passing of the ACA, especially in light of Section 3506, which specifically encourages their use and application. This section of the ACA establishes shared decision-making as an ideal means of accommodating patient preferences and assuring that care-delivered matches care-desired. Nevertheless, this ideal is yet to be consistently reached with less than

10 % of medical decisions meeting the standard for informed decision-making, (Braddock et al. 1999) and little being done to promote shared decision-making since the passing of the ACA. Assessing the success of medical care is a hallmark of the ACA and should include the assessment of patient-reported outcomes. This includes both health-related quality of life as well as satisfaction with care. We believe that the quality of consent should be assessed and that incorporation of anticipated regret will lead to increased satisfaction and trust.

Conclusions

Because patient decision aids are yet to be widely implemented, we are uniquely poised to affect the future of the shared decision-making process. The results of this pilot study suggest that incorporation of regret rates into decision aids might be a potential strategy to encourage patients to think more elaborately before making a choice. Anticipated regret may be an important element of physician-patient decision-making capable of improving the quality of medical decisions and, in turn, the value of health care delivered. Our results make a strong argument for applying this design to a larger, relevant population to investigate the validity of these findings and their potential for improving shared decision-making strategies.

Abbreviations

ACA: Affordable Care Act; IPDAS: International Patient Decision Aids Standards; WBL: Wharton Behavioral Lab.

Competing interests

The authors declare that they have no competing interests.

Authors' contributions

RMS contributed to the design, acquisition of data, data analysis and interpretation, and drafted and revised the manuscript. MDN contributed to the design, data interpretation, and drafted and revised the manuscript. KSR contributed to the design, acquisition of data, data interpretation, and drafted and revised the manuscript. BAM contributed to the design, acquisition of data, data interpretation, and revised the manuscript. LAF contributed to the design, data interpretation, and revised the manuscript. All authors read and approved the final manuscript.

Acknowledgements

Funding source

Financial support for the data collection associated with this study was provided by the internal Department of Anesthesiology and Critical Care funds. The funding agreement ensured the authors' independence in designing the study, interpreting the data, writing, and publishing the report. No study authors received salary support for this work.

Author details

[1]Department of Anesthesiology and Critical Care, Center for Pharmacoepidemiology Research and Training, University of Pennsylvania, 3400 Spruce Street, Dulles 6, Philadelphia, PA 19104, USA. [2]Evidera, 1417 4th Ave., Suite 510, Seattle, WA 98101, USA. [3]Department of Anesthesiology and Critical Care, Leonard Davis Institute, University of Pennsylvania, 3400 Spruce Street, Dulles 6, Philadelphia, PA 19104, USA. [4]Department of Psychiatry, University of Pennsylvania, 3535 Market St, Philadelphia, PA 19104, USA. [5]Department of Psychology, Department of Marketing, University of Pennsylvania, 3720 Walnut St, Philadelphia, PA 19104, USA. [6]Department of Anesthesiology and Critical Care, Center for Pharmacoepidemiology Research and Training, Leonard Davis Institute, University of Pennsylvania, 3400 Spruce Street, Dulles 6, Philadelphia, PA 19104, USA.

References

Barry MJ, Edgman-Levitan S. Shared decision making—pinnacle of patient-centered care. N Engl J Med. 2012;366(9):780–1.

Braddock 3rd CH, Edwards KA, Hasenberg NM, Laidley TL, Levinson W. Informed decision making in outpatient practice: time to get back to basics. JAMA. 1999;282(24):2313–20.

Camille N, Coricelli G, Sallet J, Pradat-Diehl P, Duhamel JR, Sirigu A. The involvement of the orbitofrontal cortex in the experience of regret. Science. 2004;304(5674):1167–70.

Canessa N, Motterlini M, Alemanno F, Perani D, Cappa SF. Learning from other people's experience: a neuroimaging study of decisional interactive-learning. Neuroimage. 2011;55(1):353–62.

Chandrasekhar PV, Capra CM, Moore S, Noussair C, Berns GS. Neurobiological regret and rejoice functions for aversive outcomes. Neuroimage. 2008;39(3):1472–84.

Coricelli G, Critchley HD, Joffily M, O'Doherty JP, Sirigu A, Dolan RJ. Regret and its avoidance: a neuroimaging study of choice behavior. Nat Neurosci. 2005;8(9):1255–62.

Fernandes-Taylor S, Bloom JR. Post-treatment regret among young breast cancer survivors. Psychooncology. 2011;20(5):506–16.

Goel V, Sawka CA, Thiel EC, Gort EH, O'Connor AM. Randomized trial of a patient decision aid for choice of surgical treatment for breast cancer. Med Decis Making. 2001;21(1):1–6.

Hayat MJ, Howlader N, Reichman ME, Edwards BK. Cancer statistics, trends, and multiple primary cancer analyses from the Surveillance, Epidemiology, and End Results (SEER) Program. Oncologist. 2007;12(1):20–37.

Hu JC, Kwan L, Saigal CS, Litwin MS. Regret in men treated for localized prostate cancer. J Urol. 2003;169(6):2279–83.

Kamenova K, Reshef A, Caulfield T. Angelina Jolie's faulty gene: newspaper coverage of a celebrity's preventive bilateral mastectomy in Canada, the United States, and the United Kingdom. Genet Med. 2014;16(7):522–8.

Lantz PM, Janz NK, Fagerlin A, et al. Satisfaction with surgery outcomes and the decision process in a population-based sample of women with breast cancer. Health Serv Res. 2005;40(3):745–67.

Lewin T. Nancy Reagan defends her decision to have mastectomy. N Y Times. 1988 March;5.

Nattinger AB, Hoffmann RG, Howell-Pelz A, Goodwin JS. Effect of Nancy Reagan's mastectomy on choice of surgery for breast cancer by US women. JAMA. 1998;279(10):762–6.

Nelissen RM, de Vet E, Zeelenberg M. Anticipated emotions and effort allocation in weight goal striving. Br J Health Psychol. 2011;16(Pt 1):201–12.

O'Connor AM, Bennett CL, Stacey D, et al. Decision aids for people facing health treatment or screening decisions. Cochrane Database Syst Rev. 2009;2009(3):CD001431.

Oshima Lee E, Emanuel EJ. Shared decision making to improve care and reduce costs. N Engl J Med. 2013a;368(1):6–8.

Reyna VF, Nelson WL, Han PK, Dieckmann NF. How numeracy influences risk comprehension and medical decision making. Psychol Bull. 2009;135(6):943–73.

Schroeck FR, Krupski TL, Sun L, et al. Satisfaction and regret after open retropubic or robot-assisted laparoscopic radical prostatectomy. Eur Urol. 2008;54(4):785–93.

Sheehan JSK, Lam T, Boyages J. Association of information satisfaction, psychological distress and monitoring coping style with post-decision regret following breast reconstruction. Psychooncology. 2007;16:342–51.

Simonson I. The influence of anticipating regret and responsibility on purchase decisions. J Consum Res. 1992;19(1):105–18.
Stacey D, Bennett CL, Barry MJ, et al. Decision aids for people facing health treatment or screening decisions. Cochrane Database Syst Rev. 2011;2011(10):CD001431.
Wennberg JE. Unwarranted variations in healthcare delivery: implications for academic medical centres. BMJ. 2002;325(7370):961–4.
Wennberg JE, Fisher ES, Skinner JS. Geography and the debate over Medicare reform. Health Aff (Milwood). 2002;Suppl Web Exclusives:W96–114.
Wennberg DE, Marr A, Lang L, O'Malley S, Bennett G. A randomized trial of a telephone care-management strategy. N Engl J Med. 2010;363(13):1245–55.
Zeelenberg M. Anticipated regret, expected feedback and behavioral decision-making. J Behav Decis Mak. 1999;12:93–106.

6

Association of intraoperative transfusion of blood products with mortality in lung transplant recipients

Denise Weber[†], Silvia R Cottini[†], Pascal Locher, Urs Wenger, Paul A Stehberger, Mario Fasshauer, Reto A Schuepbach and Markus Béchir[*]

Abstract

Background: The impact of intraoperative transfusion on postoperative mortality in lung transplant recipients is still elusive.

Methods: Univariate and multivariate analysis were performed to investigate the influence of red blood cells (RBCs) and fresh frozen plasma (FFP) on mortality in 134 consecutive lung transplants recipients from September 2003 until December 2008.

Results: Intraoperative transfusion of RBCs and FFP was associated with a significant increase in mortality with odds ratios (ORs) of 1.10 (1.03 to 1.16, $P = 0.02$) and 1.09 (1.02 to 1.15, $P = 0.03$), respectively. For more than four intraoperatively transfused RBCs multivariate analysis showed a hazard ratio for mortality of 3.8 (1.40 to 10.31, $P = 0.003$). Furthermore, non-survivors showed a significant increase in renal replacement therapy (RRT) (36.6% versus 6.9%, $P < 0.0001$), primary graft dysfunction (PGD) (39.3% versus 5.9%, $P < 0.0001$), postoperative need of extracorporeal membrane oxygenation (ECMO) (26.9% versus 3.1%, $P = 0.0019$), sepsis (24.2% versus 4.0%, $P = 0.0004$), multiple organ dysfunction syndrome (MODS) (26.9% versus 3.1%, $P < 0.0001$), infections (18.1% versus 0.9%, $P = 0.0004$), retransplantation (12.1% versus 6.9%, $P = 0.039$) and readmission to the ICU (33.3% versus 12.8%, $P = 0.024$).

Conclusions: Intraoperative transfusion is associated with a strong negative influence on outcome in lung transplant recipients.

Keywords: Lung transplantation, Mortality, Transfusion, ICU complications

Background

Liberal transfusion practice has been shown to exert negative influences on morbidity and mortality in different groups of patients due to increased incidence in viral and bacterial infections, activation of inflammatory and coagulation pathways, and immunologic reactions related to transfusion of red blood cells (RBCs) [1]. After lung transplantation the grafts are vulnerable for dysfunction because of denervation, postischemic condition, absent perfusion of bronchial arteries and lacking of lymphatic drainage system. In this context, transfusion-related acute lung injury (TRALI) and transfusion-associated circulatory overload (TACO) are more common than infectious complications, and increase morbidity and mortality [2]. Transfusion of fresh frozen plasma (FFP) may also be associated with adverse effects as transfusion of FFP has been independently associated with a higher risk of developing multiple organ dysfunction syndrome (MODS) and acute respiratory distress syndrome (ARDS) in trauma [3] and critically ill patients [4]. Recently, we demonstrated that intraoperative transfusion of more than 7 units of RBCs in liver transplant recipients was associated with increased mortality [5]. In lung transplant recipients, however, we still lack clear data on the influence of transfusion practice on outcome. To date, there is only one report demonstrating

* Correspondence: markus.bechir@usz.ch
[†]Equal contributors
Surgical Intensive Care Medicine, University Hospital of Zurich, Raemistrasse 100, CH-8091 Zurich, Switzerland

reduced survival after platelet transfusion in lung transplant recipients [6].

The present retrospective study was designed to investigate the influence of intraoperative transfusion of RBCs and FFPs on mortality in lung transplant recipients.

Methods

Following approval by the local Ethics Committee of the Canton of Zurich, Switzerland, (KEK 4), which waived the need for written informed consent for this retrospective analysis, we included a total of 134 consecutive lung transplant recipients who were treated at the ICU, University Hospital of Zurich, Zurich, Switzerland. The study period was 75 months, from September 2003 until December 2008.

Pretransplant recipient data

For baseline characteristics, we collected age, gender, height and weight. The underlying disease and the presence or absence of pulmonary hypertension (PH) was documented. Furthermore, we assessed whether the patients were admitted to transplantation from home, normal ward or an ICU.

Intraoperative data

The number of transfused units of RBCs, FFP, platelet concentrates, fibrinogen and the use of extracorporeal circulation (ECC) during the operation were recorded. The management of coagulation and transfusions practice was done according to internal guidelines. In fact a hemoglobin threshold of 7 g/dL and a coagulation management aiming at functional fibrinogen levels as assessed by thromboelastometry were used [7].

ICU data

The following data were collected: length of stay (LOS) in the ICU, ventilation days, occurrence of renal replacement therapy (RRT) and of primary graft dysfunction (PGD), postoperative use of extracorporeal membrane oxygenation (ECMO), occurrence of sepsis and MODS, frequency of readmission to the ICU, and need of retransplantation. Indications for ECMO were exactly as described previously [8] and for RRT the occurrence of risk, injury, failure, loss, end-stage renal disease (RIFLE) class 2 (injury), as we use routinely in our transplant programme [5,9].

Analyzing protocol

All of the data were extracted from the patients' charts. Endpoint of the observational period and for analysis was 31 December 2008. The patients were divided into survivors (S) and non-survivors (NS).

First, baseline and clinical data were analyzed and compared. Then, intraoperative and ICU data were analyzed and compared between the two groups.

Survival was analyzed in terms of ICU mortality and cumulative survival over the entire observation period. In addition, we performed subgroup analyses assessing cumulative survival comparing the patients that received more than four RBCs to the ones with less RBCs transfused. Finally, a multivariate analysis was done to examine whether transfusing RBCs or FFPs are independent risk factors for mortality.

Statistical analysis

Univariate analysis was done with chi-square test for nominal data; unpaired data analysis for continuous variables was performed by means of Mann–Whitney test or logistic regression. For multivariate analysis we used a Cox proportional hazards model to identify independent risk factors for mortality. Calculation of cumulative survival overall and for the subgroups was done by Kaplan–Meier analysis with log rank testing. Data are expressed as mean ± SD; different data expression is stated in the text. All calculations were done with StatView 4.5 (Abacus Concepts, Berkeley, CA, USA). Statistical significance was accepted with P <0.05 (two-sided tests).

Results

Univariate analysis

Baseline characteristics in survivors and non- survivors

Baseline characteristics of the recipients are shown in Table 1. There was no difference in the incidence of PH

Table 1 Baseline characteristics

	All (n = 134)	S (n = 102)	NS (n = 32)	*P*
Men	79 (78.9%)	58 (56.9%)	21 (65.6%)	0.56
Women	55 (41.9%)	44 (43.1%)	11 (34.4%)	0.56
Age (years)	44.8 ± 16.4 (13 to 68)	44.6 ± 16.7 (13 to 68)	45.8 ± 15.8 (18 to 66)	0.71
Weight (kg)	60.6 ± 16.6 (32 to 122)	59.9 ± 15.2 (32 to 100)	62.8 ± 20.2 (37 to 122)	0.38
Height (m)	1.67 ± 0.90 (1.42 to 1.90)	1.66 ± 0.90 (1.42 to 1.90)	1.69 ± 0.90 (1.55 to 1.88)	0.14
BMI (kg/m^2)	21.6 ± 5.0 (14.0 to 39.4)	21.6 ± 5.0 (14.0 to 36.4)	21.8 ± 6.0 (14.5 to 39.4)	0.75
Creatinine (µmol/l)	74 ± 20 (29 to 147)	74 ± 21 (29 to 147)	75 ± 18 (44 to 110)	0.86
PH (pts)	61 (45.5%)	43 (42.1%)	18 (56.2%)	0.16

Data expressed as mean ± SD (range). *BMI* body mass index, *PH* pulmonary hypertension, *pts* patients.

between survivors and non-survivors (P = 0.16). Concomitant lung disease was similar in all patients, without any statistically significant difference between the two groups (P = 0.65) (Table 2). While 104 patients were admitted from home (82 survivors, 22 non-survivors), 22 were admitted from the normal wards (14 survivors, 8 non-survivors) and 8 patients from the ICU (6 survivors, 2 non-survivors), there was no difference between the two groups (P = 0.41). Mean donor age was 42.5 ± 14.2 years (42.1 ± 14.1 years in the survivors versus 43.8 ± 15.1 years in the non-survivors group, P = 0.57). Taken together, there were no statistically significant differences between survivors and non-survivors.

Intraoperative transfusion and use of intraoperative extracorporeal circuit

Intraoperative transfusion of RBCs and FFP was associated with a significant increase in mortality with odds ratios (ORs) of 1.10 (1.03 to 1.16, P = 0.02) and 1.09 (1.02 to 1.15, P = 0.03). There were no statistically significant differences regarding transfusion of platelets (P = 0.48) and application of fibrinogen (P = 0.90). Overall, there was no difference in the use of extracorporeal circuit between the groups (P = 0.31). Details are given in the Tables 3 and 4.

ICU journey

In non-survivors, LOS in the ICU (P = 0.0007) and ventilation days (P = 0.011) were significantly prolonged compared to survivors. Furthermore, non-survivors had significantly higher incidence of RRT (P <0.0001), PGD (P <0.0001), postoperative ECMO (P = 0.002), sepsis (P <0.0001), MODS (P <0.0001), retransplantation (P = 0.040) and readmission to the ICU (P = 0.024). Details are shown in Table 5.

Table 2 Underlying lung diseases

	All (n = 134)	S (n = 102)	NS (n = 32)	*P*
CF	47 (35.0%)	38 (37.2%)	9 (28.1%)	
COPD	25 (18.6%)	19 (18.6%)	6 (18.8%)	
IPF	27 (20.1%)	19 (18.6%)	8 (25.0%)	
Alpha-1 deficiency	13 (9.8%)	12 (11.8%)	1 (3.1%)	Chi-squared test for all
Re-TPL	7 (5.3%)	5 (4.9%)	2 (6.3%)	0.65
PPH	6 (4.5%)	3 (2.9%)	3 (9.3%)	
Sarcoidosis	3 (2.2%)	2 (2.0%)	1 (3.1%)	
Others	6 (4.5%)	4 (4.0%)	2 (6.3%)	

Data expressed as absolute numbers (percentage). *CF* cystic fibrosis, *COPD* chronic obstructive pulmonary disease, *IPF* interstitial pulmonary fibrosis, *re-TPL* retransplantation, *PPH* primary pulmonary hypertension.

Table 3 Transfusion requirements

	All (n = 134)	S (n = 102)	NS (n = 32)	*P*
RBC (U)	5.8 ± 6.2 (0 to 32)	4.8 ± 5.0 (0 to 32)	8.8 ± 8.4 (0 to 29)	0.02
FFP (U)	4.1 ± 6.6 (0 to 30)	3.1 ± 5.2 (0 to 30)	7.2 ± 9.0 (0 to 29)	0.03
Platelets (10^3/μl)	0.6 ± 1.9 (0 to 16)	0.5 ± 2.1 (0 to 16)	0.8 ± 1.5 (0 to 6)	0.48
Fibrinogen (g)	1.3 ± 2.4 (0 to 12)	1.3 ± 2.4 (0 to 12)	1.4 ± 2.3 (0 to 6)	0.90

Data expressed as mean ± SD (range). *RBC* red blood cell concentrate, *FFP* fresh frozen plasma.

Mortality rate

Overall ICU mortality was 8.9% (12 out of 134 patients). Overall cumulative 1-year survival was 86% and cumulative 3-year survival was 72.8%. There was a significantly decreased cumulative 1-year survival in the group with transfusion of more than four RBCs (survival 81.2% versus 87.6%, P = 0.042). For details see Figure 1.

Multivariate analysis

Risk factors for mortality

The Cox proportional hazards model for mortality identified transfusion of more than four RBCs (P = 0.003), sepsis in the ICU (P = 0.045), PGD (P = 0.0004) and RRT in the ICU (P = 0.015) as independent risk factors for mortality. In contrast, use of cardiopulmonary bypass intraoperatively (P = 0.35), pre-existing PH (P = 0.36), transfusion of more than five FFPs (P = 0.78), age >60 years (P = 0.10), RRT 6 months after transplantation (P = 0.39), body mass index (BMI) (P = 0.09) and more than 9 days of ventilation in the ICU (P = 0.12) were not discriminated as risk factors for mortality. Details are given in Table 6.

Discussion

The main finding of this study is that intraoperative transfusions of RBCs were associated with increased mortality in lung transplant recipients.

There is a growing body of evidence that the number of intraoperative transfusions alters outcome in different patient populations. Gajic *et al.* demonstrated that 8% of transfused critically ill patients developed acute lung injury within 6 hours after transfusion [4]. In another study, Christie *et al.* showed that increased amounts of soluble receptors for advanced glycation end products (a marker for lung epithelial injury) as a consequence of transfusion was clearly associated with PGD in lung transplant recipients [10]. Furthermore,

Table 4 Intraoperative extracorporeal circuit

	All	S	NS	*P*
ECC (pts)	65 (48.5%)	47 (46.0%)	18 (56.2%)	0.31

Data expressed as absolute numbers (percentage). *ECC* extracorporeal circulation, *pts* patients.

Table 5 ICU journey

	All (n = 134)	S (n = 102)	NS (n = 32)	*P*
LOS ICU (d)	12.9 ± 24.8 (2 to 164)	8.3 ± 10.9 (2 to 62)	27.0 ± 43.8 (2 to 164)	0.0007
LOS hospital (d)	49.2 ± 40.3 (3 to 270)	45.5 ± 29.0 (24 to 238)	60.7 ± 63.1 (3 to 270)	0.075
Ventilation (d)	9.6 ± 24.3 (1 to 162)	5.0 ± 9.1 (1 to 51)	23.9 ± 43.7 (1 to 162)	0.011
CRRT (pts)	14.2% (19)	6.8% (7)	37.5% (12)	<0.0001
PGD (pts)	14.2% (19)	5.9% (6)	40.6% (13)	<0.0001
ECMO (pts)	7.4% (10)	2.9% (3)	21.9% (7)	0.002
Sepsis (pts)	9.0% (12)	4.0% (4)	25.0% (8)	<0.0001
MODS (pts)	11.2% (15)	2.9% (3)	37.5% (12)	<0.0001
Re-TPL (pts)	8.3% (11)	6.8% (7)	12.6% (4)	0.040
Readmission ICU (pts)	17.2% (23)	11.8% (12)	24.4% (11)	0.024

Data expressed as mean ± SD (range) or percentage of incidence (number of patients). *CRRT* continuous renal replacement therapy, *d* days, *ECMO* extracorporeal membrane oxygenation, *LOS ICU* length of stay in ICU, *LOS hospital* length of stay in hospital, *MODS* multiple organ dysfunction syndrome, *PGD* primary graft dysfunction, *pts* patients, *re-TPL* retransplantation.

Table 6 Cox proportional hazards model for mortality (n = 134)

Parameter	*P*	Hazard ratio	CI
Sepsis in ICU	0.045	3.8	1.02 to 14.8
PGD	0.0004	5.4	2.1 to 13.6
Transfusion >4 RBC	0.003	4.7	1.7 to 13.3
CRRT in ICU	0.015	4.0	1.3 to 12.5
>9 ventilation days	0.12	2.2	0.8 to 6.1
BMI >25 kg/m^2	0.087	1.07	0.99 to 1.13
Transfusion >5 FFP	0.78	1.14	0.5 to 2.6
Age >60 years	0.10	0.5	0.2 to 1.2
PH	0.36	1.5	0.7 to 3.3
RRT 6 months after TPL	0.39	2.2	0.4 to 13.5
ECC	0.35	0.7	0.3 to 1.6

BMI body mass index, *CI* confidence interval, *CRRT* continuous renal replacement therapy, *ECC* extracorporeal circulation, *FFP* fresh frozen plasma, *PGD* primary graft dysfunction, *PH* pulmonary hypertension, *RBC* red blood cell, *RRT* renal replacement therapy, *TPL* transplantation.

intraoperative transfusion of platelets was associated with worse outcome after lung transplantation [6]. To date, we are still lacking literature regarding the impact of transfusions on long-term outcome in lung transplant recipients. In liver transplant recipients, however, Massicotte *et al.* prospectively demonstrated that transfusion was associated with worse outcome [11].

Interestingly, in our study population there were no baseline differences between the groups; in particular, there was no influence of underlying diagnosis, intraoperative cardiopulmonary bypass use or pre-existing PH to transfusion rates, which could explain these findings. Nevertheless, we cannot exclude such a difference because of the small sample size, in which the analysis might fail revealing relevant differences between survivors and non-survivors. But, taken together, in this context our study supports the hypothesis that intraoperative transfusion might have negative impact on outcome in lung transplantation recipients. As a consequence, avoiding intraoperative transfusion of at least RBCs as much as feasible might be a beneficial strategy to improve survival in such patients.

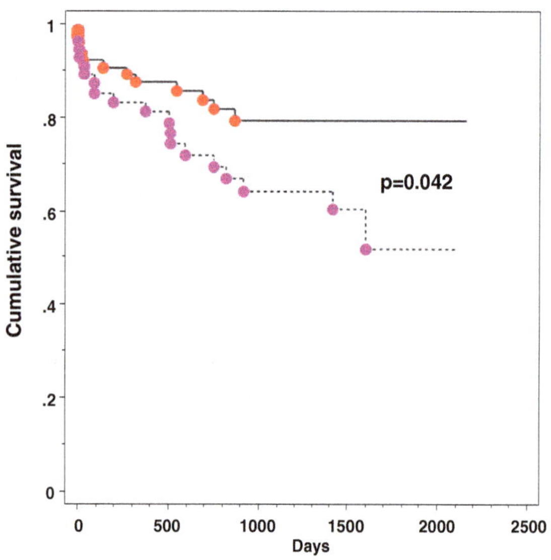

Figure 1 Kaplan-Meier analysis with log rank test. There was a significantly lower cumulative 1-year survival in the group with transfusion of more than four RBCs (dashed line). RBC, red blood cell.

A limitation of that suggestion and of this study is clearly the retrospective design. Other limitations are that we did not systematically measure comorbidities in our population and therefore we cannot exclude such an influence on the transfusion requirement. Therefore, a prospective approach in an equal design as Massicotte used in liver transplantation adapted to lung transplants would be important to strengthen or rule out the conclusions drawn from this retrospective setting. Furthermore, the sample size of the study is only moderate and therefore our results must be interpreted very carefully. However, as long as we lack data of a larger sample size or of prospective trials, we recommend being careful with intraoperative transfusion in lung transplantation.

Conclusions

Intraoperative transfusion of RBCs appears to be an independent risk factor for worsened outcome in lung transplant recipients. Therefore, transfusions should be reduced and be avoided as much as possible, at least as long as we lack results of further prospective data.

Abbreviations

ARDS: Acute respiratory distress syndrome; BMI: Body mass index; CF: Cystic fibrosis; CI: Confidence interval; COPD: Chronic obstructive pulmonary disease; CRRT: Continuous renal replacement therapy; ECC: Extracorporeal circulation; ECMO: Extracorporeal membrane oxygenation; FFP: Fresh frozen plasma; IPF: Interstitial pulmonary fibrosis; LOS: Length of stay; MODS: Multiple organ dysfunction syndrome; OR: Odds ratio; PGD: Primary graft dysfunction; PH: Pulmonary hypertension; PPH: Primary pulmonary hypertension; RBC: Red blood cell; re-TPL: Retransplantation; RIFLE: Risk, injury, failure, loss, end-stage renal disease; RRT: Renal replacement therapy; TACO: Transfusion-associated circulatory overload; TPL: Transplantation; TRALI: Transfusion-related acute lung injury.

Competing interests

The authors declare that they have no competing interests.

Authors' contributions

DW, PAS and SRC performed data analysis, interpretation and drafted the article. PL and UW undertook statistics and critical review. RAS and MF undertook data collection and critical review. MB conceived the study, and undertook interpretation and critical review. All authors read and approved the final manuscript.

References

1. Carson JL, Carless PA, Hebert PC: **Transfusion thresholds and other strategies for guiding allogeneic red blood cell transfusion.** *Cochrane Database Syst Rev* 2012, **4**:CD002042.
2. Kleinman S, Chan P, Robillard P: **Risks associated with transfusion of cellular blood components in Canada.** *Transfus Med Rev* 2003, **17**(2):120–162.
3. Watson GA, Sperry JL, Rosengart MR, Minei JP, Harbrecht BG, Moore EE, Cuschieri J, Maier RV, Billiar TR, Peitzman AB, Inflammation and Host Response to Injury Investigators: **Fresh frozen plasma is independently associated with a higher risk of multiple organ failure and acute respiratory distress syndrome.** *J Trauma* 2009, **67**(2):221–227.
4. Gajic O, Rana R, Winters JL, Yilmaz M, Mendez JL, Rickman OB, O'Byrne MM, Evenson LK, Malinchoc M, DeGoey SR, Afessa B, Hubmayr RD, Moore SB: **Transfusion-related acute lung injury in the critically ill: prospective nested case-control study.** *Am J Respir Crit Care Med* 2007, **176**(9):886–891.
5. Oberkofler CE, Dutkowski P, Stocker R, Schuepbach RA, Stover JF, Clavien PA, Béchir M: **Model of end stage liver disease (MELD) score greater than 23 predicts length of stay in the ICU but not mortality in liver transplant recipients.** *Crit Care* 2010, **14**(3):R117.
6. Zalunardo MP, Thalmann C, Seifert B, D'Cunja J, Weder W, Boehler A, Spahn DR: **Impact of preoperative right-ventricular function and platelet transfusion on outcome after lung transplantation.** *Eur J Cardiothorac Surg* 2011, **39**(4):538–542.
7. Ganter MT, Spahn DR: **Perioperative coagulation management.** *Best Pract Res Clin Anaesthesiol* 2010, **24**(1):7–8.
8. Cottini SR, Wenger U, Sailer S, Stehberger PA, Schuepbach RA, Hasenclever P, Wilhelm M, Béchir M: **Extracorporeal membrane oxygenation: beneficial strategy for lung transplant recipients.** *J Extra Corp Technol* 2013, **45**(1):16–20.
9. Wenger U, Neff TA, Oberkofler CE, Zimmermann M, Stehberger PA, Scherrer M, Schuepbach RA, Cottini SR, Steiger P, Béchir M: **The relationship between preoperative creatinine clearance and outcomes for patients undergoing liver transplantation: a retrospective observational study.** *BMC Nephrol* 2013, **14**:37.
10. Christie JD, Shah CV, Kawut SM, Mangalmurti N, Lederer DJ, Sonett JR, Ahya VN, Palmer SM, Wille K, Lama V, Shah PD, Shah A, Weinacker A, Deutschman CS, Kohl BA, Demissie E, Bellamy S, Ware LB, Lung Transplant Outcomes Group: **Plasma levels of receptor for advanced glycation end products, blood transfusion, and risk of primary graft dysfunction.** *Am J Respir Crit Care Med* 2009, **180**(10):1010–1015.
11. Massicotte L, Lenis S, Thibeault L, Sassine MP, Seal RF, Roy A: **Effect of low central venous pressure and phlebotomy on blood product transfusion requirements during liver transplantations.** *Liver Transpl* 2006, **12**(1):117–123.

7

Variability of anti-staphylococcal antibodies in healthy volunteers and pre-cardiac surgery patients

Sarka Moravcova[1], Bonnie Kyle[1], Hilary Shanahan[2], Savvas Giannaris[2], Andrew Smith[2*] and Colin Hamilton-Davies[2*]

Abstract

Background: Pre-operative antibody levels have been shown to be inversely related to development of post-operative complications. Staphylococcal infection is a major source of morbidity following surgery.

Methods: We examined the variability of anti-staphylococcal antibody levels across a group of healthy volunteers and compared this with patients scheduled to undergo cardiac surgery.

Results: Pre-operative cardiac surgical patients exhibited significantly higher levels of staphylococcal antibodies compared with healthy volunteers.

Conclusions: The relationship between pre-surgery staphylococcal antibody levels and outcome warrants further investigation.

Keywords: Staphylococcus, Antibody, Pre-operative, EndoCAb, Infection, Complication

Background

The incidence of wound infection following cardiac surgery is approximately 1–4 %, of which approximately one fifth is due to methicillin-resistant *Staphylococcus aureus* (MRSA) (Allen et al. 2014). Post-operative MRSA infection is associated with a mortality ranging from 10 to 14 % (Ridderstolpe et al. 2001). In addition, there is a considerable cost both economically and in terms of patient suffering that result from sternal wound breakdown, staphylococcal septicaemia and the associated increased length of hospital stay (Coskun et al. 2005). Kanafani demonstrated that whilst certain pre-operative characteristics were associated with an increased risk of post-operative staphylococcal sepsis, the majority of those that developed such complications had no such risk factors (Kanafani et al. 2009). These patients had no measure made of their underlying immunity to *Staphylococcus*. Similarly, in one of the largest retrospective studies of cardiac surgical patients ($n > 330{,}000$), there were again relationships drawn between pre-operative risk factors such as body mass index (BMI), diabetes, chronic renal insufficiency, increasing age and immunosuppressive therapy and development of infective complications (Fowler et al. 2005). In this study, again, no measure had been made of the patients' own underlying ability to resist infection.

The humoral immune system provides a level of protection to patients against a number of infective/inflammatory conditions and indeed our own institution has been involved in demonstrating links between low levels of pre-operative antibody against endotoxin and outcome following cardiac surgery (Hamilton-Davies et al. 1997; Bennett-Guerrero et al. 1997). It is likely that everyone has a varying level of antibodies to common infective organisms, thus maintaining a degree of circulating immunity to these organisms, and that these antibodies are functional, i.e. have neutralising or opsonizing functions.

It has been shown that the alpha-toxin fragments secreted by *Staphylococcus* can impair gut mucosal integrity and thus further worsen the potential for sepsis by enabling Gram-negative organism/endotoxin translocation from the gut lumen (Kwak et al. 2012).

* Correspondence: andrewsmith@doctors.org.uk; colin.hamilton-davies@bartshealth.nhs.uk
The work was carried out at the Department of Anaesthesia & Critical Care, University College London Hospitals NHS Foundation Trust, 235 Euston Road, London NW1 2BU.
[2]Barts Health NHS Trust, London, UK
Full list of author information is available at the end of the article

Anti-staphylococcal antibodies to a variety of epitopes can be measured by enzyme-linked immunosorbent assay (ELISA) (PhPlate AB, Stockholm, Sweden) (Colque-Navarro et al. 1998), and the levels of these antibodies are likely to vary between individuals. It is well established that there is considerable variation in antibody levels in healthy volunteers and in infected patients (Dryla et al. 2005). This is similar to the variation in levels of endogenous endotoxin antibodies, which are predictive of post-operative complications (Down et al. 2004).

We are particularly interested in those patients who develop serious *S. aureus* infections (deep-seated wound infection, serious bacteraemia, endocarditis) and examining whether there is a relationship with the patient's own immune state. We set out to determine if these antibodies were measurable in individuals (healthy volunteers and pre-operative cardiac surgical patients) and whether there was measurable variation in antibody levels in these two groups. We planned to study the younger volunteers as they were likely to have an active, healthy immune system as compared to the patient group who may be expected to exhibit a degree of immunosenescence and have lower levels of circulating antibodies.

We chose to assay for antibodies to alpha-toxin (AT), an extracellular polypeptide, and to teichoic acid (TA), a major surface antigen of the staphylococcal organism; both are present in almost all strains of *S. aureus*. A high proportion (86–95 %) of the *S. aureus* isolates in clinical infections produce an anti-alpha-toxin antibody response (Mollby 1983) (Fig. 1). In cases of serious staphylococcal infection, the levels of alpha-toxin have been demonstrated to be very high, suggesting that the antigen is highly immunogenic (Soderquist BC-N et al. 1993). Teichoic acid is particularly expressed in case of long-standing staphylococcal infection, for example, deep-seated wound infection or endocarditis (Colque-Navarro et al. 1998). These two antibody types are likely to be reliably expressed in those patients that we are most interested in studying; those that develop deep-seated staphylococcal wound infections following cardiac surgery.

The IgG class of antibody is likely to be a more reliable indicator due to the reliability in appearance and longevity of response. Peak levels of the IgM class may be missed due to its more transient nature (Barclay 1995).

This investigation formed the first part of an ongoing investigation into peri-operative staphylococcal antibody levels and clinical outcome. As this was a pilot study and we were uncertain as to the degree of variation in antibody levels within and between the groups, we did not perform power calculations. The results of this investigation will help with the prediction of sample sizes in our future studies.

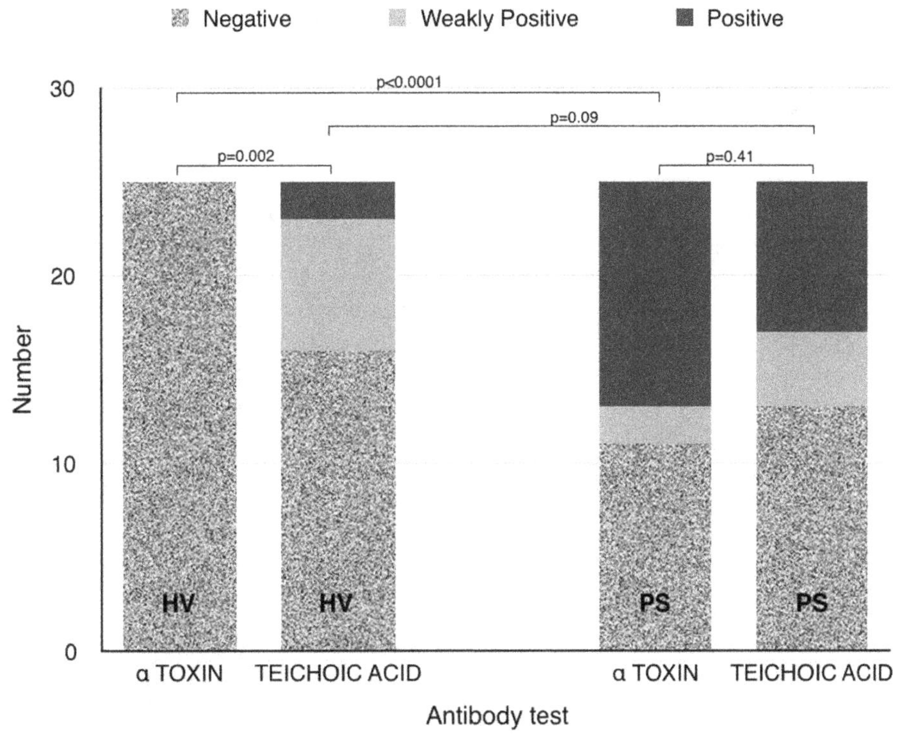

Fig. 1 Categorised antibody response (positive, weakly positive, negative) to alpha-toxin and teichoic acid domains in healthy volunteers (HV), $n = 25$, and in pre-operative cardiac surgical patients (PS), $n = 25$. Fisher's exact test (Freeman-Halton extension) used to test variability of response between groups

Hypotheses

There is a measurable intra-population and inter-population variability in anti-staphylococcal antibodies amongst different populations of individuals.

Methods

Ethical approval for this study was given by the Joint UCL/UCLH Committee on the Ethics of Human Research (Committee Alpha), REC reference 05/Q0502/72.

Prior to enrolment, verbal and written information was provided to all participants after which verbal and written consent to participate was obtained. No individual identifiable data is included in this submission.

Twenty-five healthy volunteers (HV) and 25 pre-operative cardiac surgery patients (PS) were recruited into the study, provided with study information and asked for written, informed consent for collection of 7 mL blood into a plain tube (Becton-Dickinson, Oxford, UK) for later analysis. Exclusion criteria were age under 18 years, recent or ongoing infection, pregnancy, an immunosuppressive condition and concomitant use of immunosuppressive therapy.

The patient group was consecutively recruited from a population scheduled to undergo a variety of cardiac surgical procedures. There were no refusals to participate in the study.

Sample analysis

The 7-mL blood samples were allowed to clot at room temperature for 20 min, centrifuged for 10 min at 3000 rpm and the serum removed by pipette into cryotubes for storage at −70 °C for later analysis (Thermo Scientific, MA, USA). The ELISA procedure has been detailed previously. Briefly, coating doses for the 96-well microtitration plates (Dynatech M-129B, Plochingen, Germany) with α-toxin and teichoic acid were established at 2.5 and 1 μg/mL, respectively. The working volume throughout the tests was 100 μL/well. The microtitration plates were coated with antigens diluted in phosphate-buffered saline (PBS), pH 7.4, and incubated overnight at 22 °C. The plates were washed and a serum dilution in PBS with Tween-20 0.05 % *v/v* (PBS-T) of 1 in 1000 for α-toxin and a 1 in 10,000 for teichoic acid was added to the two coated wells. Positive and negative controls were included in each plate. The plates were incubated for 1 h at room temperature (20 °C). After washing the plates, alkaline phosphatase-conjugated goat anti-human antibody (Sigma) diluted in PBS-T was added to each well, and the plates were incubated for 2 h at room temperature. After the final wash, p-nitrophenyl-phosphate substrate (Sigma) was added. Titres were read when the positive controls reached previously established values at 405 nm on a Titertek Multiskan (Flow Laboratories, Irvine, Scotland) instrument. Antibody levels were categorised to a low, intermediate and high response to the teichoic acid and alpha-toxin domains. Statistical analysis comparing the variability in proportions of response between the groups was performed using the Freeman-Halton extension of Fisher's exact test. Probabilities are two tailed.

Results

A total of 25 healthy volunteers were recruited with a mean age of 41 years (range 27–51) and included 17 males and 8 females. Twenty-five pre-operative patients were also recruited with a mean age of 62 years (range 19–78) and included 17 males and 8 females. The surgical procedures undertaken on these patients were coronary artery bypass grafts (CABG)—9, valve replacement—10, CABG+ valve—5 and atrial septal defect repair—1.

Antibody levels to both AT and TA were obtained for all participants.

The patterns of distribution of each classification (low, intermediate or high) for AT and TA antibody levels appeared to differ between the two study groups (Fig. 1). A striking element of the results was the proportion of patients in the pre-surgery group with high antibody levels to alpha-toxin (48 % vs. 0) and to teichoic acid (32 vs. 8 %) when compared with the healthy volunteer group.

The distribution of classification for alpha-toxin in the HV group (low = 25, intermediate = 0, high = 0) differed significantly from that in the PS group (11, 2, 12, respectively); $p < 0.0001$. The distribution of each classification for TA antibody level in the HV group (16, 7, 2) did not vary significantly from that of the PS group (13, 4, 8); $p = 0.09$.

Amongst the HV group, the distribution of classification of response to AT (25, 0, 0) differed from that to TA (16, 7, 2); $p = 0.002$. However, in the PS group, the distribution of response to the two tests did not differ, AT (11, 2, 12) vs. TA (13, 4, 8); $p = 0.41$.

Discussion

It is expected that antibody levels to an antigen will vary between individuals and that the response to various antigens will also vary in any given individual (Dryla et al. 2005). Both the healthy volunteers and the pre-operative patients were assumed to be in reasonable health with respect to any ongoing infection, and none were thought to have a concurrent infection at the time of study. The cohort of healthy volunteers had a significantly lower mean age than the pre-surgery group and would thus be reasonably expected to have higher antibody levels as, in general, downgraded immune responsiveness or immunosenescence is seen with advancing age (Haq and McElhaney 2014). This was not seen, and indeed, the pre-cardiac surgical group had a greater proportion of high antibody levels to both teichoic acid and alpha-toxin. Subjects with a recent infection may well have higher antibody levels than those in a non-infected group (Dryla et al. 2005). It may be that the pre-surgery group had been exposed to a significant staphylococcal challenge whereas the healthy cohort had not. Considering the different populations and looking at any obvious invasive procedure that the surgical group had undergone when compared to the healthy volunteers, we felt that cardiac catheterisation was the universally most invasive. It may be that the aseptic technique during the cardiac catheterization process, or during some other temporally related procedure such as peripheral venous cannulation, was inadequate. This hypothesis would need to be tested by comparing antibody levels before and after cardiac catheterisation procedures. There could, of course, be other factors that may lead to a differing level of antibodies between the groups. Pre-operative blood testing and venous cannulation will likely have occurred in the patient group.

It would also be interesting and useful to measure antibody levels in healthy volunteers of the same age range as pre-operative patients or perhaps measuring antibody levels in older patients not scheduled to undergo cardiac surgery. Any observed differences between these two groups may imply that another mechanism might be the cause of antibody level variation.

The variation in antibody levels in the pre-operative patient group, all of whom had a similar potential inoculative insult, may be due to a natural variation in antibody levels between individuals but also may represent variability in the individual's ability to generate an immune response. Some patients generated a high level of antibody and others generated low or no response. Do those patients with low antibody levels suffer a different level of peri-operative complication than those with higher levels?

The association between low pre-operative antibody levels and compromised outcome following cardiac surgery has already been made for endotoxin core antibodies (EndoCAb) (Hamilton-Davies et al. 1997; Bennett-Guerrero et al. 1997). In this pilot study, no outcome comparisons could be made due to small numbers and heterogeneity of both the patients and the surgical procedures. The variability in underlying immunity to both teichoic acid and alpha-toxin observed in pre-cardiac surgery patients suggests that a controlled outcome study be performed in this group. The ability of pre-operative staphylococcal antibody levels to predict post-operative infectious outcomes could be enhanced by perhaps combining with other antibody levels (e.g. EndoCAb).

If an inverse relationship between pre-operative anti-staphylococcal antibody levels and subsequent development of post-cardiac surgery complications exists, similar to that for EndoCAb, it may be possible to intervene to modify the post-procedural outcome.

It has been previously reported by Colque-Navarro and colleagues that those patients with low levels of antibodies, especially to alpha-toxin, may not mount much of a response to antigenic exposure (Colque-Navarro et al. 1998). This may reflect a more generalised immune hyporesponsiveness where active vaccination might not generate an adequate response. Passive immune therapy, such as the administration of a gammaglobulin product, may be more appropriate. It may be that for patients with a deficient pre-operative immune status, an alternative, less invasive, surgical or non-surgical intervention may be available and appropriate.

Conclusions

This demonstration of the variability in anti-staphylococcal antibody levels suggests that the relationship between pre-surgery staphylococcal antibody levels and outcome warrants further investigation. Predicting which patients are more likely to suffer a complicated course following surgery might enable either more effective redirection of those patients to other appropriate treatment modalities or targeting specific resources to those patients to give them the best chance of dealing with the surgical insult.

Abbreviations

AT: alpha-toxin; BMI: body mass index; CABG: coronary artery bypass grafts; ELISA: enzyme-linked immunosorbent assay; HV: healthy volunteers; MRSA: methicillin-resistant *Staphylococcus aureus*; PBS: phosphate-buffered saline; PS: pre-operative cardiac surgery patients; TA: teichoic acid.

Acknowledgements

The authors thank John Holton, Department of Microbiology, University College London, for kindly performing the ELISA.
Internal funding for the cost of the antibody assays was provided by the University College London Hospitals Charity-Special Trustees Fund.
No other external funding was received.

Authors' contributions

SM was involved in the recruitment, demographic data collection, results analysis and manuscript preparation. BK participated in the demographic data collection, results analysis, and manuscript preparation. HS participated in the demographic data collection results analysis, manuscript preparation. SG was involved in the patient recruitment, blood collection, sample preparation and manuscript preparation. AS helped in the study design, recruitment, blood collection, sample preparation and manuscript preparation. CHD conceived study and was involved in the study design, recruitment, blood collection, sample preparation and manuscript preparation. All authors read and approved the final manuscript.

Competing interests

The authors declare that they have no competing interests.

Author details

[1]Royal Brompton & Harefield NHS Trust, London, UK. [2]Barts Health NHS Trust, London, UK.

References

Allen KB, Fowler Jr VG, Gammie JS, et al. *Staphylococcus aureus* infections after elective cardiothoracic surgery: observations from an international randomized placebo-controlled trial of an investigational *S. aureus* vaccine. Open Forum Infect Dis. 2014;1(2):1–7.

Barclay GR. Bacterial endotoxins: lipopolysaccharides from genes to therapy. In: Levin J, Alving CR, Munford RS, Redl H, editors. Progress in clinical and biological research. New York: Wiley; 1995.

Bennett-Guerrero E, Ayuso L, Hamilton-Davies C, et al. Relationship of preoperative antiendotoxin core antibodies and adverse outcomes following cardiac surgery. JAMA. 1997;277(8):646–50.

Colque-Navarro P, Soderquist B, Holmberg H, Blomqvist L, Olcen P, Mollby R. Antibody response in *Staphylococcus aureus* septicaemia—a prospective study. J Med Microbiol. 1998;47(3):217–25.

Coskun D, Aytac J, Aydinli A, Bayer A. Mortality rate, length of stay and extra cost of sternal surgical site infections following coronary artery bypass grafting in a private medical centre in Turkey. J Hosp Infect. 2005;60(2):176–9.

Down JF, Barclay GR, Bennett-Guerrero E, et al. A descriptive study of the variation in baseline levels of antiendotoxin core antibodies between US and UK populations. J Endotoxin Res. 2004;10(3):195–6.

Dryla A, Prustomersky S, Gelbmann D, et al. Comparison of antibody repertoires against *Staphylococcus aureus* in healthy individuals and in acutely infected patients. Clin Diagn Lab Immunol. 2005;12(3):387–98.

Fowler Jr VG, O'Brien SM, Muhlbaier LH, Corey GR, Ferguson TB, Peterson ED. Clinical predictors of major infections after cardiac surgery. Circulation. 2005;112(9 Suppl):I358–65.

Hamilton-Davies C, Barclay GR, Cardigan RA, et al. Relationship between preoperative endotoxin immune status, gut perfusion, and outcome from cardiac valve replacement surgery. Chest. 1997;112(5):1189–96.

Haq K, McElhaney JE. Immunosenescence: influenza vaccination and the elderly. Curr Opin Immunol. 2014;29:38–42.

Kanafani ZA, Arduino JM, Muhlbaier LH, et al. Incidence of and preoperative risk factors for *Staphylococcus aureus* bacteremia and chest wound infection after cardiac surgery. Infect Control Hosp Epidemiol. 2009;30(3):242–8.

Kwak YK, Vikstrom E, Magnusson KE, Vecsey-Semjen B, Colque-Navarro P, Mollby R. The *Staphylococcus aureus* alpha-toxin perturbs the barrier function in Caco-2 epithelial cell monolayers by altering junctional integrity. Infect Immun. 2012;80(5):1670–80.

Mollby R. Isolation and properties of membrane damaging toxins. In: Easmon CSF, Adlam C, editors. Staphylococci and staphylococcal infections. 2. London: Academic; 1983. p. 628–30.

Ridderstolpe L, Gill H, Granfeldt H, Ahlfeldt H, Rutberg H. Superficial and deep sternal wound complications: incidence, risk factors and mortality. Eur J Cardiothorac Surg. 2001;20(6):1168–75.

Soderquist BC-N P, Blomqvist L, Olcen P, Holmberg H, Mollby R. Enzyme immunoassay for detection of ∝-toxin from staphylococcus aureus. Serodiagn Immunother Infect Dis. 1993;1:23–6.

8

Cost-effectiveness of a cardiac output-guided haemodynamic therapy algorithm in high-risk patients undergoing major gastrointestinal surgery

Zia Sadique[1], David A. Harrison[2], Richard Grieve[1], Kathryn M. Rowan[2], Rupert M. Pearse[3,4*] and for the OPTIMISE study group

Abstract

Background: The use of cardiac output monitoring to guide intra-venous fluid and inotropic therapies may improve peri-operative outcomes, but uncertainty exists regarding clinical effectiveness and robust cost-effectiveness evidence is lacking. The objective of the study was to evaluate the cost-effectiveness of peri-operative cardiac output-guided haemodynamic therapy versus usual care in high-risk patients undergoing major gastrointestinal surgery.

Methods: The study undertook a cost-effectiveness analysis using data from a multi-centre randomised trial that recruited patients from 17 hospitals in the United Kingdom. The trial compared cardiac output-guided, haemodynamic therapy algorithm for intra-venous fluid and inotrope (dopexamine) infusion during and 6 h following surgery, with usual care. Resource use and outcome data on 734 high-risk trial patients aged over 50 years undergoing major gastrointestinal surgery were used to report cost-effectiveness at 6 months and to project lifetime cost-effectiveness. The cost-effectiveness analysis used information on health-related quality of life (QoL) at randomisation, 30 days, and 6 months combined with information on vital status to report quality-adjusted life years (QALYs). Each QALY was valued using the National Institute for Health and Care Excellence (NICE) recommended threshold of willingness to pay (£20,000 per QALY) in conjunction with the costs of each group to report the incremental net monetary benefits (INB) of the treatment algorithm versus usual care.

Results: The mean [SD] quality of life at 30 days and 6 months was similar between the treatment groups (at 6 months, intervention group 0.73 [0.28] versus usual care group 0.71 [0.30]; mean gain 0.03 [95 % confidence interval (CI) −0.01 to 0.08]). At 6 months, survival, mean QALYs and mean healthcare costs (intervention group £8574 versus usual care group £8974) were also similar. At the cost-effectiveness threshold of £20,000 per QALY gained, the incremental net benefit of haemodynamic therapy over the patients' lifetime was positive (£4168 [95 % CI −£3063 to £11,398]). This corresponds to an 87 % probability that this intervention is cost-effective.

Conclusions: Cardiac output-guided haemodynamic therapy algorithm was associated with an average cost reduction and improvement in QALY and is likely to be cost-effective. Further research is needed to confirm the clinical and cost-effectiveness of this treatment.

Keywords: Cost-effectiveness analysis, Fluid therapy, Monitoring, CVS, Peri-operative care

* Correspondence: r.pearse@qmul.ac.uk
[3]Queen Mary University of London, London EC1M 6BQ, UK
[4]Adult Critical Care Unit, Royal London Hospital, Whitechapel, London E1 1BB, UK
Full list of author information is available at the end of the article

Background

More than 230 million surgical procedures are performed worldwide each year with an estimated mortality between 1 and 4 % (Pearse et al. 2012; Weiser et al. 2008). However, post-operative complications and death are much more frequent among high-risk patients, those who are older, those who have co-morbid disease and those who undergo major surgery. Importantly, patients who develop complications, but survive to leave hospital, experience a reduction in long-term survival (Pearse et al. 2011; Khuri et al. 2005). Post-operative complications increase healthcare costs significantly as a result of additional treatment and prolonged hospitals stays (Boltz et al. 2011). Implementation of new treatment strategies for this patient group therefore requires evidence of cost-effectiveness as well as clinical effectiveness.

The dose of intra-venous fluid has an important effect on patient outcomes following major gastrointestinal surgery. However, fluid is widely prescribed according to subjective criteria leading to wide variation in clinical practice (Pearse and Ackland 2012). One potential solution to this problem is the use of cardiac output monitoring to guide administration of intra-venous fluid and inotropic agents (Pearse and Ackland 2012). This approach has been recommended in a report commissioned by the Centers for Medicare and Medicaid Services in the United States of America (USA) (Agency for Healthcare Research and Quality 2007) and by the National Institute for Health and Care Excellence (NICE) in the United Kingdom (UK) (National Institute for Health and Clinical Excellence 2011). Hospitals in the UK National Health Service (NHS) receive a Commissioning for Quality and Innovation payment for each patient treated. These national policy recommendations are based on very limited health economic data. Meanwhile, the findings of a recent Cochrane review suggest that the benefit associated with this treatment may be more marginal than previously believed (Grocott et al. 2012).

In this context, the OPTIMISE trial was conducted to evaluate the clinical effectiveness of cardiac output monitoring to guide administration of intra-venous fluid and inotropic drugs as part of a haemodynamic therapy algorithm in a large, pragmatic, multi-centre and randomised controlled trial in high-risk patients undergoing major gastrointestinal surgery (Pearse et al. 2014). The aim of this analysis was to confirm whether a cardiac output-guided haemodynamic therapy algorithm is cost-effective in high-risk patients undergoing major gastrointestinal surgery.

Methods

Ethics, consent and permissions

The OPTIMISE trial protocol version 1.8 was approved by the East London and City Research Ethics Committee (chair: Dr A. Tucker) on 7 December 2009 (reference: 09/H0703/23) and by the Medical and Healthcare products Regulatory Agency (reference: 2009-009596-35). Written informed consent was obtained from all patients prior to inclusion in the trial.

Setting, patients and clinical management

OPTIMISE was a pragmatic, multi-centre, randomised and observer-blinded trial conducted in 17 NHS hospitals in the UK. The trial findings, including the study protocol, are presented in detail elsewhere (Pearse et al. 2014). Adult patients, aged 50 years or over, undergoing major gastrointestinal surgery were eligible for recruitment provided they satisfied one or more predefined high-risk criteria. The intervention period commenced with induction of anaesthesia and continued until 6 hours after surgery was completed. All patients received standard measures to maintain oxygenation ($SpO_2 \geq 94$ %), haemoglobin (>8 g/dl), core temperature (37 °C), and heart rate (<100 bpm). Five percent of dextrose was administered at 1 ml/kg/h to satisfy maintenance fluid requirements with additional fluid administered at the discretion of the treating clinician guided by pulse rate, arterial pressure, urine output, core-peripheral temperature gradient, serum lactate and base excess. Mean arterial pressure was maintained between 60 and 100 mmHg using an alpha adrenoceptor agonist or vasodilator as required. Post-operative analgesia was provided by epidural infusion (bupivacaine and fentanyl) or intra-venous infusion (morphine or fentanyl). In addition, intervention group patients received intra-venous fluid and inotropic therapy guided by a haemodynamic therapy algorithm informed by cardiac output monitoring (LiDCOrapid, LiDCO Ltd, UK). This algorithm included the use of 250 ml intra-venous fluid challenges with colloid solution, as required, in order to achieve and maintain the maximal value of stroke volume. No attempt was made to standardise the choice of colloid solution. The patients in the intervention group also received an intra-venous infusion of dopexamine at a fixed rate of 0.5 µg/kg/min (Cephalon, Welwyn Garden City, UK) either through a peripheral or central venous catheter. The dose of dopexamine was reduced if the heart rate increased above 120 % of baseline value or 100 bpm (whichever was greater) for more than 30 min despite adequate anaesthesia and analgesia. If the heart rate did not decrease despite dose reduction, then the dopexamine infusion was discontinued. The patients in the control group received usual clinical care; however, the use of a dynamic central venous pressure target was recommended. Cardiac output monitoring was not used in the control group unless specifically requested by clinical staff because of patient deterioration. All other management decisions were taken by senior clinicians who retained the discretion to alter any aspect of patient care.

Six-month outcomes

Health outcome is reported in terms of quality-adjusted life years (QALYs), which incorporate the effects of the intervention on both length of survival and quality of life. During the 6-month follow-up period, survival data were recorded by trial investigators and subsequently linked with death registrations from the Health and Social Care Information Centre (HSCIC) to give survival status and date of death for patients discharged from hospital. The patients (or their carers) were asked to complete a generic health-related quality of life questionnaire, the EuroQol (5-dimension 3-level version; EQ-5D-3L), at randomisation, 30 days and 6 months after surgery. The EQ-5D health profiles of each patient were then converted into a single summary index by applying a formula that attaches a weighting to the levels in each dimension. Patients' EQ-5D profiles were combined with health state preference values from the UK general population (Dolan et al. 1999), to derive an EQ-5D utility index score anchored on a scale from 0 (death) to 1 (perfect health). QALYs were calculated by using the area under the curve method whereby each patient's survival times is weighted by their corresponding quality of life scores at each time point (Manca et al. 2005). Patients who died between 1 and 6 months after randomisation were assigned zero quality of life scores at the corresponding time point. The base case analysis used the quality of life score at day 30 as the baseline measure rather than the score at randomisation, which for both arms may reflect the surgery itself.

Healthcare resource use and costs

Resource use data were collected prospectively for each patient including information on the surgical procedure, trial intervention, length of stay in critical care and on the surgical ward. The unit costs of the surgical procedures were estimated from the NHS Payment by Results database (Department of Health 2013). These reference costs provide an average cost of both the surgery and hospital stay. To avoid double counting associated with costs of hospital stay, the costs of average length of stay and of 1 day in a post-anaesthetic recovery unit were subtracted from the national average unit cost, for each eligible surgical procedure. Critical care bed days were costed separately according to the level of care received (levels 2 and 3). No additional staff costs were considered because the intervention was specifically designed for delivery with existing peri-operative care resources. The costs of cardiac output monitoring equipment were obtained from the manufacturer (personal communication). Use of transfused blood products and intra-venous fluids was recorded for each patient and costed using unit costs provided by the NHS Blood and Transplant and the British National Formulary (Additional file 1: Table S1) (NHS Blood and Transplant 2013; Joint Formulary Committee. British National Formulary (online) London: BMJ Group and Pharmaceutical Press (accessed on 25th October 2013)). All unit costs were reported at 2012–2013 price levels.

Six-month cost-effectiveness analysis

Cost-effectiveness analysis is based on the recognition that evidence of clinical effectiveness of interventions is necessary but not sufficient for decision making for adopting interventions. Here, it is essential to estimate the extent to which interventions represent value for money. The aim of cost-effectiveness analysis is to estimate the effect of a new treatment on the joint distribution of costs and effects. This approach can estimate the overall value of the intervention rather than accepting or rejecting value of intervention on the basis of individual tests of significance on costs and effects.

The cost-effectiveness analysis was conducted from an NHS perspective, using bivariate regression methods to correlate between costs and outcomes to report the mean (95 % confidence intervals) incremental costs and QALYs in the intervention group versus the usual care group. It needs to be highlighted that for economic analysis, the mean estimate is most required for decision-makers who will be interested in calculating the total costs of adopting an intervention and the total effects received in return for incurring these costs. The regression model was adjusted for age, gender, urgency of surgery, surgical procedure, location following surgery (critical care or standard ward), American Society of Anesthesiologists (ASA) grade, renal impairment, diabetes mellitus, risk factors for cardiac and/or respiratory disease, EQ-5D score at randomisation and included a random effect for each site. Pre-specified sub-group analyses were conducted according to urgency of surgery, surgical procedure category, and timing of patient recruitment (first ten patients recruited at each site versus all subsequent patients).

Cost-effectiveness is reported in terms of the incremental net monetary benefit (National Institute for Health and Care Excellence 2013), by valuing each incremental QALY at the relevant UK (NICE) willingness to pay threshold of £20,000 and subtracting incremental costs. A positive value of incremental net monetary benefit suggests an intervention is cost-effective. Cost-effectiveness acceptability curves were constructed by calculating the probability that the OPTIMISE intervention was cost-effective at different levels of willingness to pay for a QALY gain (from £0 to £50,000 per QALY gained) (Fenwick et al. 2004). Missing data were addressed through multiple imputation assuming that data were missing at random (Rubin 1987). Analyses were performed using STATA/IC version 13 and R version 3.0.2.

Lifetime cost-effectiveness analysis
The long-term survival for each patient was calculated from observed survival within the first 6 months following surgery and from the predicted survival after 6 months using HSCIC data. Life expectancy after 6 months was predicted for each patient by applying age-gender adjusted excess death rates for OPTIMISE patients who survived beyond 6 months compared to the age-gender-matched UK general population (Office of National Statistics 2008). The most plausible long-term survival extrapolation was selected by comparing the relative goodness of fit and excess death rates of alternative parametric survival functions (Latimer 2013). To predict long-term quality of life, we used the mean value at 6 months for patients aged 72 years (median age of OPTIMISE patients). We predicted mean quality of life between year 1 and year 2 with a linear interpolation, such that after 2 years, the mean value for the OPTIMISE patients was similar to that of the age-matched general population. We then combined these predicted values of life expectancy and quality of life to calculate the projected lifetime QALYs. Lifetime incremental costs, incremental net monetary benefit and cost-effectiveness acceptability curves were then calculated using the same methods described for the 6-month analysis. Lifetime QALYs were discounted at 3.5 %. Results were reported over all the patients randomised and for the above pre-specified subgroups.

Value of information analysis
Value of information analysis provides useful information about the economic value of further research into a given question. Value of information approaches require the estimation of the expected costs of continued uncertainty about the treatment decision (in this case, whether to introduce the haemodynamic algorithm) and then the calculation of the expected value of perfect information (EVPI), that is, of the evidence required to eliminate this uncertainty. EVPI is also the maximum that a decision-maker would be willing to pay for additional future research to inform this decision (Claxton 1999; Claxton and Posnett 1996). Here, the EVPI was calculated according to the cost-effectiveness results and according to the size of the eligible patient population estimated from the NHS Hospital Episodes Statistics database. We also assumed that future patients could be expected to benefit from the algorithm over 5 years and that the incremental net monetary benefit was normally distributed (Briggs et al. 2006), and we applied a 3.5 % discount rate (Claxton 1999).

Sensitivity analyses
The following sensitivity analyses were performed to evaluate assumptions made in the primary analysis:

(a) Analysis including additional costs of a level 2 critical care bed day and 1 h of recovery nurse time for patients who were not transferred directly to critical care after surgery.
(b) Analysis including 4.5 h of additional nurse time after surgery to deliver the intervention.
(c) Analysis using EQ-5D values measured at randomisation as opposed to 30 days after surgery.
(d) Analysis estimating QALY for decedents for the time those patients were living. For decedents between randomisation and 1 month, a linear interpolation was applied between the baseline EQ-5D and the date of death when a zero EQ-5D score was applied. For decedents between 1 and 6 months where an EQ-5D score at 1 month was available, a linear interpolation was applied between the 1-month EQ-5D and the date of death when a zero EQ-5D score was applied.
(e) Analysis assuming quality of life remained unchanged after 6 months.
(f) Analysis estimating lifetime survival by applying the most plausible parametric function to the observed data for those surviving beyond 6 months following surgery, instead of assuming survival, was the same as that of the age and gender-matched general population (Latimer 2011).

Results
Baseline characteristics and 6-month outcomes
Of 734 patients randomised to OPTIMISE, one was randomised in error and excluded from the analysis. A further seven patients formally withdrew from the trial, and two patients were lost to follow-up. Baseline risk factors and quality of life were similar between groups (Table 1). There was no significant difference in survival at 6 months (Table 2). The mean EQ-5D-3L utility index score for survivors at month 1 and month 6, and the mean QALYs up to 6 months were similar between groups (Table 2).

Healthcare resource use and costs
The mean total healthcare costs were similar in the two groups (intervention group £8574 versus usual care group £8974) (Table 3). The average cost of haemodynamic therapy during the intervention period was greater in the intervention group compared to the usual care but this cost was small compared to the total healthcare costs (intervention group £230 versus usual care group £63) (Fig. 1 and Additional file 1: Table S2). Whilst critical care utilisation and mean length of hospital stay (intervention group 13.5 days versus usual care group 14.9 days) did not differ statistically, these did contribute to the non-significant difference in total healthcare costs which more than offset the cost of the trial intervention.

Table 1 Baseline characteristics of patients recruited to the OPTIMISE trial

	Peri-operative cardiac output-guided haemodynamic therapy algorithm	Usual care
	($n = 368$)	($n = 365$)
Age (year)	71.26 (8.4)	72.20 (8.6)
Gender, male	237 (64.4)	229 (62.7)
Urgency of surgery		
Elective surgery	356 (96.7)	352 (96.4)
Non-elective surgery	12 (3.3)	13 (3.6)
Surgery†		
Upper gastrointestinal	108 (29.4)	111 (30.4)
Lower gastrointestinal	168 (45.7)	165 (45.2)
Small bowel +/− pancreas	86 (23.4)	82 (22.5)
Urological or gynaecological involving gut	5 (1.4)	4 (1.1)
No surgery performed	1 (0.3)	3 (0.8)
ASA grade[a]		
1	22 (6.0)	27 (7.4)
2	200 (54.4)	174 (47.7)
3	143 (38.9)	155 (42.5)
4	3 (0.8)	9 (2.5)
Location following surgery		
Critical care level 2	258 (70.1)	246 (67.4)
Critical care level 3	42 (11.4)	40 (11.0)
Post-anaesthetic recovery unit	10 (2.7)	9 (2.5)
General ward	58 (15.8)	70 (19.2)
Renal impairment	26 (7.1)	12 (3.3)
Diabetes mellitus	57 (15.5)	65 (17.8)
Risk factor for cardiac or respiratory disease	118 (32.1)	118 (32.3)
Baseline quality of life score[a]	0.78 (0.2)	0.77 (0.3)

Data presented as mean (SD) or *n* (%)
[a]Summaries presented after multiple imputation. †Planned surgical procedure assumed when type of surgery performed was missing for one case

Six-month cost-effectiveness analysis

At 6 months following surgery, the mean incremental costs of the intervention were negative (−£404, 95 % confidence interval (CI) −£1313 to £505), indicating that the average costs of the overall package of care were less for the trial invention versus the usual care arm (Table 4). When the QALY gain of 0.01 was valued at willingness to pay of £20,000 per QALY and the incremental cost subtracted, the incremental net monetary benefit was £580 (95 % CI −£378 to £1538) per patient (Additional file 1: Figure S1). Sub-group analyses revealed no difference in the effect of the intervention on 6-month net monetary benefits according to either urgency or type of surgery (Additional file 1: Table S3). However, in the

Table 2 Mortality, EuroQol 5-dimension (EQ-5D) and quality-adjusted life years (QALY) up to 6 months for trial participants

	Peri-operative cardiac output-guided haemodynamic therapy algorithm	Usual care	Incremental effect[a]
	($n = 368$)	($n = 365$)	
6-month mortality	28 (7.61)	42 (11.51)	−0.40 (−0.39 to 1.14)
EQ-5D for survivors at month 1	0.66 (0.30)	0.63 (0.31)	0.02 (−0.02 to 0.06)
EQ-5D for survivors at month 6	0.73 (0.28)	0.71 (0.30)	0.03 (−0.01 to 0.08)
QALY up to 6 months	0.37 (0.11)	0.36 (0.12)	0.01 (0.00 to 0.02)

Data presented as mean (SD) or mean (95 % confidence intervals)
[a]Odds ratio for death, incremental for other estimates

Table 3 Hospital resource use up to 6 months for trial participants

	Peri-operative cardiac output-guided, haemodynamic therapy algorithm (*n* = 368)	Usual care (*n* = 365)
Surgery		
Upper gastrointestinal	108 (29.4)	111 (30.4)
Lower gastrointestinal	168 (45.7)	165 (45.2)
Small bowel +/− pancreas	86 (23.4)	82 (22.5)
Urological or gynaecological involving gut	5 (1.4)	4 (1.1)
No surgery performed	1 (0.3)	3 (0.8)
Intervention		
Cardiac monitor used	364 (98.9)	31 (8.5)
Dopexamine dose infused (mg)	18.9 (8.4)	–
Intra-venous crystalloid (ml)		
During surgery	1518 (1410)	2420 (1382)
6 h following surgery	565 (254)	670 (367)
Intra-venous colloid (ml)		
During surgery	1465 (913)	708 (695)
6 h following surgery	642 (498)	226 (361)
Blood products (ml)		
During surgery	141 (723)	95 (542)
6 h following surgery	80 (555)	10 (66)
Length of stay (days)		
Critical care level 2	2.5 (3.7)	2.6 (3.4)
Critical care level 3	0.7 (2.4)	0.9 (3.8)
General surgical ward	10.3 (14.4)	11.4 (12.6)

Data presented as mean (SD) or *n* (%)

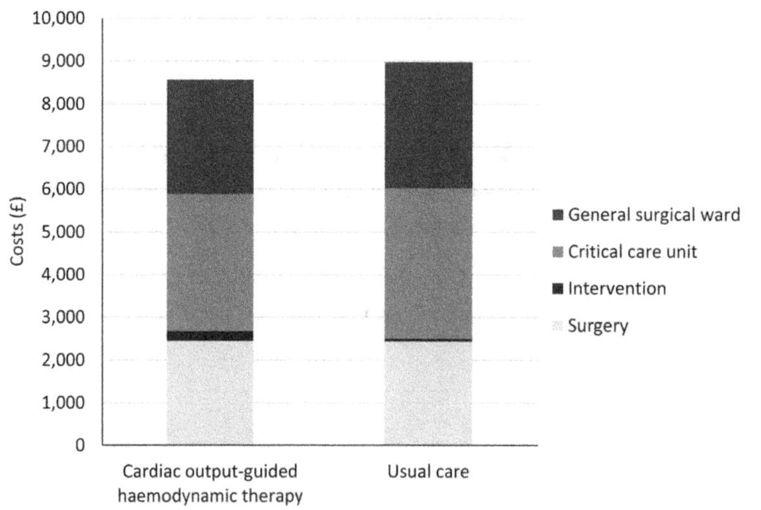

Fig. 1 Comparison of in-hospital costs up to 6 months between peri-operative cardiac output-guided haemodynamic therapy algorithm and usual care

Table 4 Hospital costs (£), quality-adjusted life years (QALY) and incremental net benefit up to 6 months and over patients' lifetime for trial participants

	Peri-operative cardiac output-guided haemodynamic therapy (*n* = 368)	Usual care (*n* = 365)	Incremental effect
Up to 6 months			
Costs (£)	8574 (6304)	8974 (7217)	−404 (−1313 to 505)
QALY	0.37 (0.11)	0.36 (0.12)	0.01 (0.00 to 0.02)
Incremental net benefit			580 (−378 to 1538)
Lifetime			
Costs (£)	8574 (6304)	8974 (7217)	−404 (−1313 to 504)
QALY	7.59 (3.34)	7.10 (3.60)	0.19 (−0.17 to 0.54)
Incremental net benefit			4168 (−3063 to 11,398)

Data presented as mean (SD) and mean (95 % confidence intervals)

sub-group of the later recruited patients (excluding the first ten patients enrolled at each site), the intervention was highly cost-effective, in line with the significant clinical benefit in this sub-group (Pearse et al. 2014).

Lifetime cost-effectiveness analysis

The Kaplan-Meier curves suggest that, when time horizon was extended beyond 6 months for those with survival data available, the probability of survival remained similar between the two groups (Additional file 1: Figure S2). When the alternative parametric specifications were applied to the OPTIMISE data, goodness of fit (lowest AIC) was similar in the various models (Additional file 1: Table S4). Compared to the general population, each of the parametric survival models tended to predict lower mortality up to year 2 and higher mortality after year 2 (Additional file 1: Table S5). It was considered implausible that the long-term mortality estimates of high-risk surgical patients would be lower than that of the general population. In the primary analysis, we therefore applied age-gender matched general population death rates after 6 months for each comparator. Of the alternative parametric functions, the Weibull was judged the most plausible, and so, we applied this extrapolation in sensitivity analysis. The small difference in long-term quality of life between the OPTIMISE patients and the general population in the first year following surgery was assumed to decline to zero within the subsequent 2 years. The intervention group patients, experienced more average lifetime QALYs and lower costs compared with usual care patients, but again, these results were not statistically significant (Table 4). However, at the willingness to pay threshold of £20,000 per QALY recommended in the UK by NICE, the incremental net monetary benefit of the intervention versus usual care was £4168 (−£3063 to £11,398) per patient, with a corresponding 87 % probability that the intervention is cost-effective when compared with usual care (Fig. 2).

Value of information analysis

A conservative estimate of the size of the NHS patient population eligible for the treatment was 270,503 eligible NHS patients over a 5-year period. At a threshold of £20,000 per QALY, the EVPI per patient is £239 and the total EVPI for the effective population is £65 million (Additional file 1: Figure S3).

Sensitivity analyses

Findings of the sensitivity analyses suggested that the primary analysis was robust to alternative approaches (Additional file 1: Table S6). The incremental net monetary benefit varied between £3979 and £4289 across the scenarios studied.

Discussion

The principal finding of this health economic evaluation was that the peri-operative, cardiac output-guided, haemodynamic therapy algorithm evaluated in the OPTIMISE trial has a high probability (87 %) of being cost-effective at the willingness to pay threshold of £20,000 per QALY gained, recommended for use in the NHS by NICE. Whereas most treatment innovations would be expected to result in a net increase in healthcare costs, lower critical care resource use and hospital stay resulted in an average cost saving amongst the intervention patients. This observation is consistent with the suggestion that improvements in the quality of peri-operative care may improve patient outcomes whilst reducing healthcare costs. The pre-specified sub-group analysis on timing of recruitment showed that the intervention was highly cost-effective in patients recruited later versus earlier at each site. This result suggests that a learning curve may have existed, consistent with expectations for trials of complex interventions. The value to the NHS of further research which would resolve the uncertainty around this treatment is £65 million, which is far greater than the likely cost of a definitive clinical trial.

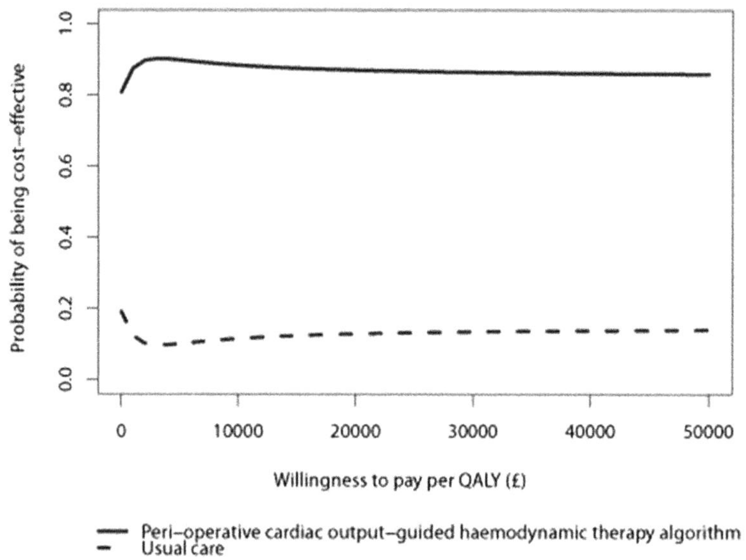

Fig. 2 Cost-effectiveness acceptability curve (all patient lifetime analysis) describing the probability that peri-operative cardiac output-guided haemodynamic therapy is cost-effective for a range of decision makers' willingness to pay thresholds per quality-adjusted life year (QALY) gained when compared with usual peri-operative care

The findings of this analysis are consistent with those of health economic analyses undertaken for previous similar trials. Cost-effectiveness analyses of data from two early single centre trials of peri-operative haemodynamic therapy suggested that this treatment resulted in a net reduction in healthcare costs and hence was cost-effective (Fenwick et al. 2002; Guest et al. 1997). However, more recent clinical trial data suggest that this treatment may only deliver more modest improvements in patient outcome and in some cases, provide only borderline evidence of clinical effectiveness (Grocott et al. 2012; Pearse et al. 2014). Whilst the findings of health economic simulations continue to suggest that peri-operative haemodynamic therapy may be cost saving and therefore cost-effective, these findings are sensitive to the size of treatment effect (Bartha et al. 2012; Ebm et al. 2014). Interestingly, economic evaluations of haemodynamic therapy in patients with early severe sepsis also indicate that the treatment may be cost-effective (Huang et al. 2007; Jones et al. 2011; Talmor et al. 2008). However, these analyses rely on the assumption of a strong treatment effect whilst the outcome of the recent major randomised trials suggest such protocols are associated with little or no clinical benefit in patients with severe sepsis (Peake et al. 2014; Yealy et al. 2014). Thus, whilst the findings of the current work are consistent with previous analyses, definitive evidence from a large clinical effectiveness trial would be required to confirm the economic impact of peri-operative cardiac output-guided haemodynamic therapy. Importantly, the findings of our value of information analysis show that such a trial would represent excellent value for money, even when confined to the NHS. This observation is consistent with a previously published estimate of EVPI for this treatment in elderly patients with hip fracture (Bartha et al. 2013).

OPTIMISE was the largest trial of a peri-operative, cardiac output-guided, haemodynamic therapy algorithm conducted to date, which addressed several methodological limitations in the existing evidence base (Pearse et al. 2014). The cost-effectiveness analysis was based on trial data with lifetime cost-effectiveness results extrapolated using appropriate methods and long-term survival data. Quality of life was assessed longitudinally allowing comparison of changes over time and comparison with the age-gender-matched general population. We calculated the cost of decision uncertainty along with traditional cost-effectiveness results. These findings will therefore inform both clinical policy and priorities for further research. However, costs and outcome data were only collected for 6 months and the lifetime cost-effectiveness analysis involved assumptions when extrapolating these data. Nonetheless, sensitivity analyses suggest the results were robust to alternative extrapolation methods. Some follow-up data were missing for the 6-month endpoints, which we addressed with a recommended approach of multiple imputation (Rubin 1987). Whilst health economic data were prospectively included in the trial dataset, the sample size calculation was based on clinical outcomes. These results should be interpreted in light of the fact that most trials are designed to detect differences in clinical effectiveness rather than cost-effectiveness. Healthcare costs are more variable than clinical outcomes, and economic evaluations may therefore lack statistical power. The primary objective of economic evaluation is not hypothesis testing but rather the estimation of incremental cost-effectiveness measures along with appropriate representation of the uncertainty surrounding those estimates. The results of this economic evaluation show that confidence interval of incremental costs, incremental QALY and incremental net monetary benefit included zero, implying considerable uncertainty surrounding these estimates. These uncertainties were summarised with the recommended use of cost-effectiveness acceptability curves, which conveys to decision-makers the strength of evidence in support of an intervention being cost-effective, at different levels of willingness to pay for a QALY gain (e.g. £20,000 or £30,000 per QALY).

Conclusions

For high-risk patients undergoing major gastrointestinal surgery, the use of a peri-operative, cardiac output-guided, haemodynamic therapy algorithm was associated with an average cost reduction and is likely to be cost-effective at the willingness to pay (cost per QALY) threshold recommended for the UK by NICE. However, a further large trial is still needed to confirm both the clinical and cost-effectiveness of this treatment approach.

Abbreviations

ASA: American Society of Anesthesiologists; EVPI: expected value of perfect information; HSCIC: Health and Social Care Information Centre; NHS: National Health Service; NICE: National Institute for Health and Care Excellence; QALY: quality-adjusted life year; UK: United Kingdom; USA: United States of America.

Competing interests

RP has received equipment loans from LiDCO Ltd and a research grant from Nestle Health Sciences. RP has performed consultancy work and/or given invited lectures for Nestle Health Sciences, Edwards Lifesciences and Massimo Inc. All other authors declare they have no conflicts of interest.

Authors' contributions

ZS, DH, RG, KR and RP were responsible for the design and conduct of this analysis. The manuscript was drafted by ZS and RP and revised following critical review by all authors. The authors received no other assistance in drafting this manuscript. All authors read and approved the final manuscript.

Author details

[1]Department of Health Services Research and Policy, London School of Hygiene and Tropical Medicine, London, UK. [2]Intensive Care National Audit & Research Centre, London, UK. [3]Queen Mary University of London, London EC1M 6BQ, UK. [4]Adult Critical Care Unit, Royal London Hospital, Whitechapel, London E1 1BB, UK.

References

Agency for Healthcare Research and Quality. Esophageal Doppler ultrasound-based cardiac output monitoring for real-time therapeutic management of hospitalized patients. 2007. http://www.cms.gov/Medicare/Coverage/DeterminationProcess/downloads/id45TA.pdf.

Bartha E, Davidson T, Hommel A, Thorngren KG, Carlsson P, Kalman S. Cost-effectiveness analysis of goal-directed hemodynamic treatment of elderly hip fracture patients: before clinical research starts. Anesthesiology. 2012;117(3):519–30.

Bartha E, Davidson T, Brodtkorb TH, Carlsson P, Kalman S. Value of information: interim analysis of a randomized, controlled trial of goal-directed hemodynamic treatment for aged patients. Trials. 2013;14:205.

Boltz MM, Hollenbeak CS, Julian KG, Ortenzi G, Dillon PW. Hospital costs associated with surgical site infections in general and vascular surgery patients. Surgery. 2011;150(5):934–42. doi:10.1016/j.surg.2011.04.006.

Briggs A, Sculpher M, Claxton K. Decision modelling for health economic evaluation. Oxford: Oxford University Press; 2006.

Claxton K. The irrelevance of inference: a decision-making approach to the stochastic evaluation of health care technologies. J Health Econ. 1999;18(3): 341–64.

Claxton K, Posnett J. An economic approach to clinical trial design and research priority-setting. Health Econ. 1996;5(6):513–24.

Department of Health. NHS reference costs 2012–2013. London: Department of Health; 2013.

Dolan P, Gudex C, Kind P, Williams A. A social tariff for EuroQoL: results from a UK general population survey. CHE Discussion Paper 138. York: Centre for Health Economics, University of York; 1999.

Ebm C, Cecconi M, Sutton L, Rhodes A. A cost-effectiveness analysis of postoperative goal-directed therapy for high-risk surgical patients. Crit Care Med. 2014;42(5):1194–203. doi:10.1097/CCM.0000000000000164.

Fenwick E, Wilson J, Sculpher M, Claxton K. Pre-operative optimisation employing dopexamine or adrenaline for patients undergoing major elective surgery: a cost-effectiveness analysis. Intensive Care Med. 2002;28(5):599.

Fenwick E, O'Brien BJ, Briggs A. Cost-effectiveness acceptability curves—facts, fallacies and frequently asked questions. Health Econ. 2004;13(5):405–15.

Grocott MP, Dushianthan A, Hamilton MA, Mythen MG, Harrison D, Rowan K, et al. Perioperative increase in global blood flow to explicit defined goals and outcomes following surgery. The Cochrane database of systematic reviews. 2012;11, CD004082. doi:10.1002/14651858.CD004082.pub5.

Guest JF, Boyd O, Hart WM, Grounds RM, Bennett ED. A cost analysis of a treatment policy of a deliberate perioperative increase in oxygen delivery in high risk surgical patients. Intensive Care Med. 1997;23(1):85–90.

Huang DT, Clermont G, Dremsizov TT, Angus DC, Pro CI. Implementation of early goal-directed therapy for severe sepsis and septic shock: a decision analysis. Crit Care Med. 2007;35(9):2090–100.

Joint Formulary Committee. British National Formulary (online) London: BMJ Group and Pharmaceutical Press; (Accessed on 25th October 2013).

Jones AE, Troyer JL, Kline JA. Cost-effectiveness of an emergency department-based early sepsis resuscitation protocol. Crit Care Med. 2011;39(6):1306–12. doi:10.1097/CCM.0b013e31821201be.

Khuri SF, Henderson WG, DePalma RG, Mosca C, Healey NA, Kumbhani DJ, et al. Determinants of long-term survival after major surgery and the adverse effect of postoperative complications. Ann Surg. 2005;242(3):326–41. discussion 41–3.

Latimer N. Survival analysis for economic evaluations alongside clinical trials—extrapolation with patient-level data. NICE DSU technical support documents: No. 14. Sheffield: University of Sheffield; 2011.

Latimer NR. Survival analysis for economic evaluations alongside clinical trials—extrapolation with patient-level data: inconsistencies, limitations, and a practical guide. Med Decis Making. 2013;33(6):743–54.

Manca A, Hawkins N, Sculpher MJ. Estimating mean QALYs in trial-based cost-effectiveness analysis: the importance of controlling for baseline utility. Health Econ. 2005;14(5):487–96.

National Institute for Health and Care Excellence. Guide to the methods of technology appraisal. London: National Institute for Health and Care Excellence; 2013.

National Institute for Health and Care Excellence. CardioQ-ODM oesophageal Doppler monitor. NICE medical technology guidance [MTG3]. 2011. https://www.nice.org.uk/guidance/mtg3.

NHS Blood & Transplant. National blood and blood products price list 2013/2014. http://www.nhsbt.nhs.uk/.

Office of National Statistics. Interim Life Tables, 2008–2010. In: Newport: Office of National Statistics. 2011. http://www.ons.gov.uk/ons/rel/lifetables/interim-life-tables/2008-2010/index.html.

Pearse RM, Ackland GL. Perioperative fluid therapy. BMJ. 2012;344, e2865. doi:10.1136/bmj.e2865.

Peake SL, Delaney A, Bailey M, Bellomo R, et al. Goal-directed resuscitation for patients with early septic shock. N Engl J Med. 2014;371(16):1496–506. doi:10.1056/NEJMoa1404380.
Pearse RM, Holt PJ, Grocott MP. Managing perioperative risk in patients undergoing elective non-cardiac surgery. BMJ. 2011;343:d5759. doi:10.1136/bmj.d5759.
Pearse RM, Moreno RP, Bauer P, Pelosi P, Metnitz P, Spies C, et al. Mortality after surgery in Europe: a 7 day cohort study. Lancet. 2012;380(9847):1059–65. doi:10.1016/S0140-6736(12)61148-9.
Pearse RM, Harrison DA, MacDonald N, Gillies MA, Blunt M, Ackland G, et al. Effect of a perioperative, cardiac output-guided hemodynamic therapy algorithm on outcomes following major gastrointestinal surgery: a randomized clinical trial and systematic review. JAMA. 2014;311(21):2181–90. doi:10.1001/jama.2014.5305.
Rubin DB. Multiple imputation for nonresponse in surveys. New York: J Wiley & Sons; 1987.
Talmor D, Greenberg D, Howell MD, Lisbon A, Novack V, Shapiro N. The costs and cost-effectiveness of an integrated sepsis treatment protocol. Crit Care Med. 2008;36(4):1168–74. doi:10.1097/CCM.0b013e318168f649.
Weiser TG, Regenbogen SE, Thompson KD, Haynes AB, Lipsitz SR, Berry WR, et al. An estimation of the global volume of surgery: a modelling strategy based on available data. Lancet. 2008;372(9633):139–44. doi:10.1016/S0140-6736(08)60878-8.
Yealy DM, Kellum JA, Huang DT, Barnato AE, Weissfeld LA, et al. A randomized trial of protocol-based care for early septic shock. N Engl J Med. 2014;370(18):1683–93. doi:10.1056/NEJMoa1401602.

9

Postoperative respiratory failure necessitating transfer to the intensive care unit in orthopedic surgery patients: risk factors, costs, and outcomes

Roman Melamed[1*], Lori L. Boland[2], James P. Normington[2], Rebecca M. Prenevost[2], Lindsay Y. Hur[3], Leslie F. Maynard[4], Molly A. McNaughton[4], Tyler G. Kinzy[2], Adnan Masood[1], Mehdi Dastrange[5] and Joseph A. Huguelet[5]

Abstract

Background: Postoperative pulmonary complications in orthopedic surgery patients have been associated with worse clinical outcomes. Identifying patients with respiratory risk factors requiring enhanced monitoring and management modifications is an important part of postoperative care. Patients with unanticipated respiratory decompensation requiring transfer to the intensive care unit (ICU) have not been studied in sufficient detail.

Methods: A retrospective case-control study of elective orthopedic surgery patients (knee, hip, shoulder, or spine, $n = 51$) who developed unanticipated respiratory failure (RF) necessitating transfer to the ICU over a 3-year period was conducted. Controls ($n = 153$) were frequency matched to cases by gender, age, and surgical procedure. Patient and perioperative care factors, clinical outcomes, and cost of care were examined.

Results: Transfer to the ICU occurred within 48 h of surgery in 73 % of the cases, 31 % required non-invasive ventilation, and 18 % required mechanical ventilation. Cases had a higher prevalence of chronic obstructive pulmonary disease (COPD), obstructive sleep apnea (OSA), and regular psychotropic medication use than controls. Cases received more intravenous opioids during the first 24 postoperative hours, were hospitalized 4 days longer, had higher in-hospital mortality, and had excess hospitalization costs of US$26,571. COPD, OSA, preoperative psychotropic medications, and anesthesia time were associated with risk of RF in a multivariate analysis.

Conclusions: Unanticipated RF after orthopedic surgery is associated with extended hospitalization, increased mortality, and higher cost of care. Hospital protocols that include risk factor assessment, enhanced monitoring, and a cautious approach to opioid use in high-risk patients may reduce the frequency of this complication.

Keywords: Respiratory failure, Orthopedic procedure, In-hospital, Critical care medicine, Intensive care unit transfer

Background

Demand for elective orthopedic procedures in the USA is expected to grow (Kurtz et al. 2007), and these procedures can be associated with serious cardiorespiratory complications (Dahl 1997). Identifying patients at high risk for postoperative pulmonary complications (PPC) and managing modifiable risk factors is essential, but effective strategies are limited (Bapoje et al. 2007). PPC develop in 7–14 % of patients undergoing spine or major joint surgery (Imposti et al. 2010; Lee et al. 2011; Lee et al. 2012; Lee et al. 2013; Ryu et al. 2010), and their occurrence is associated with longer length of stay and higher mortality (Lee et al. 2011; Lee et al. 2013; Lawrence et al. 2002; Liu et al. 2011; Smith et al. 2012). Potential PPC include pneumonia, atelectasis, pleural effusion, aspiration, airway compromise, acute respiratory distress syndrome, transfusion-related acute lung injury, fat or pulmonary embolism, opiate-related respiratory

* Correspondence: roman.melamed@allina.com
[1]Department of Critical Care Medicine, Abbott Northwestern Hospital, 800 East 28th Street, Minneapolis, MN 55407, USA
Full list of author information is available at the end of the article

depression, and respiratory arrest (Imposti et al. 2010; Lee et al. 2012; Issack et al. 2009; Raw et al. 2003; Taylor and Gropper 2006), and their occurrence may be affected by the surgical site (Miura et al. 1996; Suk et al. 2006; Yoshida et al. 2007; Sagi et al. 2002).

Risk factors for PPC include advanced age, higher American Society of Anesthesiologists (ASA) class, smoking, chronic obstructive pulmonary disease (COPD), congestive heart failure (CHF), chronic renal failure, diabetes, and obstructive sleep apnea (OSA) (Imposti et al. 2010; Lee et al. 2012; Lee et al. 2013; Liu et al. 2011; Fu et al. 2011; Gupta et al. 2001; Memtsoudis et al. 2011; Mokhlesi et al. 2013; Moller et al. 2003; Roche et al. 2005; Weis et al. 1997). Intraoperative risk factors include surgical invasiveness, longer anesthesia time, thoracic-level procedure, and increased blood loss (Imposti et al. 2010; Lee et al. 2012; Sagi et al. 2002). The use of opioids in the postoperative period is also of concern as it may suppress central respiratory drive and cough and induce a monotonous respiratory pattern (Taylor and Gropper 2006), particularly in the elderly (Egbert 1996; Petre et al. 2012). However, studies of PPC have largely focused on preoperative and intraoperative predictors, and only one has quantified postoperative opioids in orthopedic surgery patients (Petre et al. 2012).

Estimated additional total costs related to PPC range from US$5983 to US$120,579 per procedure, with higher costs associated with mechanical ventilation or tracheostomy (Sabate et al. 2014). Opioid-related PPC are associated with increased lengths of stay and costs and are associated with higher opioid doses (Oderda et al. 2007).

We conducted a case-control study of orthopedic surgery patients who were transferred from the post-anesthesia care unit (PACU) to the general orthopedic floor but subsequently developed respiratory failure (RF) requiring transfer to the intensive care unit (ICU). The study objectives were to describe the causes of RF, to investigate potential perioperative factors which can cause postoperative deterioration, and to examine outcomes such as mortality and total cost of care in cases and controls.

Methods

We conducted a retrospective frequency-matched case-control study (1:3) among adult patients who underwent major orthopedic surgery between December 1, 2010, and November 30, 2013, at Abbott Northwestern Hospital, a tertiary hospital in Minneapolis, MN, that performs approximately 4000 spine and 2000 major joint surgeries annually. The study protocol was approved by the Schulman Institutional Review Board with a waiver of informed consent.

Cases were patients who underwent elective or semi-elective spine or major joint surgery and were postoperatively initially stable (i.e., oxygen saturation >90 % while receiving supplemental oxygen via nasal cannula and not requiring respiratory or hemodynamic support beyond standard care) but then experienced unanticipated RF and were subsequently transferred to the ICU. We queried the hospital's electronic health record (EHR) for procedural codes representing specific spine or major joint surgery based on the International Classification of Diseases 9th Revision (ICD-9). For descriptive purposes, patients were grouped by anatomical site of the surgery, i.e., knee, hip, spine (cervical), spine (non-cervical), and shoulder. We then restricted this list of patients to those who were initially stable and transferred directly from the PACU to a medical/surgical unit. Instances of unanticipated RF were then identified using a two-step process. First, we identified patients who were transferred to the ICU and had any of the following ICD-9 discharge diagnosis codes: 518.81 (acute RF), 518.84 (acute and chronic RF), 518.51 (acute RF following trauma/surgery), 518.52 (other pulmonary insufficiency following trauma/surgery), 518.82 (acute pulmonary insufficiency), or 786.09 (respiratory distress). The medical records of these patients were then reviewed independently by two physicians (RM and MD) who confirmed RF if any of the following criteria were met: pO_2 <60 mmHg on room air or pCO_2 >45 mmHg; increase in pCO_2 from baseline or increase in supplemental oxygen requirements; or documentation of the patient's inability to protect airway or maintain adequate gas exchange. Controls were selected from among patients who underwent the same surgical procedures as the cases during the study timeframe but who were neither transferred to the ICU nor developed RF. Three controls were randomly selected for each case, frequency-matched on surgical procedure, gender, and 10-year age category. Patients <18 years of age or who did not provide consent for use of their EHR data for research were excluded.

Patient demographics and event details including preoperative ASA class, length of stay, and in-hospital mortality were extracted from the EHR. ICU length of stay and ventilatory support details were extracted for cases. Two physicians (RM and MD) independently reviewed patient care records to determine the primary cause of RF; conditions present on admission such as COPD, OSA, and regular use of psychotropic medications (defined as antipsychotics, antidepressants, benzodiazepines, sleep aides, or muscle relaxants); and total operative anesthesia time (minutes). Total cost of care was obtained via financial databases maintained by the hospital.

Clinicians with expertise in pain management (LYH, LFM, MAM) reviewed EHR data and quantified postoperative opioid use. Use of patient-controlled analgesia (PCA) was categorized as none, incremental dosing only, or a combination of a continuous basal rate and incremental dosing. Total morphine equivalents (milligrams) were computed for 12 consecutive 8-h intervals from the end of surgery up to 96 h after surgery or patient discharge (whichever occurred sooner) using a standardized conversion tool developed by Allina Health Pharmacy Services based on established methods (McPherson 2009). Postoperative use of other sedatives such as diazepam and lorazepam was also documented.

Analysis

Continuous variables were described using means or medians based on results of Shapiro-Wilk tests for normality, and values in cases and controls were compared using t tests or Wilcoxon-Mann-Whitney rank-sum tests accordingly. Categorical data were described using counts and proportions, with differences between cases and controls assessed using Fisher's exact test. Unconditional logistic regression models were used to estimate adjusted odds ratios and 95 % confidence intervals for associations between hypothesized risk factors and RF. All analyses were conducted using Stata 12.1 (StataCorp LP, College Station, TX).

Results

Fifty-one cases of unanticipated postoperative RF occurred among 14,465 qualifying surgical procedures performed during the study timeframe (0.4 %). The most common procedure-related diagnoses were spinal stenosis and degenerative joint disease. There was no significant difference in obesity between cases and controls, but cases had a statistically significantly higher prevalence of COPD, OSA, chronic kidney disease (CKD), and psychotropic medication use and higher ASA class (Table 1). Among the 35 patients with diagnosed OSA, 35 % of cases (5/18) and 71 % of controls ($n = 12/17$) were using continuous positive airway pressure (CPAP) at home at the time of admission ($p = 0.02$), and among 16 patients with COPD, 18 % of cases (2/11) and 20 % of controls (1/5) were using home oxygen.

The most common primary causes of RF were decreased levels of consciousness with depressed respiratory drive (with or without laboratory confirmation of hypercarbia), pneumonia, CHF, and COPD exacerbation (Table 2). There were three cases of cardiac arrest: two related to respiratory depression and one due to acute myocardial infarction. Most cases (72 %) developed RF within the first 2 postoperative days, with a median time from the end of surgery to the ICU transfer of 42 h.

Spine and shoulder surgery patients received general anesthesia while regional anesthesia was used for knee and hip procedures. Cases generally had longer anesthesia times and higher estimated blood loss than controls, but there was no significant difference between the groups with regard to transfusion requirements (data not shown). Among spine surgery patients, cases received slightly higher doses of intraoperative opioids, but this difference was not observed in major joint surgery patients (Table 3).

Overall, cases received more intravenous opioids during the first 24 postoperative hours than controls (median 110 vs 73 mg, $p = 0.006$), and opioid use was examined separately for patients with spine versus major joint procedures (Table 3). In spine surgery patients, the use of any PCA was more frequent in cases than in controls, and cases were more likely to have used a combination of continuous and incremental PCA than controls. Total postoperative opioids were generally higher in spine surgery patients than in major joint surgery patients. In major joint surgery patients, doses received in the first 8- and 24-h intervals were positively associated with the development of RF, with the median total dose in the first 8-h interval nearly three times higher in cases than in controls. Data in spine surgery patients suggest a similar pattern of higher opioid doses in cases across the 96-h postoperative interval. Use of additional sedatives during the postoperative course was associated with RF in spine surgery patients.

Among the cases and controls with previously diagnosed OSA, CPAP was started in the PACU in 11 % of cases (2/18) and 29 % of controls (5/17; $p = 0.23$). Non-invasive ventilation (NIV) was ultimately initiated in 56 % of cases who had OSA (10/18), commonly as a rescue therapy after the development of respiratory insufficiency.

Nine cases required mechanical ventilation (median hours = 56), 16 were managed with non-invasive ventilation, and in-hospital mortality was 6 % in cases and 0 % in controls ($p = 0.003$, Table 4). Average hospitalization cost was significantly higher in cases (US$46,456) than in controls ($19,885, $p < 0.001$).

Multivariate logistic regression models initially included the three matching variables and the following covariates that were statistically significant in univariate analyses ($p \leq 0.01$): ASA class, COPD, OSA, CKD, smoking, psychotropic medication use, total operative anesthesia time, estimated blood loss, and opioids in the first 24 postoperative hours. Due to collinearity with comorbidities, ASA class was omitted from the final model, the results of which are presented in Table 5. COPD, OSA, CKD, psychotropic medication use, and total anesthesia time were all independently associated with risk of RF, but opioids in the first 24 postoperative hours were not associated with RF in the presence of these other factors.

Discussion

Previous studies of PPC have been conducted in more heterogeneous groups of surgical patients and have not

Table 1 Surgical procedures, patient characteristics, and conditions present on admission

Variable	Cases ($n = 51$)	Controls ($n = 153$)	p value*
Surgical procedure type			
Knee	37 % (19)	37 % (57)	
Spine (cervical)	41 % (21)	41 % (63)	
Spine (non-cervical)	16 % (8)	16 % (24)	
Hip	4 % (2)	4 % (6)	
Shoulder	2 % (1)	2 % (3)	
Age, years	66 (34–88)	67 (32–90)	
Age category, years			
31–40	2 % (1)	2 % (3)	
41–50	6 % (3)	6 % (9)	
51–60	22 % (11)	22 % (33)	
61–70	33 % (17)	33 % (51)	
71–80	22 % (11)	22 % (33)	
81+	16 % (8)	16 % (24)	
Male	35 % (18)	35 % (54)	
Body mass index (BMI), kg/m^2			
<25	14 % (7)	17 % (26)	0.67
25.0–29.9	43 % (22)	37 % (56)	0.41
30.0–35.0	18 % (9)	25 % (38)	0.34
>35.0	26 % (13)	22 % (33)	0.57
ASA class			
1	0 % (0)	2 % (3)	0.58
2	41 % (21)	69 % (105)	<0.001
3	57 % (29)	29 % (44)	<0.001
4	2 % (1)	1 % (1)	0.44
Conditions present on admission			
Asthma	20 % (10)	10 % (16)	0.10
COPD	22 % (11)	3 % (5)	<0.001
OSA	35 % (18)	11 % (17)	<0.001
Obesity (BMI ≥ 30 kg/m^2)	43 % (22)	46 % (71)	0.75
CHF	10 % (5)	2 % (3)	0.03
CKD	22 % (11)	6 % (9)	0.002
Restrictive lung disease	4 % (2)	1 % (1)	0.16
Opioid use	41 % (21)	34 % (52)	0.40
Smoking history	57 % (29)	37 % (57)	0.01
Regular use of psychotropic medication	71 % (36)	37 % (56)	<0.001
Diabetes	18 % (9)	11 % (17)	0.23

Results are expressed as mean (range) or percent (n) unless otherwise indicated
ASA American Society of Anesthesiologists, *BMI* body mass index, *COPD* chronic obstructive pulmonary disease, *OSA* obstructive sleep apnea, *CHF* congestive heart failure, *CKD* chronic kidney disease
*Fisher's exact test; p values not shown for matched variables

Table 2 Cause of respiratory failure and timing of ICU transfer in cases

Variable	Cases ($n = 51$)
Cause of respiratory failure	
Altered LOC with respiratory depression	20 % (10)
Hypercapnic respiratory failure	18 % (9)
Pneumonia	16 % (8)
CHF	10 % (5)
COPD exacerbation	8 % (4)
Aspiration	6 % (3)
Cardiac arrest	6 % (3)
Sepsis	6 % (3)
Pulmonary embolism	4 % (2)
Upper airway edema/obstruction	4 % (2)
Fat embolism	2 % (1)
OSA/OHS	2 % (1)
Total	100 % (51)
Day transferred to ICU	
Day 0	12 % (6)
Day 1	28 % (14)
Day 2	33 % (17)
Days 3–4	20 % (10)
Days 5–6	8 % (4)
Time between end of surgery and transfer to ICU, hours	42 (4–107)

Results are expressed as mean (range) or percent (n) unless otherwise indicated
ICU intensive care unit, *LOC* loss of consciousness, *CHF* congestive heart failure, *COPD* chronic obstructive pulmonary disease, *MI* myocardial infarction, *OSA* obstructive sleep apnea, *OHS* obesity hypoventilation syndrome

distinguished between patients who were initially stable versus those who were directly transferred to the ICU after surgery. To our knowledge, this is the first case-control study of postoperative RF in orthopedic surgery patients to examine detailed information on postoperative opiate administration and to provide information on the primary causes of RF, clinical outcomes, and cost of care.

Postoperative RF is a significant complication in terms of increased mortality, length of stay, and cost (Dimick et al. 2004; Khuri et al. 2005), so there is strong interest in developing and validating tools that accurately identify high-risk patients for targeted intervention (Sabate et al. 2014; Canet and Gallart 2013). A scorecard quantifying the risk of opioid-related respiratory depression (Katie Felhofer 2013) and two scoring algorithms designed specifically for predicting postoperative RF have been proposed (Arozullah et al. 2000; Gupta et al. 2011). The demographic homogeneity of the surgical population that yielded one approach has been cited as a serious limitation (Arozullah et al. 2000), and while the score developed recently by Gupta et al. (Gupta et al.

Table 3 Intraoperative and postoperative opioid use, by spine and major joint procedures

Variable	Spine surgery			Major joint surgery		
	Cases	Controls	p value*	Cases	Controls	p value*
	n = 29	n = 87		n = 22	n = 66	
Total intraoperative opioids (ME), mg	115 (95–185)	85 (69–120)	0.006	18 (15–45)	23 (15–68)	0.77
Postoperative PCA						
Incremental only	21 % (6)	15 % (13)	0.56	0 % (0)	2 % (1)	1.00
Continuous and incremental	69 % (20)	36 % (31)	0.002	0 % (0)	3 % (2)	1.00
None	10 % (3)	49 % (106)	<0.001	100 % (22)	95 % (63)	0.57
Total postoperative opioids (ME), mg						
First 8 h	40 (0–470)	33 (0–179)	0.42	26 (0–107)	9 (0–240)	0.01
First 24 h	117 (10–1414)	87 (0–448)	0.05	109 (15–224)	64 (0–499)	0.03
First 48 h	240 (10–981)	153 (0–857)	0.37	130 (65–397)	137 (0–934)	0.97
First 72 h	416 (20–1451)	242 (15–1262)	0.33	174 (112–236)	190 (17–1480)	0.79
First 96 h	716 (408–1023)	331 (37–1667)	0.64	112 (112–112)	189 (22–2110)	0.59
Use of other sedative during postoperative course	83 % (24)	48 % (42)	0.001	64 % (14)	52 % (34)	0.46

Results are expressed as median (range) or percent (n) unless otherwise indicated
PCA patient-controlled analgesia, *ME* morphine equivalents
*Fisher's exact test or Wilcoxon rank-sum test as appropriate

2011) appears promising in terms of more generalizable use, only 4 % of the patients underwent orthopedic procedures and their criteria for RF were stricter (i.e., patients requiring intubation or mechanical ventilation for >48 h). In addition, only one of the five criteria used in this score (i.e., ASA class) would have any significant variability in the patients studied here.

Consistent with previous studies, we found that risk of RF was associated with preexisting COPD, OSA, CHF, and CKD, as well as with smoking, longer anesthesia time, and higher intraoperative blood loss (Imposti et al. 2010; Lee et al. 2011; Lee et al. 2012; Sagi et al. 2002; Gupta et al. 2001; Moller et al. 2003; Roche et al. 2005). Advanced age was a strong risk factor for PPC in previous studies (Imposti et al. 2010; Lee et al. 2012; Canet and Gallart 2013; Smetana et al. 2006), although we find it noteworthy that almost 30 % of our cases were under the age of 60.

Table 4 Hospitalization details and outcomes

Variable	Cases (n = 51)	Controls (n = 153)	p value*
Mechanical ventilation	18 % (9)		
Non-invasive ventilatory support (BiPAP)	31 % (16)		
Total ventilation time, h	56 (1–347)		
ICU length of stay, days	1.6 (0.2–17)		
Hospital length of stay, days	7 (2–41)	3 (1–8)	<0.001
In-hospital mortality	6 % (3)	0 % (0)	0.003
Cost of hospitalization, $US[a]	46,456	19,885	<0.001
Discharge destination			
Died	6 % (3)	0 % (0)	0.003
Home	55 % (28)	70 % (107)	0.046
SNF/rehabilitation	39 % (20)	30 % (46)	0.193

Results are expressed as median (range) or percent (n) unless otherwise indicated
ICU intensive care unit, *SNF* skilled nursing facility
*Wilcoxon rank-sum test, two-sample t test, or Fisher's exact test, as appropriate
[a]Mean US dollars

OSA is a common disorder associated with increased morbidity and mortality (Peppard et al. 2013; Young et al. 2009). In a large analysis of orthopedic surgery patients, OSA was present in 8.4 % and was associated with increased pulmonary and cardiac complications, use of intensive care, ventilatory support, and longer hospitalization (Memtsoudis et al. 2014). The postoperative state has been shown to exacerbate OSA symptoms and even cause sleep-disordered breathing in patients without OSA (Chung et al. 2014). In our study, cases with OSA had lower rates of compliance with home CPAP than controls. A validated OSA screening tool as described by Chung et al (Chung et al. 2016) could potentially be used to prompt earlier NIV use and enhanced postoperative monitoring in orthopedic surgical patients with diagnosed or suspected OSA.

Postoperative pain management with opioids presents significant challenges in orthopedic surgery patients (Taylor and Gropper 2006). Opioid-induced oversedation and associated respiratory depression is a principal concern, particularly in the presence of OSA, obesity, advanced age, preexisting pulmonary or cardiac disease, and longer anesthesia times (The Joint Commission 2012). But while opioid use may be an important risk factor for PPC, it is noticeably absent from the

Table 5 Adjusted odds ratios and 95 % confidence intervals of unplanned postoperative respiratory failure according to selected risk factors

Variable	OR	95 % CI
COPD	4.87	(1.24–19.21)
OSA	4.79	(1.81–12.67)
CKD	4.83	(1.36–17.17)
Regular use of psychotropic medication	4.02	(1.58–10.26)
Total operative anesthesia time	1.27	(1.10–1.48)
Total opioid dose in the first 24-h postoperative interval	1.02	(0.98–1.06)

Results from a logistic regression model that included gender, surgical procedure type, age (10-year categories), and all variables shown in the table
OR odds ratio, *CI* confidence interval, *COPD* chronic obstructive pulmonary disease, *OSA* obstructive sleep apnea, *CKD* chronic kidney disease

summarized evidence presented in two recent systematic reviews (Sabate et al. 2014; Canet and Gallart 2013). Data from the only other study that has quantified postoperative opioids when examining PPC in orthopedic surgery patients (Petre et al. 2012) suggest that higher doses of opioids may be associated with increased risk of PPC. In our study, cases had received significantly more opioids than controls in the first 8–24 postoperative hours and typically required transfer to the ICU within the first 48 h after surgery. The initial 24–48 postoperative hours thus may represent a particularly sensitive period when patients are prone to the development of respiratory insufficiency and the side effects of opioids, a theory that is supported by evidence that postoperative patients who experience analgesic-related respiratory events are more likely to have those events in the first 24 h after surgery (Taylor et al. 2005). Our finding that the use of additional sedatives during the postoperative course was also associated with RF further supports this hypothesis, but this topic requires further study.

Cases in our study remained hospitalized an average of 4 days longer than controls, and on average, total costs were US$26,571 more for their hospitalization. Nearly one in five cases in our study required mechanical ventilation, and previous studies estimate that patients requiring intubation have longer hospital stays and higher total charges (Liu et al. 2011; Gupta et al. 2001; Mokhlesi et al. 2013).

Our results highlight the need for postoperative protocols that incorporate the type and complexity of the surgical procedure, perioperative events, individual patient risk factors, and facility-specific workflow and resources. Future studies should evaluate the effect on patient outcomes of clinical pathways that include patient assessment in the immediate postoperative period and a standardized hand-off process from anesthesia to the medical team. A mechanism for alerting the entire multidisciplinary team (e.g., nursing, hospitalists, respiratory care, pharmacists, surgeons) to the patient's risk factors and pain control, respiratory support, and monitoring needs would be an essential component of such protocols. This approach may reduce the frequency of both severe cases of RF requiring ICU transfer and respiratory events of lesser severity that can be managed outside the ICU.

Limitations of this study include the fact that we did not ascertain the entire spectrum of PPC in elective orthopedic surgery patients at our facility during the study timeframe. Second, given the single-center study design and narrowly defined patient population, our results may not be applicable to other treatment centers or surgical populations. Third, a detailed evaluation of the patient's preoperative cardiorespiratory and nutritional status was limited by the retrospective study design. Fourth, we were unable to blind the clinicians who computed total opioids from the case status of patients, but we do not believe this resulted in systematic differences in the assessment given the objective nature of the computation.

Conclusions

Unanticipated RF requiring ICU transfer occurs in less than 1 % of patients who undergo elective orthopedic surgery, but despite their rarity, these events are associated with higher mortality, longer length of stay, and significantly increased hospital costs. Hospitals, and particularly high-volume orthopedic surgery centers, should consider a structured multidisciplinary team approach to postoperative management that involves systematic risk factor assessment, enhanced monitoring techniques, a judicious approach to pain management, and early identification and treatment of PPC.

Abbreviations

ASA class, American Society of Anesthesiologists physical status classification (system for assessing the fitness of patients before surgery); CHF, congestive heart failure; CKD, chronic kidney disease; COPD, chronic obstructive pulmonary disease; EHR, electronic health record; ICU, intensive care unit; LFM, Leslie F. Maynard, CNP (author); LYH, Lindsay Y. Hur, PharmD (author); MAM, Molly A. McNaughton, CNP (author); MD, Mehdi Dastrange, MD (author); OSA, obstructive sleep apnea; PACU, post-anesthesia care unit; PCA, patient-controlled analgesia; PPC, postoperative pulmonary complications; RF, respiratory failure; RM, Roman Melamed, MD (author)

Authors' contributions

All authors meet the criteria for authorship as recommended by the ICMJE. RM conceived of the study, participated in the study design and coordination, and helped to draft the manuscript. LB conceived of the study, performed the statistical analysis, participated in the study design and coordination, and helped to draft the manuscript. JN performed the statistical analysis, participated in the study design and coordination, and helped to draft the manuscript. RP performed the statistical analysis, participated in the study design, and helped to draft the manuscript. LH conceived of the study, participated in its design and coordination, and helped to draft the manuscript. LM conceived of the study, participated in its design and coordination, and helped to draft the manuscript. MM conceived of the study, participated in the study design and coordination, and helped to draft the manuscript. TK performed the statistical analysis, participated in the study design and coordination, and helped to draft the manuscript. AM conceived of the study, participated in the study design and coordination, and helped to draft the manuscript. MD conceived of the study, participated in the study design and coordination, and helped to draft the manuscript. JH participated in the study design and coordination and helped to draft the manuscript. All authors read and approved the final manuscript.

Competing interests

The authors declare that they have no competing interests.

Author details

[1]Department of Critical Care Medicine, Abbott Northwestern Hospital, 800 East 28th Street, Minneapolis, MN 55407, USA. [2]Division of Applied Research, Allina Health, 2925 Chicago Ave South, Minneapolis, MN, USA. [3]Department of Pharmacy, Abbott Northwestern Hospital, 800 East 28th Street, Minneapolis, MN, USA. [4]Chronic Pain Team, Abbott Northwestern Hospital, 800 East 28th Street, Minneapolis, MN, USA. [5]Internal Medicine Residency Program, Abbott Northwestern Hospital, 800 East 28th Street, Minneapolis, MN, USA.

References

Arozullah AM, Daley J, Henderson WG, et al. Multifactorial risk index for predicting postoperative respiratory failure in men after major noncardiac surgery. The National Veterans Administration Surgical Quality Improvement Program. Ann Surg. 2000;232:242–53.

Bapoje SR, Whitaker JF, Schulz T, et al. Preoperative evaluation of the patient with pulmonary disease. Chest. 2007;132:1637–45.

Canet J, Gallart L. Predicting postoperative pulmonary complications in the general population. Curr Opin Anaesthesiol. 2013;26:107–15.

Chung F, Liao P, Yegneswaran B, et al. Postoperative changes in sleep-disordered breathing and sleep architecture in patients with obstructive sleep apnea. Anesthesiology. 2014;120:287–98.

Chung F, Abdullah HR, Liao P. STOP-Bang Questionnaire: a practical approach to screen for obstructive sleep apnea. Chest. 2016;149:631–8.

Dahl OE. Cardiorespiratory and vascular dysfunction related to major reconstructive orthopedic surgery. Acta Orthop Scand. 1997;68:607–14.

Dimick JB, Chen SL, Taheri PA, et al. Hospital costs associated with surgical complications: a report from the private-sector National Surgical Quality Improvement Program. J Am Coll Surg. 2004;199:531–7.

Egbert AM. Postoperative pain management in the frail elderly. Clin Geriatr Med. 1996;12:583–99.

Fu KM, Smith JS, Polly Jr DW, et al. Correlation of higher preoperative American Society of Anesthesiology grade and increased morbidity and mortality rates in patients undergoing spine surgery. J Neurosurg Spine. 2011;14:470–4.

Gupta RM, Parvizi J, Hanssen AD, et al. Postoperative complications in patients with obstructive sleep apnea syndrome undergoing hip or knee replacement: a case-control study. Mayo Clin Proc. 2001;76:897–905.

Gupta H, Gupta PK, Fang X, et al. Development and validation of a risk calculator predicting postoperative respiratory failure. Chest. 2011;140:1207–15.

Imposti F, Cizik A, Bransford R, et al. Risk factors for pulmonary complications after spine surgery. Evid Based Spine Care J. 2010;1:26–33.

Issack PS, Lauerman MH, Helfet DL, et al. Fat embolism and respiratory distress associated with cemented femoral arthroplasty. Am J Orthop (Belle Mead NJ). 2009;38:72–6.

Katie Felhofer PD. Developing a respiratory depression scorecard for capnography monitoring. Innovations in Pharmacy. 2013;4:11.

Khuri SF, Henderson WG, DePalma RG, et al. Determinants of long-term survival after major surgery and the adverse effect of postoperative complications. Ann Surg. 2005;242:326–41. discussion 341–323.

Kurtz S, Ong K, Lau E, et al. Projections of primary and revision hip and knee arthroplasty in the United States from 2005 to 2030. J Bone Joint Surg Am. 2007;89:780–5.

Lawrence VA, Hilsenbeck SG, Noveck H, et al. Medical complications and outcomes after hip fracture repair. Arch Intern Med. 2002;162:2053–7.

Lee MJ, Hacquebord J, Varshney A, et al. Risk factors for medical complication after lumbar spine surgery: a multivariate analysis of 767 patients. Spine (Phila Pa 1976). 2011;36:1801–6.

Lee MJ, Konodi MA, Cizik AM, et al. Risk factors for medical complication after spine surgery: a multivariate analysis of 1,591 patients. Spine J. 2012;12:197–206.

Lee MJ, Konodi MA, Cizik AM, et al. Risk factors for medical complication after cervical spine surgery: a multivariate analysis of 582 patients. Spine (Phila Pa 1976). 2013;38:223–8.

Liu SS, Chisholm MF, Ngeow J, et al. Postoperative hypoxemia in orthopedic patients with obstructive sleep apnea. HSS J. 2011;7:2–8.

McPherson ML. Demystifying opioid conversion calculations: a guide to effective dosing. 2009.

Memtsoudis S, Liu SS, Ma Y, et al. Perioperative pulmonary outcomes in patients with sleep apnea after noncardiac surgery. Anesth Analg. 2011;112:113–21.

Memtsoudis SG, Stundner O, Rasul R, et al. The impact of sleep apnea on postoperative utilization of resources and adverse outcomes. Anesth Analg. 2014;118:407–18.

Miura Y, Mimatsu K, Iwata H. Massive tongue swelling as a complication after spinal surgery. J Spinal Disord. 1996;9:339–41.

Mokhlesi B, Hovda MD, Vekhter B, et al. Sleep-disordered breathing and postoperative outcomes after elective surgery: analysis of the nationwide inpatient sample. Chest. 2013;144:903–14.

Moller AM, Pedersen T, Villebro N, et al. Effect of smoking on early complications after elective orthopaedic surgery. J Bone Joint Surg (Br). 2003;85:178–81.

Oderda GM, Said Q, Evans RS, et al. Opioid-related adverse drug events in surgical hospitalizations: impact on costs and length of stay. Ann Pharmacother. 2007;41:400–6.

Peppard PE, Young T, Barnet JH, et al. Increased prevalence of sleep-disordered breathing in adults. Am J Epidemiol. 2013;177:1006–14.

Petre BM, Roxbury CR, McCallum JR, et al. Pain reporting, opiate dosing, and the adverse effects of opiates after hip or knee replacement in patients 60 years old or older. Geriatr Orthop Surg Rehabil. 2012;3:3–7.

Raw DA, Beattie JK, Hunter JM. Anaesthesia for spinal surgery in adults. Br J Anaesth. 2003;91:886–904.

Roche JJ, Wenn RT, Sahota O, et al. Effect of comorbidities and postoperative complications on mortality after hip fracture in elderly people: prospective observational cohort study. BMJ. 2005;331:1374.

Ryu YJ, Chun EM, Shim SS, et al. Risk factors for pulmonary complications, including pulmonary embolism, after total knee arthroplasty (TKA) in elderly Koreans. Arch Gerontol Geriatr. 2010;51:299–303.

Sabate S, Mazo V, Canet J. Predicting postoperative pulmonary complications: implications for outcomes and costs. Curr Opin Anaesthesiol. 2014;27:201–9.

Sagi HC, Beutler W, Carroll E, et al. Airway complications associated with surgery on the anterior cervical spine. Spine (Phila Pa 1976). 2002;27:949–53.

Smetana GW, Lawrence VA, Cornell JE, et al. Preoperative pulmonary risk stratification for noncardiothoracic surgery: systematic review for the American College of Physicians. Ann Intern Med. 2006;144:581–95.

Smith JS, Saulle D, Chen CJ, et al. Rates and causes of mortality associated with spine surgery based on 108,419 procedures: a review of the Scoliosis Research Society Morbidity and Mortality Database. Spine (Phila Pa 1976). 2012;37:1975–82.

Suk KS, Kim KT, Lee SH, et al. Prevertebral soft tissue swelling after anterior cervical discectomy and fusion with plate fixation. Int Orthop. 2006;30:290–4.

Taylor JM, Gropper MA. Critical care challenges in orthopedic surgery patients. Crit Care Med. 2006;34:S191–199.

Taylor S, Kirton OC, Staff I, et al. Postoperative day one: a high risk period for respiratory events. Am J Surg. 2005;190:752–6.

The Joint Commission: safe use of opioids in hospitals. Sentinel Event Alert. 2012;1:5.

Weis JC, Betz RR, Clements 3rd DH, et al. Prevalence of perioperative complications after anterior spinal fusion for patients with idiopathic scoliosis. J Spinal Disord. 1997;10:371–5.

Yoshida M, Neo M, Fujibayashi S, et al. Upper-airway obstruction after short posterior occipitocervical fusion in a flexed position. Spine (Phila Pa 1976). 2007;32:E267–270.

Young T, Palta M, Dempsey J, et al. Burden of sleep apnea: rationale, design, and major findings of the Wisconsin Sleep Cohort study. WMJ. 2009;108:246–9.

10

Association between preoperative haemoglobin concentration and cardiopulmonary exercise variables: a multicentre study

James M Otto[1,2*], Alasdair F O'Doherty[2], Philip J Hennis[2], Jackie A Cooper[3], Michael PW Grocott[2,4], Chris Snowdon[6], John B Carlisle[7], Michael Swart[7], Toby Richards[1] and Hugh E Montgomery[5]

Abstract

Background: Preoperative anaemia and low exertional oxygen uptake are both associated with greater postoperative morbidity and mortality. This study reports the association among haemoglobin concentration ([Hb]), peak oxygen uptake ($\dot{V}O_2$ peak) and anaerobic threshold (AT) in elective surgical patients.

Methods: Between 1999 and 2011, preoperative [Hb] and cardiopulmonary exercise tests were recorded in 1,777 preoperative patients in four hospitals. The associations between [Hb], $\dot{V}O_2$ peak and AT were analysed by linear regression and covariance.

Results: In 436 (24.5%) patients, [Hb] was <12 g dl^{-1} and, in 83 of these, <10 g dl^{-1}. Both AT and $\dot{V}O_2$ peak rose modestly with increasing [Hb] (r^2 = 0.24, *P* <0.0001 and r^2 = 0.30, *P* <0.0001, respectively). After covariate adjustment, an increase in [Hb] of one standard deviation was associated with a 6.7 to 9.7% increase in $\dot{V}O_2$ peak, and a rise of 4.4 to 6.0% in AT. Haemoglobin concentration accounted for 9% and 6% of the variation in $\dot{V}O_2$ peak and AT respectively.

Conclusions: To a modest extent, lower haemoglobin concentrations are independently associated with lower oxygen uptake during preoperative cardiopulmonary exercise testing. It is unknown whether this association is causative.

Keywords: Anaemia, Cardiopulmonary exercise testing, CPET, Haemoglobin concentration, Oxygen uptake, Surgery

Background

Increased mitochondrial oxygen uptake requires increased cellular oxygen delivery. When oxygen delivery, or utilization, fails to meet metabolic demand, anaerobic cytoplasmic metabolism significantly augments aerobic mitochondrial ATP generation with a consequent increase in lactic acid production and accumulation. It has been suggested that an imbalance in oxygen demand-supply contributes to the point during cardiopulmonary exercise testing (CPET) known as the anaerobic threshold (AT) [1], although this physiological underpinning is not without controversy [2,3]. Major surgery places substantial metabolic demands upon the patient and may increase resting oxygen uptake from an average preoperative value of 110 ml min^{-1} m^{-2} to approximately 170 ml min^{-1} m^{-2} [4,5]. Lower preoperative exertional oxygen uptake ($\dot{V}O_2$), both the peak and that noted at AT, are associated with postoperative morbidity and mortality [6-8].

Each gram of haemoglobin carries 1.34 ml of oxygen when fully saturated. Anaemia, commonly defined as a haemoglobin concentration ([Hb]) below 13 g dl^{-1} (males) and 12 g dl^{-1} (non-pregnant females), reduces the blood's oxygen carriage capacity. Anaemia is common amongst preoperative patients, with a prevalence ranging from 5% to 76% [9]. Anaemia and blood transfusion are associated with poor postoperative outcomes [10-16].

* Correspondence: james.otto@ucl.ac.uk
[1]Division of Surgery and Interventional Science, University College London, 21 University Street, London WC1E 6DE, UK
[2]The Portex Unit, UCL Institute of Child Health, 30 Guilford Street, London WC1N 1EH, UK
Full list of author information is available at the end of the article

Oxygen delivery limits maximal oxygen uptake during exercise under normoxic conditions [17,18]. Increases in [Hb] increase $\dot{V}O_2$ peak, whilst acute reductions in [Hb] lower $\dot{V}O_2$ peak and endurance performance [19-21]. However, the extent to which postoperative outcomes are dependent upon interactions between [Hb] and $\dot{V}O_2$ is unknown. We analysed a large multicentre dataset to explore the relationship between preoperative [Hb] and $\dot{V}O_2$.

Methods

Patient population

We analysed cardiopulmonary exercise (CPET) data collected between December 1999 and February 2011 by four centres: University College London Hospitals NHS Trust (UCLH); the Whittington Hospital NHS Trust; Torbay Hospital, South Devon Healthcare NHS Foundation Trust; and the Freeman Hospital, Newcastle Upon Tyne Hospitals NHS Foundation Trust. Patients had been routinely tested as part of the clinical service before elective surgery: maxillofacial, hepatobiliary, vascular, upper gastrointestinal, colorectal, orthopaedic, bariatric and other specialties (mainly urological).

Following discussion among the researchers and the local Research and Development and clinical governance departments, formal ethical approval was waived and confirmation of audit status granted due to the nature of the data collection.

Cardiopulmonary exercise testing

Across all testing sites, CPET was performed according to the American Thoracic Society/American College of Chest Physicians (ATS/ACCP) guidelines, under stable environmental conditions, with continuous 12 lead ECG monitoring and in the presence of a clinician [22].

Patients pedalled an electromagnetically-braked cycle ergometer (Lode BV, Groningen, Netherlands), with breath-by-breath respiratory gas analysis performed by various machines, (UCL-Cortex Biophysik, Leipzig, Germany; Torbay and Newcastle-Medical Graphics, Minnesota, USA) calibrated according to ATS/ACCP guidelines. During exercise, oxygen uptake ($\dot{V}O_2$) and carbon dioxide output ($\dot{V}CO_2$) were recorded, together with respiratory rate, tidal volume, ventilation and end-tidal gas tensions.

A 3-minute rest period followed fitting of relevant equipment, after which unloaded cycling was performed at a cadence of 60 to 70 rpm for 3 minutes. Thereafter, patients performed a symptom-limited continuous incremental exercise ramp protocol, determined by the physiologist or clinician on the basis of predictive work rate algorithms and patient-reported activity levels [23]. The test continued (usually for 8 to 12 minutes) until volitional exhaustion occurred, or the patient was unable to maintain a cadence of 40 rpm for more than 30 seconds despite encouragement. The clinician stopped the test if the patient developed a sign or symptom listed in the ATS/ACCP guidelines, which included: new arrhythmia; more than 2 mm of ST elevation or depression on the ECG; an arterial blood pressure of more than 250 mm Hg systolic or 120 mm Hg diastolic (see 2003 ATS/ACCP statement on Cardiopulmonary Exercise Testing for an exhaustive list) [23]. Following termination of CPET, patients were encouraged to perform a 'warm-down' period of unloaded cycling.

The anaerobic threshold was estimated by an exercise physiologist or consultant physician, both experienced in CPET interpretation, using a combination of the modified V-slope, ventilatory equivalents and end-tidal pressure methods [24], which improves the rigor of AT detection. The $\dot{V}O_2$ peak was recorded as the highest average $\dot{V}O_2$ over the final 30 s period [25]. The ventilatory equivalents for carbon dioxide ($\dot{V}E/\dot{V}CO_2$) and oxygen ($\dot{V}E/\dot{V}O_2$) were recorded at the AT [26].

We recorded age, sex, height, weight, body mass index (BMI, kg m^{-2}) and Lee's Revised Cardiac Risk Index (RCRI) from patients' medical histories [27]. In addition, serum creatinine, obtained from hospital electronic records systems, was used as an index of renal function. At UCLH and the Whittington Hospital, [Hb] was measured on the day of CPET (HemoCue AB, Angelholm, Sweden). Preoperative [Hb] was recorded from hospital electronic record systems within 3 days of CPET at Newcastle and at the time of pre-assessment (usually within 4 weeks of CPET) at Torbay. No patient received a blood transfusion between the [Hb] measurement and the CPET.

Statistical analysis

Statistical analysis was performed using Stata Version 11 (StataCorp, Texas, USA). Gaussian distributions of the data were verified by the Kolmogorov-Smirnov test, in conjunction with visual inspection of histogram charts. A difference between data was considered significant if $P < 0.05$. We transformed seven continuous variables with skewed distributions by taking their $\log_{10}$: weight, BMI, AT, $\dot{V}O_2$ peak, $\dot{V}E/\dot{V}CO_2$, $\dot{V}E/\dot{V}O_2$, and creatinine. These variables are presented as geometric means and approximate SD.

Historically, measurements of oxygen uptake have been indexed to body mass (ml kg^{-1} min^{-1}), as it allows comparisons between individuals [28,29]. However, this value may still vary with body mass [30-32]. We therefore adjusted the measured oxygen uptake by raising the body mass to a power determined by allometric scaling using the power function ratio (Y/X^{β}) [29,33]. Specifically, the allometric relationship between body size and performance measure (AT or $\dot{V}O_2$ peak) is determined by the allometric equation below (see equation 1), where Y is AT or $\dot{V}O_2$ peak, X is body mass, β is a scaling exponent, a is the proportionality constant (intercept), and ε is the multiplicative error term, which overcomes the problem of heteroscedasticity [34].

$$Y = aX^{\beta}\varepsilon \quad (1)$$

The allometric relationship between body mass (X) and fitness parameter (Y) is expressed using the logarithmic transformation of equation 1 so that

$$\log Y = \beta \cdot \log \text{mass} + \log a + \log \varepsilon \quad (2)$$

where β is the sample specific slope of the linear least squares regression line calculated by log-linear regression analysis (that is, scaling exponent β was 0.83 in the current study) and log a is the equivalent constant value (a) [34]. We further built models by adjustment for the determinant variable (AT and $\dot{V}O_2$ peak) to potential confounders. Three levels of increasing adjustment were used: i) a basic adjustment for testing site; ii) an extended adjustment for testing site, age and sex; and iii) a fully adjusted model for all known confounders (testing site, age, sex, revised cardiac risk index, diabetes, creatinine and operation category). Results were standardised for testing centre by the inclusion of dummy variables in the regression model.

The effect size was expressed as the percentage increase in $\dot{V}O_2$ for a 1 g dl^{-1} (or one standard deviation) increase in [Hb]. Partial correlations between [Hb] and CPET markers were performed controlling for confounding variables. Regression models assessed the associations between $\dot{V}O_2$ and [Hb] and the proportion of variance in oxygen uptake explained by variation in [Hb]. Covariance models were analysed with [Hb] as a clinically relevant categorical variable ([Hb] <10 g dl^{-1}; 10 to 12 g dl^{-1}; >12 g dl^{-1}), as similarly described [15,35]. The adjusted values for $\dot{V}O_2$ generated by the model were transformed back to the original scale to give geometric means and approximate standard deviations by [Hb] group.

Results

We analysed data from 1,777 patients (1,108 male) undergoing various operations: 549 vascular (31%), 530 colorectal (30%), 337 bariatric (19%), 75 upper gastrointestinal (4%), 66 hepatobiliary (4%), 48 maxillofacial (3%) and 172 other operations (9%). Contributions from each centre were as follows: 804 UCLH; 484 Whittington; 305 Torbay; 184 Newcastle. The mean (SD) $\dot{V}O_2$ peak and AT were 15.5 (5.9) and 11.2 (3.5) ml kg^{-1} min^{-1} respectively. The $\dot{V}E/\dot{V}O_2$ and $\dot{V}E/\dot{V}CO_2$ at AT were 25.9 (6.4) and 30.8 (6.4). The AT was not identified in 146 patients (8.2%). Mean (SD) [Hb] and creatinine were 13.2 (1.8) g dl^{-1} and 82 (30) μmol l^{-1}. Table 1 lists other physical characteristics.

Relationships between haemoglobin concentration and oxygen uptake

Figure 1 graphs the increase in unadjusted $\dot{V}O_2$ peak with [Hb], whilst Figure 2 shows the relationship between unadjusted oxygen uptake at AT and [Hb]. The $\dot{V}O_2$ peak and AT increased across each [Hb] group (Table 2). More patients awaiting colorectal surgery were anaemic: in 144/530 (27%) of these, the [Hb] was 10 to 12 g dl^{-1} and in 32/530 (6%) the [Hb] was <10 g dl^{-1}.

Haemoglobin concentration showed weak correlation with $\dot{V}O_2$ peak (r^2 0.30, P <0.0001) and AT (r^2 0.24, P <0.0001), after adjusting for weight and testing centre. Correlations between [Hb] and $\dot{V}O_2$ peak at each site were: Whittington (r^2 0.30, P <0.0001), Torbay (r^2 0.16, P = 0.004), UCLH (r^2 0.31, P <0.0001), and Newcastle (r^2 0.33, P <0.0001). Correlations between [Hb] and AT at each site were; Whittington (r^2 0.23, P <0.0001), Torbay (r^2 0.23, P <0.0001), UCLH (r^2 0.24, P <0.0001), and Newcastle (r^2 0.33, P <0.0001).

Regression models

An increase in [Hb] by one SD was associated with a 9.7% (95% CI, 8.2 to 11.3) increase in $\dot{V}O_2$ peak after adjusting for weight (P <0.0001), which was reduced to 6.7% (95% CI, 5.4 to 7.8) after adjusting for age, sex, weight and testing centre (P <0.0001). The percentage of the variance in $\dot{V}O_2$ peak explained by [Hb] was 8.9% (P <0.0001) after adjusting for weight, and 5.5% (P <0.0001) after adjusting for age, sex, weight and testing site. An increase in [Hb] by one SD was associated with a 6.0% (95% CI, 4.8 to 7.3) increase in AT after adjusting for weight P <0.0001), which was reduced to 4.4% (95% CI, 3.3 to 5.5) after adjusting for age, sex, weight and testing centre (P <0.0001). The percentage of variance in AT explained by [Hb] was 5.9% (P 0.0001) after weight adjustment, reducing to 3.5% (P <0.0001) after adjusting for age, sex, weight and testing centre.

Table 1 Physical characteristics of the whole-study cohort

	N	Mean	SD
Age (yr)	1,777	61.9	15.8
Height (cm)	1,776	169.0	9.1
Weight (kg)	1,775	83.7	23.6
BMI (kg m^{-2})	1,774	29.4	8.3
$\dot{V}O_2$ peak (ml min^{-1})	1,774	1300	500
AT (ml min^{-1})	1,631	940	300

BMI body mass index, *AT* anaerobic threshold, $\dot{V}O_2$ peak, peak oxygen uptake.

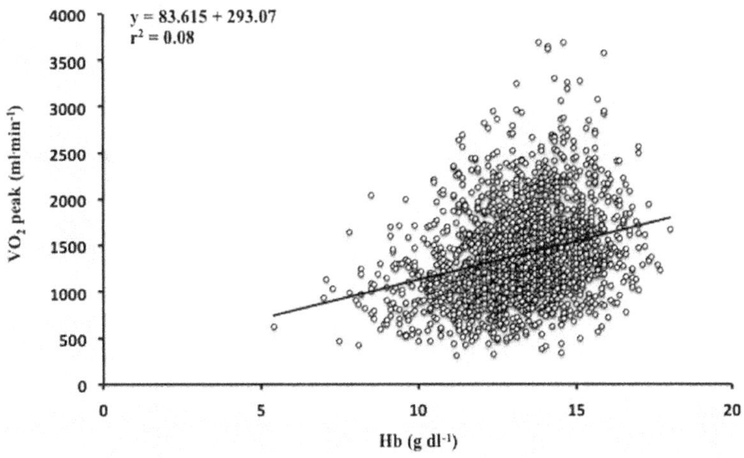

Figure 1 **Linear regression between unadjusted $\dot{V}O_2$ peak (ml min^{-1}) and haemoglobin concentration ([Hb]), n = 1,774.**

Analysis of covariance across haemoglobin group

$\dot{V}O_2$ peak and AT increased across [Hb] groups, after adjusting for confounding variables (*P* <0.0001, Table 3 and Figure 3).

We analysed allometrically scaled $\dot{V}O_2$ peak across individual surgical cohorts, with and without adjustment for confounders. $\dot{V}O_2$ peak did not differ in hepatobiliary patients across [Hb] groups. $\dot{V}O_2$ peak increased across each [Hb] group for colorectal, bariatric and other (mainly urological) patients, after adjusting for all confounders (testing centre, age, sex, weight, RCRI, diabetes, serum creatinine and operation category). $\dot{V}O_2$ peak increased across each [Hb] classification for upper gastrointestinal and vascular patients after adjustment for testing centre, age, sex and weight, but not when additional confounders (RCRI, diabetes, serum creatinine and operation category) were added. $\dot{V}O_2$ peak increased with each [Hb] group for maxillofacial patients after adjusting for testing and weight, but not when additional confounders were added to the model.

Discussion

To our knowledge, this is the largest study to explore the relationship between oxygen uptake and haemoglobin concentration in the clinical setting, and the first to control for body mass with allometric (log-linear) scaling. Oxygen uptake at peak exercise and at the anaerobic threshold (AT) increased with haemoglobin concentration [Hb], after adjusting for measured confounding variables.

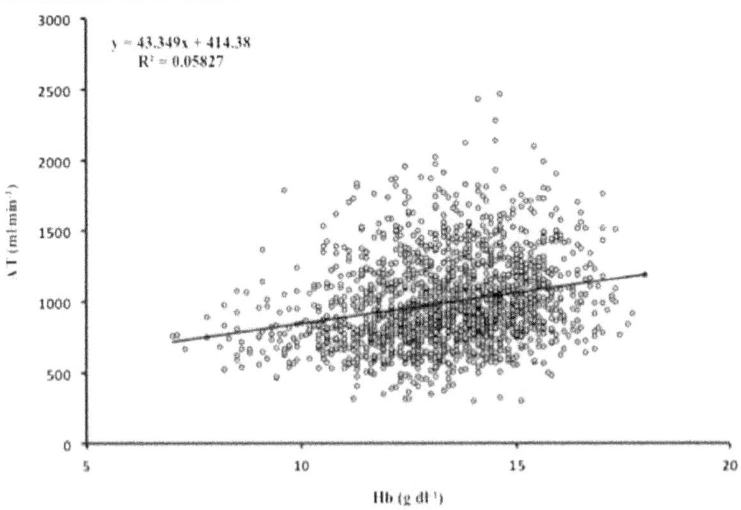

Figure 2 **Linear regression between unadjusted oxygen uptake at anaerobic threshold (AT) (ml min^{-1}) and haemoglobin concentration ([Hb]), n = 1,631.**

Table 2 Physical characteristics across haemoglobin concentration ([Hb]) group (<10 g dl^{-1}; Hb 10 to 12 g dl^{-1}; Hb >12 g dl^{-1})

	[Hb]		
	<10 g dl^{-1}	10 to 12 g dl^{-1}	>12 g dl^{-1}
N	83	353	1341
Age (yr)	63.5 (16.8)	61.8 (16.4)	61.8 (15.5)
Height (cm)	165.8 (9.2)	166.1 (9.2)	170.0 (8.9)
Weight (kg)	73.3 (22.1)	78.9 (23.7)	85.7 (23.3)
BMI (kg m^{-2})	26.8 (8.1)	28.7 (8.7)	29.7 (8.2)
Creatinine (μmol l^{-1})	79.8 (39.0)	78.7 (29.5)	83.4 (28.9)
$\dot{V}O_2$ peak (ml min^{-1})[a]	960 (330)	1150 (430)	1380 (500)
$\dot{V}O_2$ peak (ml kg^{-1} min^{-1})[b]	13.0 (4.5)	14.5 (5.4)	16.1 (5.8)
$\dot{V}O_2$ peak (ml $kg^{-0.83}$ min^{-1})[c, g]	27.8 (6.9)	31.5 (8.1)	34.3 (8.1)
AT (ml min^{-1})[d]	760 (190)	860 (260)	970 (310)
AT (ml kg^{-1} min^{-1})[e]	10.3 (2.5)	10.9 (3.2)	11.3 (3.6)
AT (ml $kg^{-0.83}$ min^{-1})[f, g]	21.3 (4.3)	23.5 (4.8)	24.4 (4.8)
$\dot{V}E/\dot{V}O_2$	26.7 (4.8)	25.3 (5.4)	26.0 (6.8)
$\dot{V}E/\dot{V}CO_2$	31.7 (5.9)	30.2 (5.9)	31.0 (6.6)

BMI body mass index, $\dot{V}E/\dot{V}O_2$ and $\dot{V}E/\dot{V}CO_2$, ventilatory equivalents for oxygen and carbon dioxide at the AT; AT, anaerobic threshold; $\dot{V}O_2$ peak, peak oxygen uptake. Values are mean (SD). [a]ANOVA, $P < 0.0001$; linear trend, $P < 0.0001$. [b]ANOVA, $P < 0.0001$; linear trend, $P < 0.0001$. [c]ANOVA, $P < 0.0001$; linear trend, $P < 0.0001$; [d]ANOVA, $P < 0.0001$; [e]linear trend, $P < 0.0001$; [f]linear trend, $P < 0.0001$; [g]Adjusted for weight, testing site, age, sex, revised cardiac risk index, diabetes, creatinine and operation category.

The [Hb] was 10 to 12 g dl^{-1} in 353 patients (20%) and <10 g dl^{-1} in 83 (5%) patients. Other studies have reported rates of anaemia between 5% and 76%, a range partly dependent upon the indication for surgery and definition of anaemia [9]. The American College of Surgeons' National Surgical Quality Improvement Program (ACS NSQIP) recently reported a similar prevalence of preoperative anaemia (30.4%) [15].

The mean AT of 11 ml kg^{-1} min^{-1} is similar to that reported by other studies of preoperative populations [7,36,37]. However, this value is 2 to 3 ml kg^{-1} min^{-1} less than gender-specific reference values for age and height [38]. The mean $\dot{V}O_2$ peak in our population, 15.5 ml kg^{-1} min^{-1}, is 11 ml kg^{-1} min^{-1} less than gender-specific reference values for age and height [38,39]. The aim of allometric scaling is to appropriately account for body size (that is, the scaled variable no longer varies with body size) [40]. Oxygen uptake is usually reported per unit body mass, ml kg^{-1} min^{-1}, a scale that requires further adjustment for body size [41]. In the obese, oxygen uptake expressed as ml kg^{-1} min^{-1} underestimates fitness and overestimates risk [42]. In the cachectic patient this scale overestimates fitness and underestimates risk [43].

Both AT and $\dot{V}O_2$ peak increased with [Hb], for the whole population, across individual testing sites and across all groups, except hepatobiliary surgery. However, this relationship was weak and although being highly statistically significant does not necessarily reflect a magnitude of clinical association. Nonetheless, an increase in [Hb] by one standard deviation (that is, 1.8 g dl^{-1} rise in [Hb]) was associated with a 9.7% and 6.0% increase in weight-adjusted $\dot{V}O_2$ peak and AT. The [Hb] explained 9% and 6% of the variance in $\dot{V}O_2$ peak and AT respectively. The increase in AT and $\dot{V}O_2$ peak with [Hb] may be due to increased oxygen-carrying capacity, or patients who are not anaemic exercising more than patients who are anaemic, or due to confounding. For instance, sick patients may be both anaemic and less fit. In addition, differences in AT, to some extent (although probably small), may be explained by inherent variations in measurement and/or interpretation or physiological context [44].

The cause of anaemia may be important. The most common cause is reported to be chronic disease, the severity of which being related to the degree of systemic inflammation [45,46]. Features of anaemia due to chronic disease include reduced red cell survival, impaired erythropoiesis, and impaired iron metabolism, all of which may reduce AT and $\dot{V}O_2$ peak, directly or in combination [47]. Iron status was not routinely assessed

Table 3 Allometrically scaled oxygen uptake

	Haemoglobin concentration			*P*-value	
	<10 g dl^{-1}	10 to 12 g dl^{-1}	>12 g dl^{-1}	ANOVA	Trend
$\dot{V}O_2$ peak (ml $kg^{-0.83}$ min^{-1})	26.7 (7.8) 83	29.9 (8.4) 352	34.4 (10.1) 1339	<0.0001	<0.0001[a]
	27.8 (7.1) 83	31.2 (8.2) 352	34.0 (8.7) 1333	<0.0001	<0.0001[b]
	27.8 (6.9) 64	31.5 (8.1) 291	34.3 (8.1) 1136	<0.0001	<0.0001[c]
AT (ml $kg^{-0.83}$ min^{-1})	20.9 (4.6) 67	22.7 (5.0) 307	24.4 (5.2) 1257	<0.0001	<0.0001[a]
	21.3 (4.5) 67	23.2 (4.9) 307	24.3 (5.1) 1251	<0.0001	<0.0001[b]
	21.3 (4.3) 49	23.5 (4.8) 252	24.4 (4.8) 1068	<0.0001	<0.0001[c]

$\dot{V}O_2$ peak and AT, mean (SD) number of patients, by haemoglobin classification. *AT* anaerobic threshold, *[Hb]* haemoglobin concentration, $\dot{V}O_2$ peak, peak oxygen uptake.
[a]Adjusted for weight and testing site.
[b]Adjusted for weight, testing site, age, sex.
[c]Adjusted for weight, testing site, age, sex, revised cardiac risk index, diabetes, creatinine and operation category.

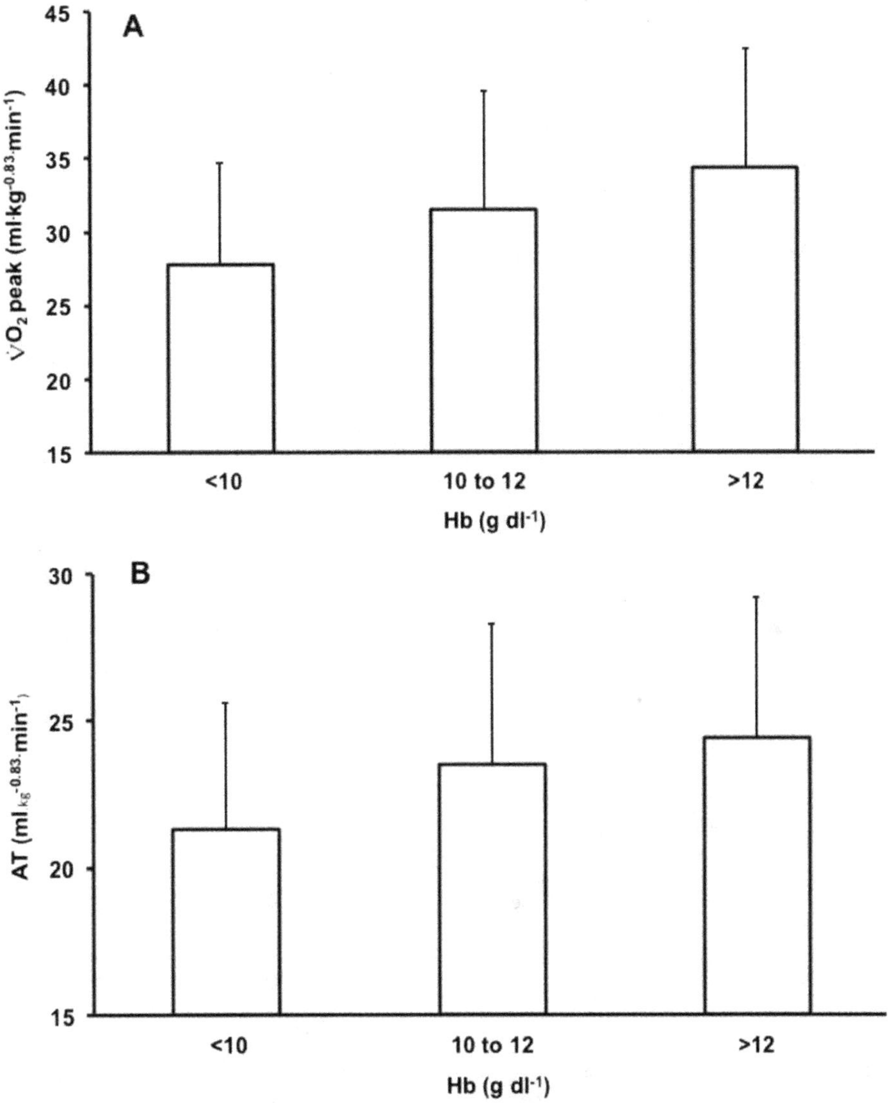

Figure 3 Allometrically scaled oxygen uptake (ml kg$^{-0.83}$ min^{-1}) across [Hb] group (<10 g dl^{-1}, 10 to 12 g dl^{-1}, >12 g dl^{-1}); $\dot{V}O_2$ peak (A) and at the anaerobic threshold (AT) (B). Mean +/- SD values adjusted for weight, testing site, age, sex, revised cardiac risk index, diabetes, creatinine and operation category. *P* <0.0001 (ANOVA) and trend (*P* <0.0001) for both measures. Hb, haemoglobin concentration.

in our cohort but may independently influence fitness markers in the absence of anaemia. For example, iron deficiency with or without anaemia is associated with reduced fitness [48-50].

This study had some limitations. The observational, cross-sectional and retrospective nature of the data generates causative hypotheses but does not test them [51]. It would have been valuable to assess the association of overall survival and critical care use with both anaemia and oxygen uptake. The [Hb] may be an imprecise measure of blood oxygen carrying capacity, given that its value is influenced by disease- or therapy-related contractions or expansions in plasma volume. For instance, oxygen-carrying capacity may be normal if [Hb] is low due simply to an increase in intravascular volume. A better measure of oxygen-carrying capacity may thus be total mass of haemoglobin (tHb-mass). The tHb-mass displays a higher correlation with $\dot{V}O_2$ peak (r^2 = 0.79) than either blood volume (r^2 = 0.76) or [Hb] [52,53]. The relatively small explained variance in AT and $\dot{V}O_2$ peak by [Hb] (oxygen carrying capacity) in the current study suggests that other factors may play an important role in determining aerobic capacity. For example, other physiological factors that may limit $\dot{V}O_2$ peak include pulmonary diffusing capacity, cardiac output and skeletal muscle limitations [54]. Although it is suggested that the AT reflects an imbalance in oxygen demand-supply, that is, that AT reflects onset of anaerobiosis, this is a much-debated and controversial concept [44,55]. In addition, variations in the AT, to some extent may be explained by inherent discrepancies in its measurement and/or interpretation [44].

Future studies of preoperative cardiopulmonary exercise testing should include [Hb] with long-term survival and quality of life as outcomes as well as considering alternative endpoints measured during exercise testing such as metabolic efficiency and the oxygen pulse [44].

Conclusions

In conclusion, anaemia is common in preoperative patients undergoing elective major surgery. There is an association between haemoglobin concentration and oxygen uptake during exercise, both $\dot{V}O_2$ peak and AT, even after adjusting for measured confounding variables. Future studies may wish to address whether reversing anaemia before surgery improves these values, and thereby increases postoperative survival and function.

Abbreviations

AT: Anaerobic threshold; BMI: Body mass index; CPET: Cardiopulmonary exercise testing; [Hb]: Hemoglobin concentration; RCRI: Revised cardiac risk index; tHb-mass: Total haemoglobin mass; $\dot{V}CO_2$: Carbon dioxide; $\dot{V}E/\dot{V}O_2$: Ventilatory equivalent for oxygen; $\dot{V}E/\dot{V}CO_2$: Ventilatory equivalent for carbon dioxide; $\dot{V}O_2$: Oxygen uptake; $\dot{V}O_2$ peak: peak oxygen uptake.

Competing interests

JM Otto: JMO is receiving an Impact PhD Studentship part-funded by VIFOR (INTERNATIONAL) Inc. Total funding £32,534 over 3 years.
MPW Grocott: MPWG has received honoraria for speaking and / or travel expenses from: Edwards Lifescience, Fresenius-Kabi, BOC Medical (Linde Group), Ely-Lilly Critical Care, Cortex GmBH.
MPWG has received research grants from: National Institute of Health Research, National Institute of Academic Anaesthesia, Intensive Care Society, Association of Anaesthetists of Great Britain and Ireland, Sir Halley Stuart Trust, Francis and Augustus Newman Foundation. MPWG is the R&D Lead for Division A, University Hospitals Southampton NHS Foundation Trust; Director, National Institute of Academic Anaesthesia Health Services Research Centre; Specialty Group Lead (Critical Care and Anaesthesia), Hampshire and Isle of Wight Comprehensive Local Research Network, NIHR Comprehensive Research Network.
MPWG leads the Xtreme-Everest hypoxia research consortium and the group have received unrestricted research grant funding from: BOC Medical (Linde Group), Ely-Lilly Critical Care, Smiths Medical, Deltex Medical, London Clinic, Rolex. MPWG runs a number of educational meetings and these meetings have sponsorship from multiple industry partners declared on a meeting-bymeeting basis.
MPWG: Board and Research Council member of the National Institute of Academic Anaesthesia, Co-Chairman of Evidence Based Perioperative Medicine (annual scientific meeting), Co-Chairman of Current Controversies in Anaesthesia and Perioperative Medicine (annual scientific meeting), Co-chairman of National Perioperative CPET Meeting (annual scientific meeting), Co-chairman of KnO2wledge (annual scientific meeting), Member organising group, UK Perioperative Clinical Research Forum (annual scientific meeting), Faculty of Perioperative CPET course, Executive faculty of UK-UIAA Diploma in Mountain Medicine, Editor in Chief of Extreme Physiology and Medicine, Editorial board of Perioperative Medicine and British Journal of Hospital Medicine, Member of the Improving Surgical Outcomes Group. All remaining authors declare that they have no competing interests.

Authors' contributions

JMO, AFO, PJH, CS, JBC, and MS were responsible for data collection, drafting and revising the article and final approval of the version to be published. JAC was responsible for statistical analyses, revising the article and final approval of the version to be published. MPWG was responsible for substantial contribution to conception and design and facilitating acquisition of data, revising the article and final approval of the version to be published. TR and HEM were responsible for substantial contribution to conception and design, revising the article and final approval of the version to be published. All authors read and approved the final manuscript.

Author details

[1]Division of Surgery and Interventional Science, University College London, 21 University Street, London WC1E 6DE, UK. [2]The Portex Unit, UCL Institute of Child Health, 30 Guilford Street, London WC1N 1EH, UK. [3]Department of Medicine, Centre of Cardiovascular Genetics, University College London, 5 University Street, London WC1E 6JF, UK. [4]Integrative Physiology and Critical Illness Group, Division of Clinical and Experimental Science, Faculty of Medicine, University of Southampton, University Road, Southampton SO17 1BJ, UK. [5]UCL Institute for Human Health and Performance, c/o 4th Floor, Rockefeller Building, 21 University Street, London WC1E 6DE, UK. [6]Newcastle Upon Tyne NHS Foundation Trust, Freeman Hospital, Freeman Road, High Heaton, Newcastle Upon Tyne NE7 7DN, UK. [7]Torbay Hospital, South Devon Healthcare NHS Foundation Trust, Torbay Hospital, Lawes Bridge, Torquay TQ2 7AA, UK.

References

1. Wasserman K, Koike A: **Is the Anaerobic Threshold Truly Anaerobic?** *Chest* 1992, **101**(5 Suppl):S211–S218.
2. Myers J, Ashley E: **Dangerous curves. A perspective on exercise, lactate, and the anaerobic threshold.** *Chest* 1997, **111**:787–795.
3. Brooks GA: **Anaerobic threshold: review of the concept and directions for future research.** *Med Sci Sports Exerc* 1985, **17**:22–34.
4. Older P, Smith R: **Experience with the preoperative invasive measurement of haemodynamic, respiratory and renal function in 100 elderly patients scheduled for major abdominal surgery.** *Anaesth Intensive Care* 1988, **16**:389–395.
5. Shoemaker WC, Appel PL, Kram HB, Waxman K, Lee TS: **Prospective trial of supranormal values of survivors as therapeutic goals in high-risk surgical patients.** *Chest* 1988, **94**:1176–1186.
6. Carlisle J, Swart M: **Mid-term survival after abdominal aortic aneurysm surgery predicted by cardiopulmonary exercise testing.** *Br J Surg* 2007, **94**:966–969.
7. Older P, Hall A, Hader R: **Cardiopulmonary exercise testing as a screening test for perioperative management of major surgery in the elderly.** *Chest* 1999, **116**:355–362.
8. Snowden CP, Prentis JM, Anderson HL, Roberts DR, Randles D, Renton M, Manas DM: **Submaximal cardiopulmonary exercise testing predicts complications and hospital length of stay in patients undergoing major elective surgery.** *Ann Surg* 2010, **251**:535–541.
9. Shander A, Knight K, Thurer R, Adamson J, Spence R: **Prevalence and outcomes of anemia in surgery: a systematic review of the literature.** *Am J Med* 2004, **116**(Suppl 7A):58S–69S.
10. Horwich TB, Fonarow GC, Hamilton MA, MacLellan WR, Borenstein J: **Anemia is associated with worse symptoms, greater impairment in functional capacity and a significant increase in mortality in patients with advanced heart failure.** *J Am Coll Cardiol* 2002, **39**:1780–1786.
11. Dunne JR, Malone D, Tracy JK, Gannon C, Napolitano LM: **Perioperative anemia: an independent risk factor for infection, mortality, and resource utilization in surgery.** *J Surg Res* 2002, **102**:237–244.
12. Beattie WS, Karkouti K, Wijeysundera DN, Tait G: **Risk associated with preoperative anemia in noncardiac surgery: a single-center cohort study.** *Anesthesiology* 2009, **110**:574–581.
13. Karkouti K, Wijeysundera DN, Beattie WS: **Risk associated with preoperative anemia in cardiac surgery: a multicenter cohort study.** *Circulation* 2008, **117**:478–484.
14. Kulier A, Levin J, Moser R, Rumpold-Seitlinger G, Tudor IC, Snyder-Ramos SA, Moehnle P, Mangano DT: **Impact of preoperative anemia on outcome in patients undergoing coronary artery bypass graft surgery.** *Circulation* 2007, **116**:471–479.
15. Musallam KM, Tamim HM, Richards T, Spahn DR, Rosendaal FR, Habbal A, Khreiss M, Dahdaleh FS, Khavandi K, Sfeir PM, Soweid A, Hoballah JJ, Taher AT, Jamali FR: **Preoperative anaemia and postoperative outcomes in non-cardiac surgery: a retrospective cohort study.** *Lancet* 2011, **378**:1396–1407.
16. Ferraris VA, Davenport DL, Saha SP, Austin PC, Zwischenberger JB: **Surgical**

outcomes and transfusion of minimal amounts of blood in the operating room. *Arch Surg* 2012, **147**:49–55.
17. Saltin B, Strange S: **Maximal oxygen uptake: "old" and "new" arguments for a cardiovascular limitation.** *Med Sci Sports Exerc* 1992, **24**:30–37.
18. Wagner PD: **Muscle O_2 transport and O_2 dependent control of metabolism.** *Med Sci Sports Exerc* 1995, **27**:47–53.
19. Ekblom B, Goldbarg AN, Gullbring B: **Response to exercise after blood loss and reinfusion.** *J Appl Physiol* 1972, **33**:175–180.
20. Berglund B, Ekblom B: **Effect of recombinant human erythropoietin treatment on blood pressure and some haematological parameters in healthy men.** *J Intern Med* 1991, **229**:125–130.
21. Calbet JA, Lundby C, Koskolou M, Boushel R: **Importance of hemoglobin concentration to exercise: acute manipulations.** *Respir Physiol Neurobiol* 2006, **151**:132–140.
22. ATS/ACCP: **ATS/ACCP Statement on cardiopulmonary exercise testing.** *Am J Respir Crit Care Med* 2003, **167**:211–277.
23. Wasserman K, Hansen JE, Sue DY, Stringer WW, Whipp BJ: *Principles of Exercise Testing and Interpretation Including Pathophysiology and Clinical Applications.* Philadelphia: Lippincott Williams & Wilkins; 2005.
24. Beaver WL, Wasserman K, Whipp BJ: **A new method for detecting anaerobic threshold by gas exchange.** *J Appl Physiol* 1986, **60**:2020–2027.
25. Midgley AW, McNaughton LR, Carroll S: **Effect of the VO_2 time-averaging interval on the reproducibility of VO_{2max} in healthy athletic subjects.** *Clin Physiol Funct Imaging* 2007, **27**:122–125.
26. Wasserman K: **The anaerobic threshold: definition, physiological significance and identification.** *Adv Cardiol* 1986, **35**:1–23.
27. Lee TH, Marcantonio ERM CM, Thomas EJ, Polanczyk CA, Cook EF, Sugarbaker DJ, Donaldson MC, Poss R, Ho KK, Ludwig LE, Pedan A, Goldman L: **Derivation and prospective validation of a simple index for prediction of cardiac risk of major noncardiac surgery.** *Circulation* 1999, **100**:1043–1049.
28. Nevill AM, Holder RL: **Modelling health-related performance indices.** *Ann Hum Biol* 2000, **27**:543–559.
29. Nevill AM, Ramsbottom R, Williams C: **Scaling physiological measurements for individuals of different body size.** *Eur J Appl Physiol Occup Physiol* 1992, **65**:110–117.
30. Tanner JM: **Fallacy of per-weight and per-surface area standards, and their relation to spurious correlation.** *J Appl Physiol* 1949, **2**:1–15.
31. Toth MJ, Goran MI, Ades PA, Howard DB, Poehlman ET: **Examination of data normalization procedures for expressing peak VO_2 data.** *J Appl Physiol* 1993, **75**:2288–2292.
32. Winter EM, Brookes FB, Hamley EJ: **Maximal exercise performance and lean leg volume in men and women.** *J Sports Sci* 1991, **9**:3–13.
33. Batterham AM, Vanderburgh PMM MT, Jackson AS: **Modeling the influence of body size on VO_2 peak: effects of model choice and body composition.** *J Appl Physiol* 1999, **87**:1317–1325.
34. Nevill AM, Holder RL: **Scaling, normalizing, and per ratio standards: an allometric modeling approach.** *J Appl Physiol* 1995, **79**:1027–1031.
35. Wu WC, Schifftner TL, Henderson WG, Eaton CB, Poses RM, Uttley G, Sharma SC, Vezeridis M, Khuri SF, Friedmann PD: **Preoperative hematocrit levels and postoperative outcomes in older patients undergoing noncardiac surgery.** *JAMA* 2007, **297**:2481–2488.
36. Wilson RJ, Davies S, Yates D, Redman J, Stone M: **Impaired functional capacity is associated with all-cause mortality after major elective intra-abdominal surgery.** *Br J Anaesth* 2010, **105**:297–303.
37. Hennis PJ, Meale PM, Hurst RA, O'Doherty AF, Otto J, Kuper M, Harper N, Sufi PA, Heath D, Montgomery HE, Grocott MP: **Cardiopulmonary exercise testing predicts postoperative outcome in patients undergoing gastric bypass surgery.** *Br J Anaesth* 2012, **109**:566–571.
38. Davis JA, Storer TW, Caiozzo VJ: **Prediction of normal values for lactate threshold estimated by gas exchange in men and women.** *Eur J Appl Physiol Occup Physiol* 1997, **76**:157–164.
39. Koch B, Schaper C, Ittermann T, Spielhagen T, Dorr M, Volzke H, Opitz CF, Ewert R, Glaser S: **Reference values for cardiopulmonary exercise testing in healthy volunteers: the SHIP study.** *Eur Respir J* 2009, **33**:389–397.
40. Albrecht GH, Gelvin BR, Hartman SE: **Ratios as a size adjustment in morphometrics.** *Am J Phys Anthropol* 1993, **91**:441–468.
41. Welsman JR, Armstrong N: **Statistical Techniques for Interpreting Body Size-Related Exercise Performance During Growth.** *Pediatr Exerc Sci* 2000, **12**:112–127.
42. Milano GE, Rodacki A, Radominski RB, Leite N: **Scale of VO_2 peak in obese and non-obese adolescents by different methods.** *Arq Bras Cardiol* 2009, **93**:554–557. 598-602.
43. Donohoe CL, Ryan AM, Reynolds JV: **Cancer cachexia: mechanisms and clinical implications.** *Gastroenterol Res Pract* 2011, **2011**:601434.
44. Hopker JG, Jobson SA, Pandit JJ: **Controversies in the physiological basis of the 'anaerobic threshold' and their implications for clinical cardiopulmonary exercise testing.** *Anaesthesia* 2011, **66**:111–123.
45. Weiss G: **Pathogenesis and treatment of anaemia of chronic disease.** *Blood Rev* 2002, **16**:87–96.
46. Cartwright GE: **The anemia of chronic disorders.** *Semin Hematol* 1966, **3**:351–375.
47. Means RT Jr: **Advances in the anemia of chronic disease.** *Int J Hematol* 1999, **70**:7–12.
48. Celsing F, Blomstrand E, Werner B, Pihlstedt P, Ekblom B: **Effects of iron deficiency on endurance and muscle enzyme activity in man.** *Med Sci Sports Exerc* 1986, **18**:156–161.
49. Klingshirn LA, Pate RR, Bourque SP, Davis JM, Sargent RG: **Effect of iron supplementation on endurance capacity in iron-depleted female runners.** *Med Sci Sports Exerc* 1992, **24**:819–824.
50. Newhouse IJ, Clement DBT JE, McKenzie DC: **The effects of prelatent/latent iron deficiency on physical work capacity.** *Med Sci Sports Exerc* 1989, **21**:263–268.
51. Mann CJ: **Observational research methods. Research design II: cohort, cross sectional, and case-control studies.** *Emerg Med J* 2003, **20**:54–60.
52. Kanstrup IL, Ekblom B: **Blood volume and hemoglobin concentration as determinants of maximal aerobic power.** *Med Sci Sports Exerc* 1984, **16**:256–262.
53. Schmidt W, Prommer N: **Effects of various training modalities on blood volume.** *Scand J Med Sci Sports* 2008, **18**(Suppl 1):57–69.
54. Bassett DR Jr, Howley ET: **Limiting factors for maximum oxygen uptake and determinants of endurance performance.** *Med Sci Sports Exerc* 2000, **32**:70–84.
55. Whipp BJ, Ward SA: **The physiological basis of the 'anaerobic threshold' and implications for clinical cardiopulmonary exercise testing.** *Anaesthesia* 2011, **66**:1049–1050.

11

The maintenance and monitoring of perioperative blood volume

Takehiko Iijima[1], Birgitte Brandstrup[2], Peter Rodhe[3], Audrius Andrijauskas[4] and Christer H Svensen[3*]

Abstract

The assessment and maintenance of perioperative blood volume is important because fluid therapy is a routine part of intraoperative care. In the past, patients undergoing major surgery were given large amounts of fluids because health-care providers were concerned about preoperative dehydration and intraoperative losses to a third space. In the last decade it has become clear that fluid therapy has to be more individualized. Because the exact determination of blood volume is not clinically possible at every timepoint, there have been different approaches to assess fluid requirements, such as goal-directed protocols guided by invasive and less invasive devices.
This article focuses on laboratory volume determination, capillary dynamics, aspects of different fluids and how to clinically assess and monitor perioperative blood volume.

Keywords: Fluid therapy, Blood volume, Blood volume assessment, Monitoring, Fluid responsiveness

Review

Fluid therapy is a routine part of intraoperative anesthetic and surgical practice, and there is increasing evidence that fluid therapy can affect perioperative outcomes [1-5]. The goals of perioperative fluid management are to restore and maintain blood volume, secure adequate perfusion to pertinent tissues, and avoid excessive administration of fluids. Traditionally, fluid therapy consisted of infusing large volumes of crystalloids, which often resulted in postoperative body weight gain [6]. This treatment was based on the premise that patients were hypovolemic due to fasting and bowel preparation. Furthermore, it was believed, based on questionable tracer methods, that surgery caused extracellular contraction that needed replacement [7-9]. In recent years, fasting rules and patient preparation have changed and the idea that one must replace fluid allocated to the third space has mostly been abandoned [10]. Care providers are also now more prone to administer vasopressors instead of fluids to offset the hypotension caused by general or neuraxial anesthesia [11-13]. Several randomized clinical trials have tested the efficacy of different fluid protocols [14-16], and many protocols aim to achieve either zero fluid balance or a near maximum stroke volume using both invasive and minimally invasive devices [17].

This article focuses on laboratory volume determination, capillary dynamics, different fluids and how to clinically assess and monitor perioperative blood volume.

Body fluid compartments

The amount of water found in the body, total body water (TBW), can be assessed indirectly by any method capable of measuring body fat or fat-free mass such as hydrodensitometry, dual-energy x-ray absorptiometry or total body potassium levels. The amount of body fat thus influences the TBW: the more fat gives relatively less water [18]. The anatomical view of fluid distribution is usually represented as distinct compartments with fixed volumes. TBW comprises approximately 60% of the lean body mass, or the equivalent of 42 L in a normal-sized adult man. This volume can be subdivided into an intracellular fluid space (ICF), which consists of approximately 28 L, and an extracellular fluid volume (ECV), which occupies approximately 14 L. The ECV consists of the plasma volume (PV, 3 L) and the interstitial fluid space (ISF, 11 L). The blood volume (BV, 5 L) consists of the PV and the red cell mass or blood cells (2 L). The red blood cell mass is usually expressed as a percentage of the total blood volume and is referred to as the hematocrit (Figure 1). The osmolality in the ECV is 290 mosmol/kg. The ECV

* Correspondence: christer.svensen@sodersjukhuset.se
[3]Karolinska Institutet, Department of Clinical Science and Education, Section of Anesthesiology and Intensive Care, Södersjukhuset, Stockholm, Sweden
Full list of author information is available at the end of the article

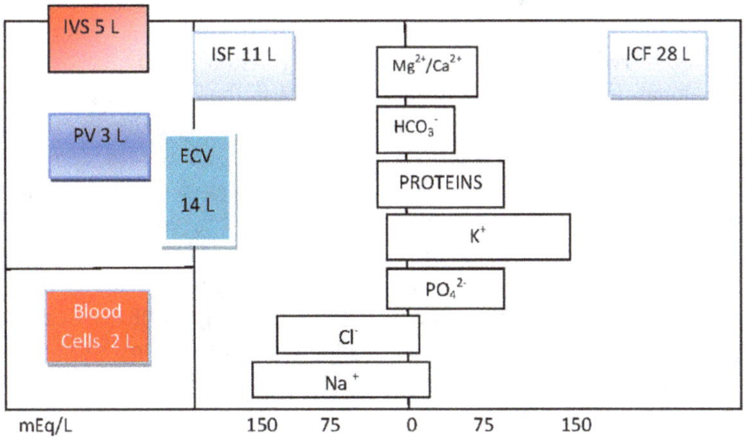

Figure 1 Body fluid compartments. Amounts in liters. mEq/L is milliequivalents per liter. Reproduced with permission [19]. ECV: extracellular volume (PV + ISF); ICF: intracellular fluid space; ISF: interstitial fluid space; IVS: intravascular space; PV: plasma volume.

and ICF differ primarily in their concentrations of sodium (Na^+) and potassium (K^+). The high Na^+ (142 mmol/L) and low K^+ (4.3 mmol/L) concentrations in the ECV are responsible for maintaining the ECV, while the high K^+ (139 mmol/L) and low Na^+ (12 mmol/L) concentrations in the ICF are required for maintaining an electric potential across cell membranes. The capillary endothelial wall, however, is readily permeable to electrolytes. Oncotically active molecules together with an intact wall are necessary to create and maintain a colloid osmotic pressure (COP) of 25 mm Hg inside the vascular lumen. Because the interstitial COP is approximately 5 mm Hg, the intravascular volume remains intact. This will be discussed further in the section on the capillary wall and the glycocalyx.

Estimation of body compartment volumes

TBW can be estimated with isotopically labeled water using deuterium or tritium. The ECV can be estimated using isotopes of bromide ($^{82}Br^-$) or sulfate ($^{35}SO_4^{2-}$) and the ICF is obtained as the difference between TBW and the ECV. The PV can be estimated using either isotope-labeled albumin or different dyes. The red cell mass, or the hematocrit, can be estimated using ^{51}Cr-labeled red cells. Together the PV and the hematocrit make up the total BV. The ISF is the result of subtracting the BV from the ECV. These are static measurements, with isotopes taking different times to equilibrate and can hardly be used for clinical purposes.

Plasma volume

The PV can be estimated using radio-iodinated serum albumin (RISA) with the ^{125}I isotope [19,20]. The drawback of this method, besides its high level of radioactivity, is that albumin leaks through the capillaries into the interstitial fluid and this tends to give an overestimation of the distribution volume. Variation coefficients are between 3% and 4% [21]. Other commonly used agents for measuring the PV are Evans Blue, a dye that binds to albumin, and indocyanine green (ICG), a dye that binds to globulin [22]. The main advantage of these dyes is that they are non-radioactive and can achieve the same level of precision as that obtained with ^{125}I, although they are not without their own drawbacks.

Blood volume

BV is defined as the total volume of blood in the body, and includes blood stored in the spleen, liver and bone marrow. Of the total circulating BV, 70% to 80% is contained in the venous circulation and in the visceral organs in particular. In 1854, Welcker bled animals to death, washed out the blood vessels and determined the hemoglobin content of the blood that had been obtained. He concluded that the blood constituted one-thirteenth of the total body weight in mammals. Many textbooks state that BV is approximately 75 mL/kg for adult men and 65 mL/kg for adult women, or 7% to 8% of body weight [23], and that the BV is slightly higher per kilogram in younger subjects [24]. Formulas based solely on body weight, however, can be misleading. Nadler included height in the estimate defining formulas that have been used frequently [23]. Prediction of BV based on body surface area may be more accurate in that this method compensates for differences in adiposity, and the International Council for Standardization in Haematology recommends formulas based on this value [25].

Blood volumes vary considerably, both between individuals and within the same individual [26,27]. Guyton and Hall showed that BV varies between individuals depending on gender and weight [28]. Furthermore, BV can vary within an individual according to oxygen consumption, as has been shown in sports medicine [29] and Iijima and co-workers used ICG to show that BV varies when patients are subjected to anesthesia [30].

Hemorrhage consists of both red cells and plasma water. It is compensated for by an initial resetting of the precapillary and postcapillary sphincters leading to the transcapillary refill state that transports fluid and protein from the interstitial space to the intravascular space [31]. Furthermore, cells become resistant to insulin resulting in hyperglycemia [32]. This causes an osmotic gradient and water flows through the cell membranes to maintain the BV while albumin is transported from the interstitium to the intravascular space through lymph channels [32-35]. Jacob *et al.* found that BV did not change significantly after fasting [13]. Previous work that has examined changes in fluid spaces following thoracic surgery has shown that there is a postoperative decrease in BV of 6% to 19% compared to preoperative values [36-39]. Results from abdominal surgery, in contrast, have been inconsistent. Shires *et al.* found that postoperative BV decreased compared to the preoperative volume, but in this study the lost blood was not replaced [9]. Ariel found that the preoperative BV was higher than the BV immediately following surgery, but had returned to preoperative levels the following morning [40]. In abdominal and orthopedic surgery, BV does not change significantly from the preoperative value [41-48]. All the above-mentioned trials of patients undergoing thoracic, abdominal or orthopedic surgery used ^{51}Cr to measure red cell volume and albumin labeled with ^{131}I or ^{125}I to measure plasma volume. Rehm and co-workers, using a dye method for measurement, found that the PV was unchanged despite excessive infusions of crystalloid, and they confirmed that, for patients undergoing surgery for ovarian cancer, albumin leaves the circulation in ways other than direct blood loss [48].

Hormones in control of regulation of volume

BV and the volumes of various other compartments are also controlled by several hormones such as antidiuretic hormone (ADH), catecholamines, the renin-angiotensin-aldosterone system (RAAS), natriuretic peptides (ANP), erythropoietin and locally active neurohormonal factors. These hormones are secreted in response to the stimulation of sensors located in the kidneys and other sites such as the atria and ventricles of the heart. The distribution of water between the intravascular and extravascular spaces is regulated by modified Starling forces in combination with alteration of the vascular endothelial glycocalyx lining [15]. The sympatho-adreno-medullary axis and the hypothalamic periventricular nucleus are activated by increases in stressful stimuli [49]. The former facilitates the release of catecholamines and activates the sympathetic nervous system and the latter increases the secretion of cortisol and adrenocorticotropic hormone. These signals trigger the anterior pituitary gland to stimulate ADH secretion, which is the most potent hormone for maintaining fluid homeostasis. Catecholamines have an impact on the heart and on the regulation of peripheral vessels. Iijima *et al.* described a pediatric patient with pheochromocytoma in whom the BV increased by more than 1.2 L, from a baseline value of 2.83 L, after resection of the tumor [50]. Such catecholamine-dependent changes in BV have been confirmed in patients with pheochromocytoma after alpha-blocker therapy. Norepinephrine is a potent α-adrenergic agonist and less potent β-vasoconstrictor, and it is used as a first-line treatment for the maintenance of blood pressure in low pressure states and septic shock [51]. The impact of norepinephrine on BV, however, is not conclusive. Shibuya *et al.* used a method with ^{51}Cr-labeled erythrocytes to investigate the effect of norepinephrine infusions during minor surgical procedures. In that study, blood pressure increased by 30% and PV decreased by 12% [52]. Hifumi *et al.* examined the correlation between norepinephrine and PV in hypertensive patients with high catecholamine levels using ^{131}I-labeled albumin and found that norepinephrine was correlated with a low PV [53]. However, Rector *et al.* showed that high norepinephrine levels are correlated with high BV levels in cirrhosis patients with ascites [54]. ANP is secreted primarily by ventricular myocytes in response to wall stress that has been induced by volume load and increased pressure, and ANP secretion is stimulated by the rapid infusion of a fluid bolus. Some studies have failed to find a correlation between BV and ANP [55-57], while others have shown that the secretion of ANP decreases BV probably due to a diuretic effect [58-60]. More interestingly, however, ANP induces shedding of the glycocalyx, which facilitates translocation of fluid to the interstitial space [61]. Vane *et al.* showed that isoproterenol, a non-specific β-adrenergic agonist, and dopamine, a mixed β-adrenergic and dopaminergic agonist, increased PV while phenylephrine, a pure α-adrenergic agonist, decreased PV [62]. Kinsky *et al.* showed that esmolol, a β-adrenergic antagonist, decreased PV and increased extravascular volume [63,64]. Phenylephrine is commonly used for perioperative support of blood pressure but reduces global cardiac output, increases myocardial wall stress, and increases myocardial oxygen requirements and should be reserved for hypertrophic subaortic stenosis, tetralogy of Fallot, and pregnancy where it results in less fetal acidosis compared to ephedrine [65].

Dynamics of capillaries

As seen in Figure 2, there are two important barriers to the distribution of fluids. First, there is the cell membrane, which keeps the interior of the cell intact. Second, there is the vascular endothelial barrier between the intravascular and the extracellular spaces. Fluid movement across the cell membrane is controlled mainly by osmotic forces and

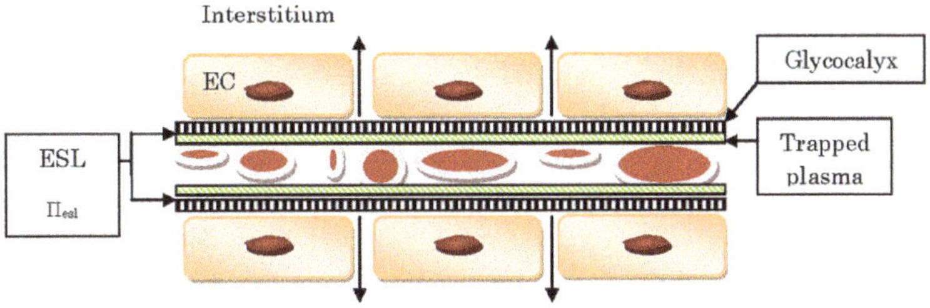

Figure 2 Capillary with red blood cells and endothelial cells (EC). The inner lining of the glycocalyx and trapped plasma together form the endothelial surface layer (ESL). A revised Starling formula would be as follows: $J_v = K_f\,([P_c - P_i] - \Omega[\Pi_{esl} - \Pi_b])$ where J_v is the net filtration, K_f is the filtration coefficient, P_c is the capillary hydrostatic pressure, P_i is the interstitial hydrostatic pressure, Ω is the reflection coefficient, Π_{esl} is the oncotic pressure within the endothelial surface layer and Π_b is the oncotic pressure beneath the endothelial surface layer. Within the ESL there is practically no circulation [15]. EC: endothelial cell; ESL: endothelial surface layer.

the forces governing fluid movement across the endothelial (capillary) wall were first described by Starling in 1896 [66]. These forces describe an outward movement of fluid due to the hydrostatic pressure on the arterial side of the capillary while there is a slight inward movement on the venous side. This is due to the colloid osmotic pressure within the vessels produced by the protein content of the plasma. Plasma hydrostatic and colloid osmotic pressures are counteracted by weak interstitial hydrostatic and colloid osmotic pressures. The vascular wall is permeable to water and small molecules but not to proteins or other large molecules. If isotonic solutions are given, there are no movements of fluid across the cell membrane and fluids remain in the extracellular space. Under normal conditions with an intact vascular barrier, there is a flow of fluid and albumin across the barrier with fluid and albumin returning via the lymph vessels.

Glycocalyx

The approach taken by Starling to describe the movement of fluids across the endothelial wall is now known to be too simplistic. The endothelium consists of a thin layer of cells with an inner fragile layer, the endothelial glycocalyx (EG), containing glycosaminoglycans (Figure 2). The glycocalyx binds plasma proteins to form the endothelial surface layer (ESL), which has a high internal oncotic pressure. The low net flux passing through the EG has low concentrations of proteins so the oncotic pressure beneath this layer is low. The EG creates a barrier that binds proteins and this prevents some erythrocytes from moving close to it. Thus, there is a zone where almost no circulation occurs and non-circulating protein-rich plasma predominates. The intravascular volume can, therefore, be considered to consist of circulating red cells and plasma volume as well as a non-circulating plasma volume. The function of the glycocalyx appears to be the maintenance of an effective colloid osmotic pressure close to 70% of the luminal osmotic pressure while keeping the colloid concentration outside the endothelium equal to that inside the lumen of the microvessel [67]. Thus, transcapillary fluid exchange seems to depend not on the difference between the hydrostatic and oncotic pressures between blood and tissue but, rather, between the blood and the small space underneath the endothelial glycocalyx but still within the lumen of the capillary. Destruction of the glycocalyx, which can occur during trauma and septicemia, will eventually cause a change in the global difference between hydrostatic and oncotic pressures and this will lead to a situation that is best described by the concepts developed by Starling. If the interstitial colloid osmotic pressure then equals that of the plasma, interstitial edema will occur. Reduction or destruction of the EG leads to platelet aggregation, leukocyte adhesion and increased permeability, all of which are hallmarks of interstitial edema. Factors that can cause destruction of the EG are proteases, ischemia/reperfusion, tumor necrosis factors, oxidized low density lipoproteins and atrial natriuretic peptide triggered by hypervolemia [15,67]. A goal for the clinician should be to maintain normovolemia during surgery to protect the EG and minimize shifts to the interstitium. Factors that have been shown experimentally to protect the endothelium are hydrocortisone, antithrombin and sevoflurane [68-70].

To determine fluid responsiveness during different conditions, it is important to understand the impact of different fluids. Over the past several decades, there has been a debate as to whether clinicians should use crystalloids or colloids. This disagreement is based mostly on tradition and local agreement on how fluid deficits should be handled and seldom on an understanding of the reason for the underlying pathophysiology. In deciding the best course of treatment, fluids should be considered as efficient drugs with their own unique impacts on patients in regard to their pharmaceutical properties, indications, contraindications and side effects.

Different fluids

Crystalloids

Crystalloids have a long history of use in clinical settings. In the 1830 s saline solutions were occasionally given during the cholera outbreak in the UK. In 1881, Landerer is credited with having established the technique of giving crystalloids in clinical practice. Ringer published groundbreaking papers in 1882 verifying the importance of certain ions such as calcium and ammonium to make saline solutions more physiological. Hartmann later added buffered ions to Ringer's solution to offset its acidity.

Crystalloids are defined as solutions containing molecules smaller than 30 kDa and thus lacking oncotic components. When glucose is administered, the glucose is metabolized in the liver leaving only water to be distributed to the ECV and ICF, and only 7% of the infused fluid will remain in the intravascular space (IVS). Isotonic crystalloids are distributed within the ECV and urine production and insensible perspiration are the primary avenues by which water is lost from the ECV. Insensible perspiration does not amount to more than 0.5 mL/kg/h in awake adults [71]. Isotonic crystalloids, preferably in a balanced form to avoid acid–base disorders [15], should theoretically be ideal for replacing losses from the ECV. Because there is a 1:5 volume ratio between the plasma space and ISF, it is estimated that 20% to 25% of an infused crystalloid will reside in the plasma space. The 1:5 distribution may only occur after a fluid bolus has been entirely equilibrated throughout the ECV during normal conditions, and provided that it still resides in the body and has not been partially eliminated. This means, however, that a crystalloid load may initially show a substantial volume effect during an ongoing infusion [72]. The hydration status of the body also influences the distribution of crystalloid solutions. This phenomenon is used in the recently introduced volume loading test, which is used to assess the hydration status of individual patients [73,74]. Tatara *et al.* showed that a 75 mL/kg crystalloid infusion after hemorrhage momentarily restored BV during the infusion. When the infusion was stopped, however, BV decreased rapidly to a volume lower than it had been before the infusion [75]. This finding supports a concept developed using homeostatic blood states theory that a physiologic target BV will change according to changes in red cell volume; for example, a decrease of red cells after hemorrhage decreases the physiologic target BV by the volume of lost red cells [73].

Volume kinetics is used to study the effect of an infused bolus over time, and is similar to pharmacokinetic methods for studying drug effects. This method uses an endogenous tracer, hemoglobin, to calculate fractional changes in plasma dilution over time [76]. Repeated sampling of hemoglobin will produce a dilution curve. When such a curve has been established for an individual patient, the values can be fitted to a non-linear equation that will give estimates of the rate constants for distribution and clearance in a similar manner to pharmacokinetics. The method has been criticized, however, for being based on calculations of estimated initial values of hemoglobin and for assessing changes only in the circulating part of the BV [15]. Presumably, the method does not account for the non-circulating part of the BV. However, volume kinetics is a pharmacokinetic tool measuring functional, not anatomical, volumes and it is a useful tool to describe fluid movement between spaces. An infused bolus of a crystalloid will allocate initially in central well-perfused spaces of the body (V_c, approximately 3 L to 4 L). This space may or may not correspond to the anatomical plasma space. Subsequently, the fluid load will be transferred to a more peripheral volume (V_t, 6 L to 8 L), which will be smaller than the anatomical interstitial space (Figure 3). V_c becomes slightly larger if based on arterial rather than on venous hemoglobin values [15]. The volume of V_t is 6 L to 8 L in adult males weighing 70 kg to 80 kg. In contrast to earlier estimations using isotopes of sodium and bromide, volume kinetics measures changes only in spaces that are able to expand upon infusion of the fluid. There are spaces, such as bone tissue, that cannot be expanded by an infused fluid. Studying volume kinetics, it is also easy to see that under ideal conditions in awake, healthy volunteers, an infused crystalloid is readily eliminated and thus it is distributed based on a one-volume model. This is in contrast to situations during trauma and hemorrhage where the fluid has a tendency to stay in the body and a two-volume model with little or no elimination is more appropriate.

The volume kinetics models, however, are hampered by two limitations. First, they require frequent and precise hemoglobin sampling, which is not feasible clinically.

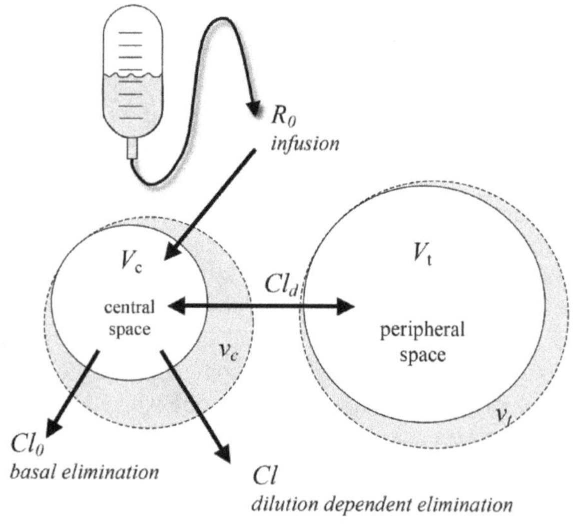

Figure 3 Functional volumes in a two-fluid space model. R_0 is the infusion rate in mL/min, V_c is the central fluid space, v_c is the expanded central fluid space in liters, V_t is the peripheral fluid space, v_t is the expanded peripheral space in liters, Cl_0 is the basal elimination in mL/min, Cl_d is the interfluid space constant in mL/min and Cl is the dilution dependent elimination in mL/min.

Second, they require a rather large and rapid infusion to generate substantial dilution curves. For the moment, volume kinetics is a research tool for bettering our understanding of fluid movement. In the future, accurate non-invasive measurement of hemoglobin levels may permit the clinical use of volume kinetics methods. An example of the kinetic profile of an infused crystalloid is given in Figure 4.

Colloids

There are a wide variety of colloids including starches, dextrans, gelatines and albumin. Artificial colloids are large macromolecules that consist of a variety of polysaccharides or polypeptides and are derived from either plant or animal sources. The artificial colloids are mainly diluted in either 0.9% saline or a balanced solution such as acetated Ringer's solution. These are in contrast to albumin, which is a more heterogeneous colloid derived from plasma. The main reason for using colloids is to replace intravascular deficits due to events such as hemorrhage or fluid shifting [15]. Colloid infusions persist in the IVS for longer periods than crystalloid infusions because it is more difficult for large molecules to transverse an intact vascular barrier. Supposedly, the colloids can contribute to hemodynamic stability with less fluid in a shorter time. This is probably true in healthy people. In sick patients, however, the endothelial glycocalyx is often damaged leading to a leaking capillary wall [15,77]. In studies of normovolemic hemodilution, Rehm and co-workers showed that volume loading with colloids in normovolemia resulted in reduced volume persistence (68%) than if blood had already been removed (90%) [78]. Furthermore, it has been shown in clinical studies that during leakiness the volume effects of colloids are similar to that of crystalloids [79]. The ratio could actually vary from 1: 1,2-1,4 for crystalloids to colloids during these conditions [80]. The earliest evidence of renal toxicity from hydroxyethylstarch (HES) solutions came from case reports of osmotic nephrosis [81]. Several clinical studies addressing this issue have been inconclusive in critically ill patients [82-84]. Recently, two large randomized clinical studies addressed this issue in patients with sepsis and septic shock [80,85]. The Scandinavian Starch for Severe Sepsis/Septic Shock Trial (6S) was an investigator-initiated, multicenter, blinded, stratified, parallel-group clinical study with randomization. Subjects received a study fluid in a 1:1 ratio for fluid resuscitation with either HES 130/0.42 in a balanced solution or Ringer's acetate. The study enrolled 800 patients with sepsis or septic shock in 26 centers in Scandinavia. The primary outcome was death or a need for renal replacement therapy (RRT) at 90 days after randomization. The study showed an increased mortality and also a clear renal toxicity in the HES group. The amount of trial fluid was approximately 3,000 mL in each group. However, the intervention came after the patients had been initially resuscitated, and you could argue that the patients received an unnecessary amount of HES [80]. The Crystalloid versus Hydroxyethyl Starch Trial (CHEST) enrolled 7,000 patients (including 1,937 with sepsis) and randomly assigned them to receive either HES 130/0.4 in 0.9% saline or 0.9% saline alone for all fluid resuscitation until discharge, death or 90 days. The primary outcome was death within 90 days and secondary outcomes included RRT or acute kidney injury (AKI). The inclusion criteria were quite similar to 6S but in CHEST the HES group received approximately 30% less fluid, had a faster increase in central venous pressure (CVP) and a lower incidence of cardiac failure. There was no significant difference in mortality at 90 days; however, in CHEST, HES was linked with a greater use of RRT. Of note, however, is that CHEST found a lower incidence of AKI with HES than with saline. When it comes to AKI by RIFLE criteria, CHEST favors saline as regards to creatinine while it favors HES in connection with increased urinary output [85]. However, low molecular weight colloids are widely used in goal-directed fluid protocols to reach a predetermined response for elective patients in surgical settings. Giving small aliquots of colloids up to a predetermined target volume allows fluids to be administered in a manner that more closely mimics natural physiological processes, and takes into consideration individual differences between patients [86-88]. This has improved the outcome for patients although this comparison

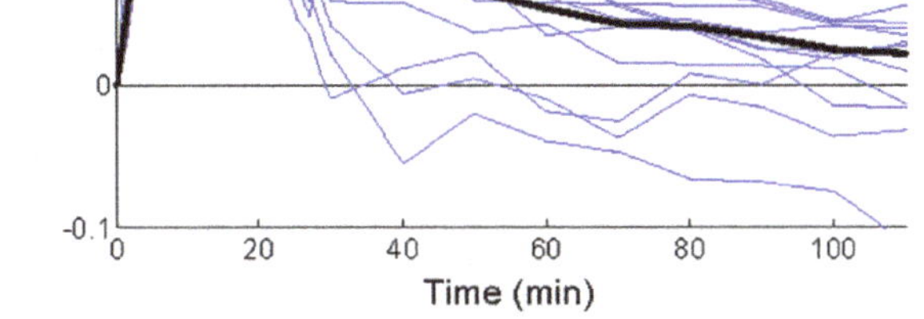

Figure 4 Dilution curves (%, thin lines) for individuals. A non-linear equation is, after iteration, fitted to the data generating a mean dilution curve (thick line) from which parameter estimates for distribution (V_c, V_t) and clearance (Cl) can be calculated [76]. The initial dilution effect of the infused bolus is approximately 25% (0.25 on the y-axis) but the effect is transient. The fluid is almost completely eliminated from the central space after 2 hours. The y-axis is the percentage dilution and the x-axis is time in minutes. In these individuals, infusion times were 10 minutes and the experiment lasted for 120 minutes.

has mostly been made with standard-of-care protocols. Whether starch solutions cause long-term renal toxicity for these patients is a question to be answered. There is currently no clinical or scientific indication that they do but there have been no long-term follow-ups from this perspective [89,90].

Can blood volume be measured?

Estimation of BV is difficult in the clinical setting and the clinician is often faced with unspecific clinical signs of hypovolemia and dehydration. Evaluation of skin turgor, blood pressure, heart rate and urinary output are not reliable and are unsuited for guiding fluid therapy protocols. Invasive measurements such as pulmonary artery pressure, central venous pressure and blood pressure are all unreliable for detecting a fluid deficit [91]. Standard pressure preload measurements such as central venous pressure and pulmonary capillary wedge pressure may not reflect the true preload pressure [92]. Over the past several years, thermodilution and echocardiographic preload determination parameters have been shown to be superior to measurements of the pulmonary capillary wedge pressure [93,94]. In particular, the global end diastolic volume measured by transpulmonary thermodilution, the right ventricular end diastolic volume assessed by a continuous thermodilution catheter, and the left ventricular end diastolic volume assessed by echocardiography are superior methods for determining preload [92]. Many clinicians tend to look at urinary output to guide fluid therapy but this is a highly nonspecific measurement. The passive leg-raising test is an easy, and probably reliable, method to test for hypovolemia [95]. A semi-automated blood volume analyzer, the BVA-100 (Daxor Corporation, NY, USA), uses a radioisotope to measure BV at the bedside. This system is used in conjunction with a single-use diagnostic kit, which uses a flow chamber and an albumin ^{131}I injectate [21]. A determination of BV, PV and red cell volume with this device takes about 30 minutes and has an accuracy of ±2.5%. Another interesting method is transcutaneous pulse dye densitometry, which employs an optical probe similar to that used in pulse oximetry to measure infused intra-arterial ICG concentrations [30].

Zero-balanced protocols

When it became clear that aggressive fluid loading with crystalloids was harmful for perioperative fluid management [96], a more restrictive approach became apparent. In thoracic surgery, fluid restriction became standard practice, but in the general surgical population this was more dependent on the discretion of the clinician. In 2003, Brandstrup and co-workers published a randomized multicenter study comparing liberal and restrictive fluid management strategies in colorectal surgery [1]. The number of postoperative patients with complications was significantly reduced in those receiving more restrictive fluid therapies. This study looked at anastomotic leakage, wound infection, and cardiovascular and pulmonary complications, all of which were reduced when perioperative fluid was limited. Postoperative weight gain was determined to be a negative factor from these limited treatment protocols. This study has been widely cited and counts as a major landmark study in its field, but it has been pointed out that the restrictive group received more colloids compared to the saline standard-of-care group. Several studies have since addressed this topic and it can be concluded that fluid amounts in groups considered restrictive and liberal vary considerably. What is restrictive in one study can very well be liberal in another and the types of surgery also vary considerably in these studies. Some studies have been performed on day surgical cases where the endpoints (well-being, less nausea, vomiting and dizziness) are different compared to more high-risk surgical patients where length of hospital stay and mortality are more relevant as endpoints. Healthy subjects undergoing short procedures seem to benefit from a moderate infusion of a crystalloid to prevent postoperative nausea [97] while patients undergoing colorectal surgery have benefited from zero-balanced protocols with a restrictive goal-directed protocol pattern, even though the total amount of fluid could exceed that administered during day surgery protocols due to the length of surgery.

Individualized goal-directed therapy

Individualized fluid therapy is likely the best course of action because patients differ in underlying pathology, size and responsiveness to different physiological perturbations. Therefore, it would be beneficial to be able to determine the baseline hydration status for each individual. This task is, indeed, a challenge for the clinician and significant amounts of research are directed towards methods for finding the baseline hydration status of an individual on the day of surgery. Intermittent estimations of BV and the fluid status in different compartments using an experimental tracer or dilution methods are not clinically feasible. Instead, an ideal therapy would measure responsiveness, which is the deviation of target parameters induced by a fluid bolus. However, fluid responsiveness requires a dynamic assessment. The Frank–Starling curve describes the relationship between diastolic myocardial tension (preload) and systolic cardiac function (Figures 5 and 6).

An increase in preload should cause an increase in cardiac output. From the curve, it is possible to analyze which patients are responders and which are non-responders to fluid therapy in the context of cardiovascular performance [17]. Functional hemodynamic parameters such as stroke volume variation (SVV) and pulse pressure variation could possibly

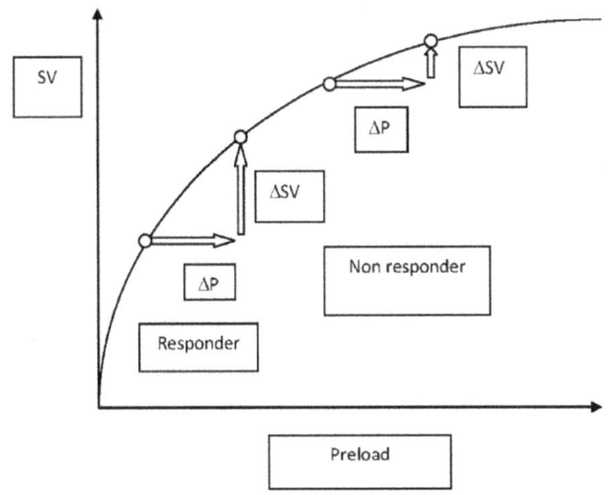

Figure 5 The Frank–Starling curve showing the relationship between diastolic myocardial tension (preload) and systolic cardiac function (stroke volume). An increase in preload results in a corresponding increase in stroke volume. Using the curve, it is possible to analyze who is a responder and who is a non-responder to fluid therapy. P: preload; SV: stroke volume.

be used to guide fluid therapy [17,98]. Both of these parameters are dependent on the interaction between the heart and the lungs (pulse contour analysis). In a spontaneously breathing patient, inspiration will reduce the intrathoracic pressure, which will augment venous return and the preload thereby increasing stroke volume. In a mechanically ventilated patient, the opposite conditions will persist. This can be observed clinically by studying the arterial waveform during mechanical ventilation and seeing how the curve moves. The movement of the curve can actually show the

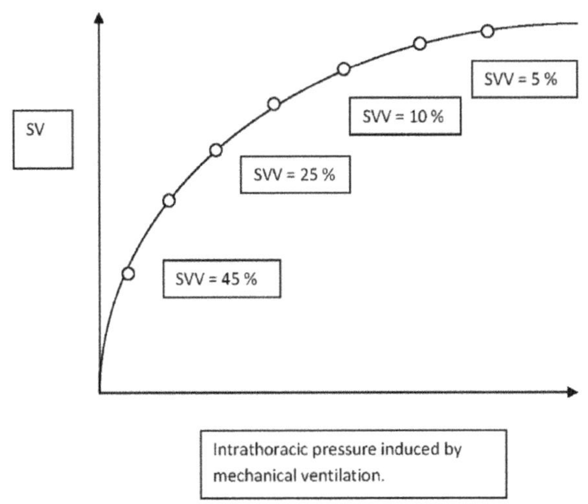

Figure 6 The correlation between stroke volume variation (SVV) and the Frank–Starling curve. Round circles indicate changes in SVV as more fluid is given. When SVV is below 10% to 12%, the patient is said to be a non-responder. SV: stroke volume; SVV: stroke volume variation.

degree of hypovolemia. Variations imposed on the Frank–Starling curve can result in major alterations if imposed in the lower part of the curve, but only minor alterations will occur if imposed on the flatter part.

Different monitoring systems

An example of an invasive device is the PiCCO (Pulsion Medical Systems, Munich, Germany), which enables continuous hemodynamic monitoring using a femoral or axillary arterial catheter and a central venous catheter. Employing patented algorithms based on the assumption that the area under the systolic part of the aortic pressure waveform corresponds to the stroke volume curve, PiCCO combines real-time continuous monitoring through pulse contour analysis with intermittent thermodilution measurement via the transpulmonary method. This device is able to give measurements of the transpulmonary cardiac output, intrathoracic blood volume, extravascular lung water and cardiac function. The latter parameters require a central venous line for injection of a cold bolus. The system, however, requires recalibrations, especially when rapid changes occur [99].

The LiDCO technique (LiDCO Ltd, London, UK) is another pulse contour method (or pulse power method), based on a purported linear relationship between net power and net flow in the vascular system provided that no major change in vascular compliance or resistance occurs. The LiDCO plus technique requires lithium dilution and gives a reliable assessment of cardiac output and stroke volume provided the restrictions mentioned above are met. The LiDCO rapid version does not require calibration and is used solely for monitoring cardiac output and stroke volume deviations from baseline [100].

The FloTrac and Vigileo (Edwards Inc., Irvine, CA) systems requires a sensor attached to an arterial line. The system continually displays cardiac output (CO) and SVV, which can be correlated to the Frank–Starling curve as seen in Figure 6. For the Vigileo system, the standard deviation of pulse pressure is correlated with a normal stroke volume based on an underlying database. Aortic impedance is also derived from historic data, but actual vascular compliance and resistance are determined using arterial waveform analysis. The device does not require calibration and is fairly easy to use but is hampered by the fact that it is less reliable when vasopressors are used [101]. Even the latest software, version 3, is not accurate when a common vasopressor such as phenylephrine is used. Furthermore, an optimal arterial signal is needed for valid cardiac output measurement. SVV measurements are also limited by the requirement of mechanical ventilation with a tidal volume of at least 8 ml/kg [91]. A new device package, the EV 1000 (Edwards Inc., Irvine, CA), combines the FloTrac system with the PreSep/PediaSet oximetry catheters to provide central venous oxygen saturation measurements ($S_{cv}O_2$), and gives both hemodynamic and volumetric data. The use of this device has recently been approved by the FDA in the US. All of these devices require optimal arterial signals and are unreliable when the patient has arrhythmias or is undergoing intra-aortic balloon pump treatment.

Recently, non-invasive methods have been presented such as plethysmographic systolic pressure variation and the plethysmographic variability index (Masimo Inc., Irvine, CA). These methods also require the patient to be mechanically ventilated. However, this could enhance perioperative monitoring [102].

Esophageal Doppler-guided therapy (ED) uses Doppler ultrasound technology to analyze the blood flow in the descending aorta. A single-use probe is inserted into the esophagus and positioned to measure the blood flow for each heartbeat. The waveform is then compared to biometric data and gives the stroke volume. Because the catheter is inserted in the lower esophagus, approximately 70% of the circulating blood flow is accounted for in the calculations. Various algorithms are used to measure fluid responsiveness. Most algorithms use small aliquots of colloids (2 to 3 mL/kg). The primary goal of the technique is to optimize the stroke volume according to the Frank–Starling curve. The stepwise fluid infusion is continued until the patient is considered a non-responder to fluid. Usually this happens when stroke volume or cardiac output deviation becomes <10%. This has been validated against standard-of-care protocols; reduced morbidity and reduced length of hospital stay have been shown [87,103-106]. The ED technique has been used in high-risk and colorectal surgery, but recent studies showed no differences between ED and a fixed protocol in more healthy patients or patients undergoing laparoscopic procedures [107,108].

Conclusions and clinical guidelines

To conclude, the evidence-based recommendations are that intraoperative fluid therapy should aim to administer an adequate and timely volume-preserving flow to pertinent organs. Healthy subjects undergoing short procedures seem to benefit from a moderate infusion of a crystalloid [97]. This will offset minor postoperative complications such as nausea and vomiting.

High-risk patients, on the other hand, benefit from a carefully monitored fluid regimen based on individualized goal-directed therapy. This can be done in several different ways. The term restrictive is purposefully avoided because this is dependent on where on the Frank–Starling curve one starts the fluid regimen. It is important, therefore, to determine the patient's responsiveness to fluid therapy. This means that fluid therapy should be moderate and individually tailored to each patient's needs. Goal-directed therapy using the esophageal doppler technique has been widely popular, and even nationally recommended in the UK, but compared to modest regimens it has been difficult to show improvements in outcome with this technique [106]. A combination of SVV-guided fluid therapy and oximetric guidance (PreSep/$S_{cv}O_2$) is probably more useful for high-risk surgery provided that the arterial waveform is readable. This should be accompanied by a moderate crystalloid infusion (1 to 2 mL/kg/h).

The choice of whether crystalloids or colloids should be used is probably less important. Crystalloids should mainly be used for losses from the ECV and colloids for losses from the IVS. However, low molecular starches should be avoided when patients have damaged endothelium as in sepsis [85]. There is currently no full consensus but albumin may be a better choice for these patients [107].

Abbreviations

6S: Scandinavian Starch for Severe Sepsis/Septic Shock Trial; ADH: Antidiuretic hormone; AKI: Acute kidney injury; ANP: Atrial natriuretic peptide; BV: Blood volume; CHEST: Crystalloid versus Hydroxyethyl Starch Trial; Cl: Dilution-dependent clearance (elimination) in mL/min; Cl_0: Basal clearance (elimination) in mL/min; Cl_d: Interfluid space constant in mL/min; CO: Cardiac output; COP: Colloid osmotic pressure; CVP: Central venous pressure; EC: Endothelial cell; ECV: Extracellular fluid volume; ED: Esophageal Doppler-guided therapy; EG: Endothelial glycocalyx; ESL: Endothelial surface layer; HES: Hydroxyethyl starch; ICF: Intracellular fluid space; ICG: Indocyanine green; ISF: Interstitial fluid space; IVS: Intravascular space; P: Preload; PV: Plasma volume; R_0: Infusion rate in mL/min; RAAS: Renin angiotensin aldosterone system; RIFLE: Risk, injury, failure, loss, end stage kidney disease; RISA: Radio-iodinated serum albumin; RRT: Renal replacement therapy; $S_{cv}O_2$: Central venous oxygen saturation; SV: Stroke volume; SVV: Stroke volume variation; TBW: Total body water; V_c: Central volume in L; v_c: Expanded central volume in L; V_t: Peripheral volume in L; v_t: Expanded peripheral volume in L.

Competing interests

Takehiko Iijima receives lecture fees from Fresenius KABI Co. Ltd., Japan, and Otsuka Pharmaceutical Co. Ltd., Japan.

Audrius Andrijauskas received a consultant's fee from Masimo Corp. of Irvine, CA, USA. Audrius Andrijauskas is an inventor on US Patent No. 7,788,045 B2, PCT International patent application PCT/US2011/057,362, and US provisional patent application No. 61/692,904.

Christer Svensen receives lecture fees from Fresenius KABI, Uppsala, Sweden, and has intermittently been a member of the Masimo Inc. Advisory Board. There are no other competing interests.

Authors' contributions

TI came up with the original idea for this manuscript. He contributed to the design and helped to draft the manuscript. BB, PR and AA contributed to the design and helped to draft the manuscript. CS contributed to the design, helped to draft the manuscript and was also responsible for the final revision of the text. All authors read and approved the final manuscript.

Author details

[1]Department of Perioperative Medicine, Division of Anesthesiology, School of Dentistry, Showa University. [2]Department of Surgical Gastroenterology, Hvidovre University Hospital, Copenhagen, Denmark. [3]Karolinska Institutet, Department of Clinical Science and Education, Section of Anesthesiology and Intensive Care, Södersjukhuset, Stockholm, Sweden. [4]Clinic of Anesthesiology and Intensive Care, Vilnius University, Vilnius, Lithuania.

References

1. Brandstrup B, Tønnesen H, Beier-Holgersen R, Hjortsø E, Ørding H, Lindorff-Larsen K, *et al*: **Effects of intravenous fluid restriction on postoperative complications: comparison of two perioperative fluid regimens.** *Ann Surg* 2003, **238**:641–648.
2. Holte K, Sharrock NE, Kehlet H: **Pathophysiology and clinical implications of perioperative fluid excess.** *Br J Anaesth* 2002, **89**:622–632.
3. Nisanevich V, Felsenstein I, Almogy G, Weissman C, Einav S, Matot I: **Effect of intraoperative fluid management on outcome after intraabdominal surgery.** *Anesthesiology* 2005, **103**:25–32.
4. Wiedemann HP, Wheeler AP, Bernard GR, Thompson BT, Hayden D, DeBoisblanc B, *et al*: **Comparison of two fluid-management strategies in acute lung injury.** *N Engl J Med* 2006, **354**:2564–2575.
5. Jacob M, Chappell D, Rehm M: **Clinical update: perioperative fluid management.** *Lancet* 2007, **369**:1984–1986.
6. Brandstrup B: **Fluid therapy for the surgical patient.** *Best Pract Res Clin Anaesthesiol* 2006, **20**:265–283.
7. Crenshaw CA, Canizaro PC, Shires GT, Allsman A: **Changes in extracellular fluid during acute hemorrhagic shock in man.** *Surg Forum* 1962, **13**:6–7.
8. Shires GT, Coln D, Carrico J, Lightfoot S: **Fluid therapy in hemorrhagic shock.** *Arch Surg* 1964, **88**:688–693.
9. Shires GT, Williams J, Brown F: **Acute changes in extracellular fluid associated with major surgical procedures.** *Ann Surg* 1961, **154**:803–810.
10. Brandstrup B, Svensen C, Engquist A: **Hemorrhage and surgery cause a contraction of the extracellular space needing replacement – evidence and implications?** *Surgery* 2006, **139**:419–432.
11. Jackson R, Reid JA, Thorburn J: **Volume preloading is not essential to prevent spinal-induced hypotension at Caesarean section.** *Br J Anaesth* 1995, **75**:262–265.
12. Norberg A, Brauer KI, Prough DS, Gabrielsson J, Hahn RG, Uchida T, *et al*: **Volume turnover kinetics of fluid shifts after hemorrhage, fluid infusion, and the combination of hemorrhage and fluid infusion in sheep.** *Anesthesiology* 2005, **102**:985–994.
13. Jacob M, Chappell D, Conzen P, Finsterer U, Rehm M: **Blood volume is normal after pre-operative overnight fasting.** *Acta Anaesthesiol Scand* 2008, **52**:522–529.
14. Bundgaard-Nielsen M, Holte K, Secher NH, Kehlet H: **Monitoring of peri-operative fluid administration by individualized goal-directed therapy.** *Acta Anaesthesiol Scand* 2007, **51**:331–340.
15. Chappell D, Jacob M, Hofmann-Kiefer K, Conzen P, Rehm M: **A rational approach to perioperative fluid management.** *Anesthesiology* 2008, **109**:723–740.
16. Holte K, Foss NB, Andersen J, Valentiner L, Lund C, Bie P, *et al*: **Liberal or restrictive fluid administration in fast-track colonic surgery: a randomized, double-blind study.** *Br J Anaesth* 2007, **99**:500–508.
17. Hofer CK, Cannesson M: **Monitoring fluid responsiveness.** *Acta Anaesthesiol Taiwan* 2011, **49**:59–65.
18. Sheng HP, Huggins RA: **A review of body composition studies with emphasis on total body water and fat.** *Am J Clin Nutr* 1979, **32**:630–647.
19. Dworkin HJ, Premo M, Dees S: **Comparison of red cell and whole blood volume as performed using both chromium-51-tagged red cells and iodine-125-tagged albumin and using I-131-tagged albumin and extrapolated red cell volume.** *Am J Med Sci* 2007, **334**:37–40.
20. Ertl AC, Diedrich A, Raj SR: **Techniques used for the determination of blood volume.** *Am J Med Sci* 2007, **334**:32–36.
21. Fairbanks VF, Klee GG, Wiseman GA, Hoyer JD, Tefferi A, Petitt RM, *et al*: **Measurement of blood volume and red cell mass: re-examination of ^{51}Cr and ^{125}I methods.** *Blood Cells Mol Dis* 1996, **22**:169–186.
22. Bradley EC, Barr JW: **Determination of blood volume using indocyanine green (cardio-green) dye.** *Life Sci* 1968, **7**:1001–1007.
23. Nadler SB, Hidalgo JU, Bloch T: **Prediction of blood volume in normal human adults.** *Surgery* 1962, **51**:224–232.
24. Morgan GE, Mikhail MS, Murray MJ: *Clinical Anesthesiology.* New York: Lange Medical Books/McGraw Hill; 2005.
25. Pearson TC, Guthrie DL, Simpson J, Chinn S, Barosi G, Ferrant A, *et al*: **Interpretation of measured red cell mass and plasma volume in adults: Expert Panel on Radionuclides of the International Council for Standardization in Haematology.** *Br J Haematol* 1995, **89**:748–756.
26. Bremer F, Schiele A, Sagkob J, Palmaers T, Tschaikowsky K: **Perioperative monitoring of circulating and central blood volume in cardiac surgery by pulse dye densitometry.** *Intensive Care Med* 2004, **30**:2053–2059.
27. Jones JG, Holland BM, Hudson IR, Wardrop CA: **Total circulating red cells versus haematocrit as the primary descriptor of oxygen transport by the blood.** *Br J Haematol* 1990, **76**:288–294.
28. Guyton AC, Hall JE: *Textbook of Medical Physiology.* 9th edition. Philadelphia: W.B. Saunders; 1996:123–148.
29. Convertino VA: **Blood volume response to physical activity and inactivity.** *Am J Med Sci* 2007, **334**:72–79.
30. Iijima T, Iwao Y, Sankawa H: **Circulating blood volume measured by pulse dye-densitometry. Comparison with 131I-HSA analysis.** *Anesthesiology* 1998, **89**:1329–1335.
31. Hahn R, Brauer LP, Rodhe P, Svensen C, Prough DS: **Isoflurane inhibits transcapillary compensatory volume expansion.** *Anesth Analg* 2006, **103**:350–358.
32. Järhult J, Holmberg J, Lundvall J, Mellander S: **Hyperglycemic and hyperosmolar responses to graded hemorrhage.** *Acta Physiol Scan* 1976, **97**:470–475.
33. Zollinger RM Jr: **Plasma volume and protein restoration after hemorrhage: role of the left thoracic duct versus transcapillary refilling.** *J Surg Res* 1972, **12**:151–160.
34. Drucker WR, Chadwick CDJ, Gann DS: **Transcapillary refill in hemorrhage and shock.** *Arch Surg* 1981, **116**:1344–1353.
35. Rieger A: **Changes in blood volume and plasma proteins after trauma and immediate substitution with different substitutes.** *Bibl Haematol* 1969, **33**:159–170.
36. Breckenridge IM, Digerness SB, Kirklin JW: **Validity of concept of increased extracellular fluid after open heart surgery.** *Surg Forum* 1969, **20**:169–171.
37. Breckenridge IM, Digerness SB, Kirklin JW: **Increased extracellular fluid after open intracardiac operation.** *Surg Gyn Obst* 1970, **131**:53–56.
38. Cohn LH, Angell WW: **Relative extracellular fluid deficits in patients undergoing coronary artery bypass.** *Surg Forum* 1971, **22**:151–152.
39. Cleland J, Pluth JR, Tauxe WN, Kirklin JW: **Blood volume and body fluid compartment changes soon after closed and open intracardiac surgery.** *J Thorac Cardiovasc Surg* 1966, **52**:698–705.
40. Ariel IM: **Metabolic alterations induced by intra-abdominal operations.** *Ann Surg* 1953, **138**:186–202.
41. Roth E, Lax LC, Maloney JV: **Ringer's lactate solution and extracellular fluid volume in the surgical patient: a critical analysis.** *Ann Surg* 1969, **169**:149–164.
42. Reid DJ: **Intracellular and extracellular fluid volume during surgery.** *Br J Surg* 1968, **55**:594–596.
43. Gutelius JR, Shizgal HM, Lopez G: **The effect of trauma on extracellular water volume.** *Arch Surg* 1968, **97**:206–214.
44. Ladegaard-Pedersen HJ, Engell HC: **A comparison between the changes in the distribution volumes of inulin and [51Cr]EDTA after major surgery.** *Scand J Clin Lab Invest* 1975, **35**:109–113.
45. Nielsen OM, Engell HC: **Extracellular fluid volume and distribution in relation to changes in plasma colloid osmotic pressure after major surgery. A randomized study.** *Acta Chir Scand* 1985, **151**:221–225.
46. Fukuda Y, Fujita T, Shibuya J, Albert SN: **The distribution between the intravascular and interstitial compartments of commonly utilized replacement fluids.** *Anesth Analg* 1969, **48**:831–838.
47. Rehm M, Orth V, Kreimeier U, Thiel M, Haller M, Brechtelsbauer H, *et al*: **Changes in intravascular volume during acute normovolemic hemodilution and intraoperative retransfusion in patients with radical hysterectomy.** *Anesthesiology* 2000, **92**:657–664.
48. Rehm M, Haller M, Brechtelsbauer H, Akbulut C, Finsterer U: **Extra protein loss not caused by surgical bleeding in patients with ovarian cancer.** *Acta Anaesthesiol Scand* 1998, **42**:39–46.
49. Chapman CR, Tuckett RP, Song CW: **Pain and stress in a systems perspective: reciprocal neural, endocrine, and immune interactions.** *J Pain* 2008, **9**:122–145.
50. Iijima T, Takagi T, Iwao Y: **An increased circulating blood volume does not prevent hypotension after pheochromocytoma resection.** *Can J Anaesth* 2004, **51**:212–215.
51. Vincent JL, Gottin L: **Type of fluid in severe sepsis and septic shock.** *Minerva Anestesiol* 2011, **77**:1190–1196.
52. Shibuya J, Bageant W, Gonzalez P, Small F, Albert S: **Comparison of effect of norepinephrine and angiotensin on blood volume and viscosity.** *Anesthesiology* 1964, **25**:109–110.
53. Hifumi S, Morise T, Honjo A, Fujimura A, Uchida K, Saito Z, *et al*: **Total blood volume in essential and secondary hypertension.** *Nihon Naibunpi Gakkai Zasshi* 1982, **58**:790–795.

54. Rector WG Jr, Hossack KF: **Pathogenesis of sodium retention complicating cirrhosis: is there room for diminished 'effective' arterial blood volume?** *Gastroenterology* 1988, **95:**1658–1663.
55. Katzarski KS, Randmaa I, Bergstrom J: **Influence of hemodialysis on intravascular volume and vasoactive hormones.** *Clin Nephrol* 1999, **52:**304–311.
56. Morishita Y, Ando Y, Ishii E, Arisaka M, Kusano E: **Comparison of markers of circulating blood volume in hemodialysis patients.** *Clin Exp Nephrol* 2005, **9:**233–237.
57. Krieger JE, Cowley AW Jr: **Prevention of salt angiotensin II hypertension by servo control of body water.** *Am J Physiol* 1990, **258:**H994–H1003.
58. Trippodo NC, Cole FE, Frohlich ED, MacPhee AA: **Atrial natriuretic peptide decreases circulatory capacitance in areflexic rats.** *Circ Res* 1986, **59:**291–296.
59. Jespersen B, Eiskjaer H, Pedersen EB: **Effect of atrial natriuretic peptide on blood pressure, guanosine 3':5'-cyclic monophosphate release and blood volume in uraemic patients.** *Clin Sci (Lond)* 1990, **78:**67–73.
60. Wijeyaratne CN, Moult PJ: **The effect of alpha human atrial natriuretic peptide on plasma volume and vascular permeability in normotensive subjects.** *J Clin Endocrinol Metab* 1993, **76:**343–346.
61. Bruegger D, Jacob M, Rehm M, Loetsch M, Welsch U, Conzen P, *et al*: **Atrial natriuretic peptide induces shedding of endothelial glycocalyx in coronary vascular bed of guinea pig hearts.** *Am J Physiol Heart Circ Physiol* 2005, **289:**H1993–H1999.
62. Vane LA, Prough DS, Kinsky MA, Williams CA, Grady JJ, Kramer GC: **Effects of different catecholamines on the dynamics of volume expansion of crystalloid infusion.** *Anesthesiology* 2004, **101:**1136–1144.
63. Kinsky MP, Vaid SU, Vane LA, Prough DS, Kramer GC: **Effect of esmolol on fluid therapy in normovolaemia and hypovolaemia.** *Shock* 2008, **30:**55–63.
64. Stephens CT, Uwaydah N, Kramer GC, Prough DS, Salter M, Kinsky MP: **Vascular and extravascular volume expansion of dobutamine and norepinephrine in normovolemic sheep.** *Shock* 2011, **36:**303–311.
65. Thiele RH, Nemergut EC, Lynch C III: **The clinical implications of isolated alpha(1) adrenergic stimulation.** *Anesth Analg* 2011, **113:**297–304.
66. Starling EH: **On the absorption of fluids from the connective tissue spaces.** *J Physiol* 1896, **19:**312–326.
67. Chappell D, Jacob M, Paul O, Mehringer L, Newman W, Becker BF: **Impaired glycocalyx barrier properties and increased capillary tube haematocrit.** *J Physiol* 2008, **586:**4585–4586.
68. Bruegger D, Rehm M, Abicht J, Paul JO, Stoeckelhuber M, Pfirrmann M, *et al*: **Shedding of the endothelial glycocalyx during cardiac surgery: on-pump versus off-pump coronary artery bypass graft surgery.** *J Thorac Cardiovasc Surg* 2009, **138:**1445–1447.
69. Becker BF, Chappell D, Bruegger D, Annecke T, Jacob M: **Therapeutic strategies targeting the endothelial glycocalyx: acute deficits, but great potential.** *Cardiovasc Res* 2010, **87:**300–310.
70. Annecke T, Chappell D, Chen C, Jacob M, Welsch U, Sommerhoff CP, *et al*: **Sevoflurane preserves the endothelial glycocalyx against ischaemia-reperfusion injury.** *Br J Anaesth* 2010, **104:**414–421.
71. Lamke LO, Nilsson GE, Reithner HL: **Water loss by evaporation from the abdominal cavity during surgery.** *Acta Chir Scand* 1977, **143:**279–284.
72. Svensen C, Hahn RG: **Volume kinetics of Ringer solution, dextran 70, and hypertonic saline in male volunteers.** *Anesthesiology* 1997, **87:**204–212.
73. Andrijauskas A: *Homeostatic blood states theory*, Thesis. Vilnius University Clinic of Anaesthesiology and Intensive Care; 2006. http://www.dissertation.com/book.php?method=ISBN&book=1599426536.
74. Andrijauskas A, Svensen C, Ivaskevicius J, Porvaneckas N, Kvederas G, Marmaite U: **Goal directed fluid therapy revised: indirect monitoring of interstitial fluid accumulation during mini fluid challenges with crystalloids.** *Open Conf Proc J* 2012, **3:**42–51.
75. Tatara T, Tsunetoh T, Tashiro C: **Crystalloid infusion rate during fluid resuscitation from acute hemorrhage.** *Br J Anaesth* 2007, **99:**212–217.
76. Hahn RG: **Volume kinetics for infusion fluids.** *Anesthesiology* 2009, **113:**470–481.
77. Schortgen F, Lacherade JC, Bruneel F, Cattaneo I, Hemery F, Lemaire F, *et al*: **Effects of hydroxyethylstarch and gelatin on renal function in severe sepsis: a multicentre randomised study.** *Lancet* 2001, **357:**911–916.
78. Rehm M, Haller M, Orth V, Kreimeier U, Jacob M, Dressel H, *et al*: **Changes in blood volume and haematocrit during acute preoperative volume loading with 5% albumin or 6% hetastarch solutions in patients before radical hysterectomy.** *Anesthesiology* 2001, **95:**849–856.
79. Reinhart K, Hartog CS: **Hydroxyethyl starch in patients with trauma.** *Br J Anaesth* 2012, **108:**321–322.
80. Perner A, Haase N, Guttormsen AB, Tenhunen J, Klemenzson G, Åneman A, *et al*: **Hydroxyethyl starch 130/0.4 versus Ringer's acetate in severe sepsis.** *N Engl J Med* 2012, **367:**124–134.
81. Dickenmann M, Oettl T, Mihatsch MJ: **Osmotic nephrosis: acute kidney injury with accumulation of proximal tubular lysosomes due to administration of exogenous solutes.** *Am J Kidney Dis* 2008, **51:**491–503.
82. Guidet B, Martinet O, Boulain T, Philippart F, Poussel JF, Maizel J, *et al*: **Assessment of hemodynamic efficacy and safety of 6% hydroxyethylstarch 130/0.4 versus 0.9% NaCl fluid replacement in patients with severe sepsis: The CRYSTMAS study.** *Crit Care* 2012, **16:**R94.
83. Brunkhorst FM, Engel C, Bloos F, Meier-Hellmann A, Ragaller M, Weiler N, *et al*: **Intensive insulin therapy and pentastarch resuscitation in severe sepsis.** *N Engl J Med* 2008, **358:**125–139.
84. Brunkhorst FM, Schortgen F: **Effects of hydroxyethyl starch in critically ill patients.** *Br J Anaesth* 2007, **98:**842–843.
85. Myburgh JA, Finfer S, Bellomo R, Billot L, Cass A, Gattas D, *et al*: **Hydroxyethyl starch or saline for fluid resuscitation in intensive care.** *N Engl J Med* 2012, **367:**1901–1911.
86. Gan TJ, Soppitt A, Maroof M, El-Moalem H, Robertson KM, Moretti EW, *et al*: **Goal-directed intraoperative fluid administration reduces length of hospital stay after major surgery.** *Anesthesiology* 2002, **97:**820–826.
87. Wakeling H, McFall M, Jenkins C, *et al*: **Intraoperative oesophageal Doppler guided fluid management shortens postoperative hospital stay after major bowel surgery.** *Br J Anaes* 2005, **95:**634–642.
88. Hamilton MA, Cecconi M, Rhodes A: **A systematic review and meta-analysis on the use of preemptive hemodynamic intervention to improve postoperative outcomes in moderate and high-risk surgical patients.** *Anesth Analg* 2011, **112:**1392–1402.
89. Van Der Linden P, James M, Mythen M, Weiskopf RB: **Review article: safety of modern starches used during surgery.** *Anesth Analg* 2013, **116:**35–48.
90. Martin C, Jacob M, Vicaut E, Guidet B, Van Aken H, Kurz A: **Effect of waxy maize-derived hydroxyethyl starch 130/0.4 on renal function in surgical patients.** *Anesthesiology* 2013, **118:**387–394.
91. Manoach S, Weingart SD, Charchaflieh J: **The evolution and current use of invasive hemodynamic monitoring for predicting volume responsiveness during resuscitation, perioperative, and critical care.** *J Clin Anesth* 2012, **24:**242–250.
92. Hofer CK, Furrer L, Matter-Ensner S, Maloigne M, Klaghofer R, Genoni M, *et al*: **Volumetric preload measurement by thermodilution: a comparison with transoesophageal echocardiography.** *Br J Anaesth* 2005, **94:**748–755.
93. Marik PE, Baram M, Vahid B: **Does central venous pressure predict fluid responsiveness? A systematic review of the literature and the tale of seven mares.** *Chest* 2008, **134:**172–178.
94. Sandham JD, Hull RD, Brant RF, Knox L, Pineo GF, Doig CJ, *et al*: **A randomized, controlled trial of the use of pulmonary-artery catheters in high-risk surgical patients.** *N Eng J Med* 2003, **348:**5–13.
95. Monnet X, Rienzo M, Osman D, Anguel N, Richard C, Pinsky MR, *et al:* **Passive leg raising predicts fluid responsiveness in the critically ill.** *Crit Care Med* 2006, **34:**1402–1407.
96. Moore FD, Shires GT: **Moderation.** *Ann Surg* 1967, **166:**300–301.
97. Holte K, Klarskov B, Christensen D, Lund C, Nielsen K, Bie P, *et al*: **Liberal vs restrictive fluid administration to improve recovery after laparoscopic cholecystectomy: a randomised, double-blind study.** *Ann Surg* 2004, **240:**892–899.
98. Michard F, Boussat S, Chemla D, Anguel N, Mercat A, Lecarpentier Y, *et al*: **Relation between respiratory changes in arterial pulse pressure and fluid responsiveness in septic patients with acute circulatory failure.** *Am J Respir Crit Care Med* 2000, **162:**134–138.
99. Hofer CK, Ganter MT, Zollinger A: **What technique should I use to measure cardiac output?** *Curr Opin Crit Care* 2007, **13:**308–317.
100. Mora B, Ince I, Birkenberg B, Skhirtladze K, Pernicka E, Ankersmit HJ, *et al*: **Validation of cardiac output measurement with the LiDCO pulse contour system in patients with impaired left ventricular function after cardiac surgery.** *Anaesthesia* 2011, **66:**675–681.
101. Meng L, Tran NP, Alexander BS, Laning K, Chen G, Kain ZN, *et al*: **The impact of phenylephrine, ephedrine, and increased preload on third-generation Vigileo-FloTrac and esophageal Doppler cardiac output measurements.** *Anesth Analg* 2011, **113:**751–757.
102. Cannesson M, Desebbe O, Rosamel P, Delannoy B, Robin J, Bastien O, *et al*: **Pleth variability index to monitor the respiratory variations in the pulse oximeter plethysmographic waveform amplitude and predict fluid responsiveness in the operating theatre.** *Br J Anaesth* 2008, **101:**200–206.

103. Mythen MG, Webb AR: **Intra-operative gut mucosal hypoperfusion is associated with increased post-operative complications and cost.** *Intensive Care Med* 1994, **20**:99–104.
104. Sinclair S, James SA, Singer M: **Intraoperative intravascular volume optimisation and length of hospital stay after repair of proximal femur fracture: randomised controlled trial.** *BMJ* 1997, **315**:909–912.
105. Venn R, Steele A, Richardson PL, Poloniecki JD, Grounds M, Newman PJ: **Randomized controlled trial to investigate influence of the fluid challenge on duration of hospital stay and perioperative morbidity in patients with hip fractures.** *Br J Anaesth* 2002, **88**:65–71.
106. Abbas SM, Hill AG: **Systematic review of the literature for the use of oesophageal Doppler monitor for fluid replacement in major abdominal surgery.** *Anaesthesia* 2008, **63**:44–51.
107. Brandstrup B, Svendsen PE, Rasmussen M, Belhage B, Rodt SA, Hansen B, *et al*: **Which goal for fluid therapy during colorectal surgery is followed by the best outcome: near-maximal stroke volume or zero fluid balance?** *Br J Anaesth* 2012, **109**:191–199.
108. Challand C, Struthers R, Sneyd JR, Erasmus PD, Mellor N, Hosie KB, *et al*: **Randomized controlled trial of intraoperative goal-directed fluid therapy in aerobically fit and unfit patients having major colorectal surgery.** *Br J Anaesth* 2012, **108**:53–62.

12

Sarcopenia and sarcopenic obesity: do they predict inferior oncologic outcomes after gastrointestinal cancer surgery?

Kimberly L. Mei[1], John A. Batsis[2,3,4], Jeannine B. Mills[2] and Stefan D. Holubar[2,3*]

Abstract

Sarcopenia, or loss of skeletal muscle mass and quality, has been studied as part of aging and adverse health outcomes in elderly patients but has only recently been evaluated as a separate condition in cancer patients and important indicator of adverse outcomes. Currently, its definition and method of assessment are still being debated. Sarcopenia within an increasingly obese population has led to a subgroup with sarcopenic obesity, at even higher risk of adverse outcomes. Yet, sarcopenia often goes undiagnosed in these patients, hidden beneath higher body mass index. Identifying sarcopenic and sarcopenic obese subpopulations would allow for more effective treatment plans and potential avoidance of suboptimal outcomes, as well as the chance to intervene and combat these modifiable risk factors. This review will examine available literature on the definition and methods of evaluating sarcopenia and sarcopenic obesity, summarize the effectiveness of sarcopenia and sarcopenic obesity as predictors of outcomes after gastrointestinal cancer surgery, including colorectal cancer resection, liver resection, and pancreatic resection, and outline strategies to minimize the impact of sarcopenia. It is clear that untreated sarcopenia and sarcopenic obesity can be associated with suboptimal post-operative outcomes, especially infections and disease-free or overall survival.

Keywords: Body composition, Obesity, Oncologic, Sarcopenia, Surgery, Surgical oncology, Colorectal cancer, Pancreatic cancer, Hepatectomy, Malnutrition

Background

Sarcopenia, the loss of skeletal muscle mass and quality that occurs as part of natural aging, can be exacerbated by systemic illnesses. Within the last 10 years, this geriatric syndrome has received increasing attention as a possible predictor of adverse outcomes after surgery (Lentine et al. 2011; Mueller et al. 2015). Traditional oncological therapies and perioperative nutritional assessments that focus on weight loss and markers such as serum albumin have overlooked sarcopenia as a determinant of prognosis after oncological surgery. Presently, there is no practical, objective, or easily accessible measure of individual frailty, a general concept that encompasses age-related decline across physiologic systems as well as in psychological and social well-being, resulting in impaired homeostatic reserve (Clegg et al. 2013; Bauer and Sieber 2008; Singh et al. 2014). Sarcopenia, considered a more reproducible signal of frailty, often precedes its development and could more effectively identify patients at higher risk of suboptimal benefit from systemic chemotherapy and surgery (Peng et al. 2011; van Vledder et al. 2012; Buettner et al. 2016).

With the increased prevalence of obesity, those with both sarcopenia and obesity (sarcopenic obesity (SO)) are at higher risk of adverse outcomes, including disability (Baumgartner et al. 2004) and mortality (Batsis et al. 2014a). These associations have not been well investigated in relation to many cancer surgeries. Sarcopenia is often underdiagnosed (Fielding et al. 2011; Prado et al. 2008), as it is not always easily characterized from overall weight loss alone or decreased body mass index (BMI), especially in obese patients (Batsis et al. 2014b). Establishing standard criteria is critical to accurately evaluate and make use of its prognostic abilities.

* Correspondence: Stefan.Holubar@dartmouth.edu
[2]Dartmouth-Hitchcock Medical Center, Lebanon, NH, USA
[3]Geisel School of Medicine at Dartmouth, Hanover, NH, USA
Full list of author information is available at the end of the article

In this review, we aim to summarize recent literature regarding the impact and effectiveness of sarcopenia and SO as predictors of gastrointestinal (GI) oncologic surgery outcomes, including colorectal cancer resection, liver resection, and pancreatic resection, and promising methods by which these risk factors can be modified.

Defining sarcopenia, cancer cachexia, and SO

Early definitions of sarcopenia rely upon measures of muscle mass and neglect a functional specification. Evidence suggests the relationship between low muscle mass and adverse outcomes is not linear or direct; rather, they are linked when low muscle mass is associated with muscle weakness (Cruz-Jentoft et al. 2010; Studenski et al. 2014). Recent definitions have evolved to additionally include measures of muscle performance or strength (Table 1).

In 2010, the European Working Group on Sarcopenia in Older People established a working clinical definition of sarcopenia as the presence of *both abnormally low muscle mass and low muscle function*, either physical performance or strength, in the form of low gait speed or low handgrip strength (Cruz-Jentoft et al. 2010).

In 2014, the Foundation for the National Institutes of Health alternatively defined sarcopenia as a "differential diagnosis" reached through sequential screening for poor physical function, muscle weakness, and low muscle mass. Low gait speed manifested poor physical performance, and inability to rise from a chair (without using arms) or time required to complete five chair stands were also useful standards. Muscle strength was assessed through unadjusted grip strength and muscle mass via body mass-adjusted appendicular lean mass (Studenski et al. 2014).

Sarcopenia is further distinguished from general cancer-related cachexia, "a multifactorial syndrome characterized by an ongoing loss of skeletal muscle mass (with or without loss of fat mass) that cannot be fully reversed by conventional nutritional support and leads to progressive functional impairment," which encompasses varying levels of body fat and muscle loss (Dodson et al. 2011; Fearon et al. 2006; Fearon et al. 2011; Fouladiun et al. 2005). Sarcopenia specifically denotes muscle loss (Peng et al. 2012). While cancer cachexic patients experience weight loss and diminished BMI, sarcopenic patients can have normal or increased BMI. As a result, it is still important to screen cancer surgery patients for sarcopenia (Fearon et al. 2011).

During aging and malignancy, lean body mass is lost while fat mass remains constant or increases, possibly leading to SO. SO is defined by subjects who fulfill the combination of criteria for sarcopenia and a given measure of adiposity, such as BMI, waist circumference (WC), computerized tomography (CT)-derived total body fat (TBF), or dual x-ray energy absorptiometry (DXA)/bioelectric impedance analysis (BIA)-derived body fat (Batsis et al. 2013; Lieffers et al. 2012) (Table 1). Metrics of adiposity more precise than BMI, which fluctuates with changes in both muscle and adiposity, may predict cancer outcomes more accurately. Traditional BMI cutoffs have poor diagnostic accuracy when identifying obesity, especially in older populations (Batsis et al. 2016; Romero-Corral et al. 2008).

Previously, decreases in muscle mass were considered largely responsible for muscle weakness and mobility impairment in patients with SO, but current research suggests that deterioration of muscle quality (evidenced by phenomena such as "marbling" or fat infiltration into muscle) is an overlooked contributor (Cruz-Jentoft et al. 2010). Both aging and obesity are associated with decline in muscle quality and higher rates of fat infiltration (Zamboni et al. 2008). Studies find that although obese elderly subjects often acquire a higher absolute muscle mass than non-obese frail and normal counterparts to compensate for body habitus (Visser et al. 2002), they have the poorest muscle quality and strength and, like the non-obese frail, exhibit reduced functional status, aerobic capacity, strength, balance, and gait speed (Villareal et al. 2004). This suggests that sarcopenia and SO may be seriously underdiagnosed, since previous definitions largely ignore muscle quality and the retrospective nature of many existing studies investigating sarcopenia and cancer surgery limits them to criteria relying on muscle mass. Moreover, there remains variability within cutoffs used across studies and uncertainty regarding the applicability of these criteria to all ethnic groups (Studenski et al. 2014).

Diagnosing sarcopenia and SO

Various morphometric measures are used to quantify muscle mass (Table 1), including *appendicular skeletal muscle (ASM) index* (the sum of lean soft-tissue masses for the arms and legs adjusted by height) (Fig. 1) (Baumgartner et al. 1998) and those of core muscles such as total skeletal muscle cross-sectional area at the level of the third lumbar vertebrae (L3mi) (Prado et al. 2008), total psoas area (TPA) (Peng et al. 2011), and psoas density (PD) (Sabel et al. 2011).

Muscle mass has traditionally been measured using BIA or DXA (Chien et al. 2008), but presently, CT and magnetic resonance imaging (MRI) are considered the gold standard methods of assessing body composition in research (Cruz-Jentoft et al. 2010; Bonekamp et al. 2008; Malafarina et al. 2012). CT and MRI are not routinely used in clinical practice for sarcopenia assessment or adiposity assessment, due to concerns about radiation and high cost (Cruz-Jentoft et al. 2010). DXA is inexpensive, most precise for measuring appendicular muscle

Table 1 Definitions and cutoffs for sarcopenia and sarcopenic obesity assessment

Sarcopenia definition	Study	Functional component of definition	Body composition analysis method	Muscle mass definition	Pros	Cons	Obesity definition	Pros	Cons
ASM index >2 SDs below sex-specific means of Rosetta study reference data (Gallagher et al. 1997)	Baumgartner (Baumgartner et al. 1998)	–	DXA	ASM/m^2 (Heymsfield et al. 1990)	–	No functional component	% body fat	Measures have been experimentally validated in comparison with BMI (Gallagher et al. 2000) Highly correlated with estimates from DXA (Baumgartner et al. 1998)	–
Low gait speed or low handgrip strength with low muscle mass	Cruz-Jentoft (Cruz-Jentoft et al. 2010)	Gait speed ≤0.8 m/s or >0.8 m/s with handgrip strength below sex-specific cutoffs	–	–	Contains functional component, capturing more of sarcopenia due to poor muscle quality/ fat infiltration	–	–	–	–
Low gait speed or inability to rise from chair with low handgrip strength and body mass-adjusted ASM below sex-specific cutoffs	Studenski (Studenski et al. 2014)	Gait speed ≤0.8 m/s or inability to rise from a chair with handgrip strength below sex-specific cutoffs (men <26 kg, women <16 kg)	DXA	ASM/BMI	Contains functional component, capturing more of sarcopenia due to poor muscle quality/ fat infiltration Recommendations based on the largest, most diverse samples to have been studied	–	BMI	Most common and widely available measure, easy to evaluate	Inaccurate, fluctuates with changes in both muscle and fat
L3mi below sex-specific cutoffs associated with mortality in cohort obtained through optimum stratification	Prado (Prado et al. 2008), Lieffers (Lieffers et al. 2012) Dello (Dello et al. 2013) Voron (Voron et al. 2015) Levolger (Levolger et al. 2015)	–	Secondary analysis of CT images (Mitsiopoulos et al. 1998; Shen et al. 2004)	L3mi	–	No functional component	BMI	–	–
	van Vledder (van Vledder et al. 2012)						Intra-abdominal fat (Yoshizumi et al. 1999)	Significantly associated with disease-free survival in men undergoing resection of colorectal liver metastases (van Vledder et al. 2012)	–
	Harimoto (Harimoto et al. 2013)						–	–	–
	Lodewick (Lodewick et al. 2015)						% body fat	–	–

Table 1 Definitions and cutoffs for sarcopenia and sarcopenic obesity assessment *(Continued)*

L3mi in the lowest sex-specific quartile	Miyamoto (Miyamoto et al. 2015)	–	Secondary analysis of CT images	L3mi	–	No functional component	–	–	–
No specific cutoffs established (lower density reflects more frailty)	Sabel (Sabel et al. 2013)	–	Secondary analysis of CT images	PD	A measure of muscle quality or fat infiltration	No functional component	VF, SFD, TBF, or BMI	VF: risk factor for developing colorectal cancer and significantly associated with increased tumor recurrence in colorectal cancer patients (Moon et al. 2008) SFD: significant predictor of wound infection following colectomy for colon cancer (Sabel et al. 2013) TBF: significant predictor of outcome following colectomy for colon cancer (Sabel et al. 2013)	–
TPA/m^2 equal to or below cutoff obtained through optimum stratification	Peng (Peng et al. 2011)	–	Secondary analysis of CT images	TPA/m^2	–	No functional component	BMI	–	–
TPA/m^2 in the lowest sex-specific quartile	Peng (Peng et al. 2012) Amini (Amini et al. 2015) Joglekar (Joglekar et al. 2015)	–	Secondary analysis of CT images	TPA/m^2	–	No functional component	BMI	–	–
TPV/m^2 in the lowest sex-specific quartile	Amini (Amini et al. 2015)	–	Secondary analysis of CT image	TPV/m^2	Volumetric measure rather than cross-sectional assessment and which may be more accurate at assessing a larger sample of muscle mass	No functional component	BMI	–	–
HUAC in the lowest sex-specific quartile	Joglekar (Joglekar et al. 2015)	–	Secondary analysis of CT image	HUAC	A measure of muscle quality or fat infiltration	No functional component	BMI	–	–

To determine ASM, the sum of lean soft-tissue masses for the arms and legs is computed from CT scans and adjusted by height. To determine L3mi, two consecutive CT images are taken from the L3 to the iliac crest, and cross-sectional areas of the sum of all the muscles in these regions are computed and adjusted by body surface area. To determine PD, CT scans of the left and right psoas muscles at the level of the fourth lumbar vertebrae are used. To determine TPA, measure the cross-sectional area of the right and left psoas muscles from CT images at the level of L3 where both vertebral spinae are clearly visible. To determine TPV, take three manual measurements at the level of L3 on the first slice where both iliac crests were visible to assess a total of 55 cm total psoas length and normalize for height. To determine HUAC, compute (right Hounsfield unit calculation + left Hounsfield unit calculation)/2, where the right Hounsfield unit calculation = (right Hounsfield unit*right psoas area)/(total psoas area) and left Hounsfield unit calculation = (left Hounsfield unit*left psoas area)/(total psoas area) from evaluation of both the right and left psoas at the L3 level

ASM appendicular skeletal muscle, *SD* standard deviation, *L3mi* L3 skeletal muscle index, or total skeletal muscle cross-sectional area at the level of the third lumbar vertebrae normalized for stature, *Intra-abdominal fat* total cross-sectional area of visceral adipose tissue, *TPA* total psoas muscle area, measured at the level of the L3, *TPV* total psoas volume, measured at the level of the L3, *HUAC* Hounsfield unit average calculation, measure of radiation attenuation or muscle density and fatty infiltration, measured at the level of the L3, *PD* psoas density or muscle attenuation (average radiodensity), measured at the cross-sectional areas of the left and right psoas muscles at the level of the L4, *VF* visceral fat, visceral anterior-to-posterior distance, or the average distance between the anterior aspect of the vertebra and the linea alba, *SFD* subcutaneous fat distance, or the average distance between the linea alba and the anterior skin along T-12 to L4, *TBF* total body fat or total AP distance, the sum of the SFD and VF

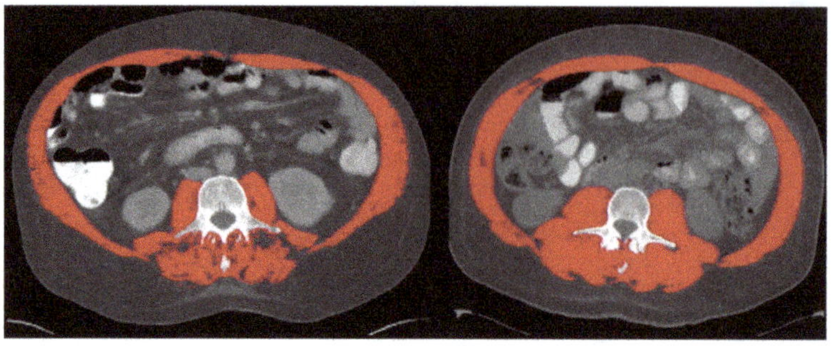

Fig. 1 Comparison of sarcopenic and non-sarcopenic computed tomography images at the third lumbar vertebral level. A comparison of two cirrhotic patients with identical BMI (32 kg/m^2). *Red color* indicates skeletal muscle: rectus abdominis, oblique and lateral abdominal muscles, psoas, and paraspinal muscles. The patient on the *left* is sarcopenic with L3mi of 49.82 cm^2/m^2; the patient on the *right* is not sarcopenic with L3mi of 70.8 cm^2/m^2. In their study of 112 cirrhotic patients, Montano-Loza et al. used abdominal CT images taken at the third lumbar vertebrae and cutoffs provided by Baumgartner et al. in 1998

mass, and exposes patients to minimal radiation but is not portable nor widely available for sarcopenia assessment or adiposity assessment (Bauer and Sieber 2008; Cruz-Jentoft et al. 2010). BIA is an inexpensive, readily reproducible, portable alternative, but results are easily confounded by a number of factors, especially fluid status, and is not preferred for adiposity assessment (Bauer and Sieber 2008).

New image analysis software packages can be used with CT or MRI to streamline segmentation and obtain more consistent body composition measures for sarcopenia assessment. Semi-automated processes like SliceOmatic, NIHImageJ, Analyze, and EasyVision have yielded similar results in terms of reproducibility, while only HippoFat, a fully automated program, has shown to be slightly inferior (Bonekamp et al. 2008). While SliceOmatic segments fastest, NIHImageJ and HippoFat are free. Overall, these software packages have comparable results in analyzing MRI (Bonekamp et al. 2008) and CT images (Irving et al. 2007) but have yet to be incorporated into routine clinical practice.

Functional implications of SO

In patients >65, SO was associated with a two to three times higher chance of reporting an instrumental activities of daily living (IADL) disability than lean sarcopenic, non-sarcopenic obese, or patients with normal body composition (Baumgartner et al. 2004). While non-sarcopenic obesity and SO were both associated with lower physical activity than non-obese sarcopenic and normal body types, only SO was significantly associated with onset of IADL disability, and low physical activity was not associated with IADL disability in the absence of SO. Thus, SO is considered a worst-case scenario compounding health risks of obesity and depleted lean mass (i.e., malnutrition) (Villareal et al. 2004; Kyle et al. 2005; Roubenoff 2004; Davison et al. 2002), and cancer patients with SO are at higher risk of oncologic treatment-related toxicities and mortality (Tsai 2012).

Impact of sarcopenia and SO on patient outcome

Colorectal cancer resection

Sarcopenia has been shown to predict complications and length of stay following colorectal surgery (Lieffers et al. 2012). Moreover, with rising levels of obesity in Western society, sarcopenia may be "hidden beneath" higher BMI.

A 2012 study of stage II–IV colorectal cancer patients undergoing primary colorectal resection found that sarcopenic patients had longer index hospitalization length of stays and post-operative length of stay, especially in those >65 (Table 2) (Lieffers et al. 2012). Sarcopenia was associated with increased infection risk, especially in those >65. Sarcopenic patients required more inpatient rehabilitation, and co-morbidities including cardiac arrhythmias, diabetes, hypertension, and deficiency anemia were more common. In patients >65, sarcopenia independently predicted post-operative infection and need for rehabilitation facility care but did not predict these or longer length of stay in younger patients. Though no explanation was provided, this may be because younger patients are healthier overall (more active, with fewer and less severe conditions and better physiological reserve) and exhibit smaller discrepancies in outcomes. The study provides strong evidence for sarcopenia as a predictor of short-term outcomes in colorectal cancer resection.

A 2015 retrospective study found significant associations between sarcopenia and long-term outcomes (Miyamoto et al. 2015). Sarcopenia was independently associated with higher disease recurrence, shorter recurrence-free survival, and shorter overall survival. Sarcopenia was also independently associated with shorter cancer-specific survival.

Another retrospective study on colon cancer patients undergoing colectomy obtained various morphometric measures to compare their effectiveness as predictors of post-operational outcomes to that of Charlson co-morbidity index scores (Sabel et al. 2013). The single

Table 2 Association between sarcopenia or sarcopenic obesity (SO) and oncological surgery outcomes

Study	Cancer type	Association with short-term oncological outcomes?		Association with long-term oncological outcomes?	
		Sarcopenia	SO	Sarcopenia	SO
Prado (Prado et al. 2008)	Respiratory or GI tract	–	Unclear, but associated with poorer functional status than in non-sarcopenic obese	Yes, independently predicted median survival	Yes, independently predicted survival
Lieffers (Lieffers et al. 2012)	Colorectal (stages II–IV)	Yes, independently predicted post-operative infection risk, longer inpatient rehabilitation, associated with higher risk of obstruction, longer index hospitalization length of stay, longer mean length of stay overall	–	–	–
Sabel (Sabel et al. 2013)	Colon	Yes, independently predicted surgical complications and infectious complications, associated with infectious post-operative complications	Unclear, but SFD is the best predictor of post-operative wound infections, and associated with infectious complications	No, not an independent predictor of disease-free or overall survival	Unclear, but TBF independently predicted disease-free survival
Miyamoto (Miyamoto et al. 2015)	Colorectal (stages I–III)	–	–	Yes, independently associated with disease recurrence rate, overall mortality, cancer-specific mortality, recurrence-free survival, overall survival, cancer-specific survival	–
van Vledder (van Vledder et al. 2012)	Colorectal liver metastases	–	–	Yes, independently predicted disease-free survival and overall survival	–
Dello (Dello et al. 2013)	Colorectal liver metastases	Yes, independently predicted disproportionally small total functional liver volume	Unclear, but fat-free body mass and body surface area independently predicted disproportionally small total function liver volume	–	–
Peng (Peng et al. 2011)	Colorectal liver metastases	Yes, independently predicted major post-operative complications, associated with risk of post-operative complications, overall morbidity risk, longer hospital stays, extended ICU stays	Yes, associated with major post-operative complications, longer hospital stays, extended ICU stays	No, not associated with recurrence-free survival, overall survival or risk of recurrence	No, not associated with overall survival or recurrence-free survival
Lodewick (Lodewick et al. 2015)	Colorectal liver metastases	No, not significantly associated with risk of major post-operative complications, presence of liver surgery-specific composite endpoint[a] (LSSCEP) items	No, not significantly associated with risk of major post-operative complications, occurrence of one or more of the LSSCEP items	No, not significantly associated with initial hospital length of stay, readmission rates, median disease-free survival, or overall survival	Yes, not predictive of initial hospital length of stay, disease-free survival, or overall survival, but significantly associated with readmission rates
Harimoto (Harimoto et al. 2013)	Liver	Yes, independent predictor of liver dysfunction	–	Yes, independent predictor of overall and recurrence-free survival	–
Voron (Voron et al. 2015)	Liver	No, not associated with severe post-operative complication rate, post-operative mortality or morbidity rates	–	Yes, independently associated with overall and disease-free survival	–
	Liver	Yes, associated with major post-operative complication (Clavien-Dindo grade ≥IIIa) and	–	Yes, associated with overall survival, but not associated with disease-free survival	Yes, associated with shorter median survival

Table 2 Association between sarcopenia or sarcopenic obesity (SO) and oncological surgery outcomes *(Continued)*

Levolger (Levolger et al. 2015)		treatment-related mortality (within 90 days post-treatment)			
Peng (Peng et al. 2012)	Pancreatic	No, not associated with overall morbidity, major post-operative complications, length of hospital stays, length of ICU stays, or hazard of 90-day death	–	Yes, independent predictor of 3-year mortality	–
Amini (Amini et al. 2015)	Pancreatic	Yes, TPA-sarcopenia not associated with morbidity, but TPV-sarcopenia associated with post-operative complications, major complications, and length of hospital stay. TPV-sarcopenia also independently associated with post-operative complications	Yes, TPV-SO associated with post-operative complications	Yes, TPV-sarcopenia associated with risk of death, and independently associated with risk of death	–
Joglekar (Joglekar et al. 2015)	Pancreatic	Yes, HUAC independently predicted length of stay, ICU stay, major grade III post-operative complications, incidence of any complications. TPA independently predicted length of stay	–	No, HUAC did not predict post-operative overall survival	–

[a]The liver surgery-specific composite endpoint (LSSCEP) is composed of ascites, post-resectional liver failure, bile leakage, intra-abdominal hemorrhage, intra-abdominal abscess, and mortality and was used to assess liver surgery-specific morbidity

best predictor of any surgical or infectious complications was PD. When considering PD, Charlson scores, age or BMI, or specific co-morbidities were not statistically significant.

After final multivariate models controlled for age and Charlson score, PD was not significantly associated with disease-free or overall survival, but TBF was. The authors concluded that PD-sarcopenia is mainly predictive of non-colorectal cancer deaths in the population and hypothesized that frailty, or immunologic correlates, contributes less to the natural progression of colorectal cancer than it may to other cancers, such as melanoma, which an earlier study by the same authors suggested (Sabel et al. 2011).

A separate cross-sectional study found that SO in patients with solid tumors of the respiratory tract, colon, rectum, or other GI sites was significantly related to worse functional status and independently predicted survival (Prado et al. 2008).

More research is needed to clarify the most effective method of sarcopenia assessment in regard to colorectal cancer resection outcomes. Sarcopenia's effectiveness as a predictor of long-term outcomes following colorectal cancer resection is unclear, as well as the associations between SO and short- and long-term outcomes.

Colorectal liver metastases and hepatectomy

Sarcopenia has also been investigated in relation to liver resection. In 2012, a study on patients undergoing colorectal cancer liver metastases determined that sarcopenia was significantly associated with disproportionally small total functional liver volume (TFLV) and impaired short-term outcomes after surgery (Dello et al. 2013). Significant correlation was also found between fat-free body mass and TFLV.

In a separate retrospective analysis, sarcopenia predicted short-term outcomes, but not long-term ones (Peng et al. 2011). Peng et al. found that sarcopenia was strongly univariately associated with increased risk of post-operative complications and overall morbidity, with sarcopenic patients >3 times more likely to develop a major (Clavien grade ≥3) complication (Clavien et al. 2009). Neither TPA nor sarcopenia was predictive of recurrence-free survival, long-term overall survival, or risk of recurrence. While sarcopenic patients had longer hospital stays and higher chances of extended ICU stay (>2 days), SO patients were at even higher risk of both. In addition, SO was associated with an even greater risk of Clavien grade ≥3 complications.

Patients with SO tended to have shorter median overall survival than other patients but, like sarcopenic patients, did not have significant differences in recurrence-free survival compared to the entire cohort. These observations support conclusions from Sabel et al. that perhaps sarcopenia has a less significant impact on the natural progression of colorectal cancer than for other cancers and thus predicts short-term outcomes following surgery in colorectal cancer, but not long-term survival.

However, in another retrospective study, sarcopenic patients had shorter median disease-free survival and lower 1-, 3-, and 5-year disease-free survival rates compared to non-sarcopenic patients (Fig. 2) (van Vledder et al. 2012). They also had decreased median overall survival and diminished 1-, 3-, and 5-year overall survival rates. Ultimately, sarcopenia independently predicted worse survival.

Most recently, however, a 2015 study found neither sarcopenia nor SO to be associated with short-term outcomes such as risk of major post-operative complications or morbidity (Lodewick et al. 2015). Moreover, sarcopenia was not significantly associated with long-term outcomes, including readmission rates or disease-free or overall survival. Interestingly, Lodewick et al. observed that sarcopenic patients had significantly higher percentage body fat and investigated SO in relation to outcomes. SO predicted higher readmission rates but no other long-term outcomes.

van Vledder et al.'s findings thus conflict with Peng et al.'s that sarcopenia does not predict long-term survival outcomes, and Lodewick et al. conflict with both on sarcopenia's association with short- and long-term outcomes. While multiple studies have supported an association between sarcopenia and short-term outcomes following hepatectomy of colorectal liver metastases, uncertainty remains about this association and surrounding sarcopenia's relation to long-term outcomes.

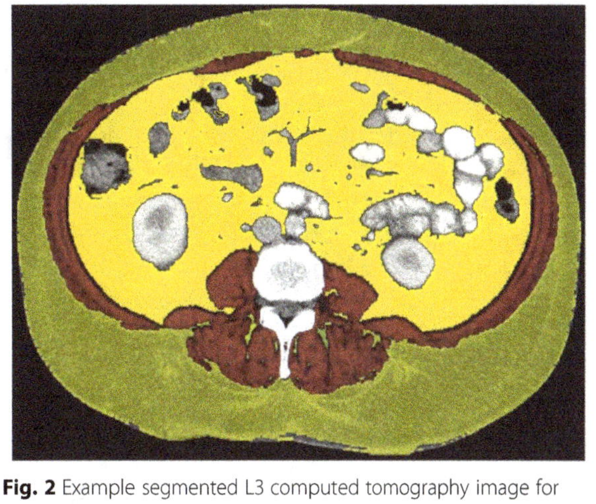

Fig. 2 Example segmented L3 computed tomography image for skeletal muscle assessment of patient undergoing hepatic resection. L3mi computed tomogram shows highlighted areas of subcutaneous (*green*) and intra-abdominal fat (*yellow*) and skeletal muscle mass (*red*). van Vledder et al. found a variety of body compositions within their population of 196 patients who underwent hepatic resection for colorectal liver metastases

Hepatocellular carcinoma and hepatectomy

A 2013 retrospective study on partial hepatectomy in patients with hepatocellular carcinoma (HCC) noted that there is currently no objective, accessible, accurate measure of a patient's condition before undergoing hepatectomy (Harimoto et al. 2013). While the American Society of Anesthesiologists' (ASA) grading estimates functional status, it is subjective (Makary et al. 2010). Child-Pugh scores are not always reliable metrics of hepatic reserve, and Model for End-Stage Liver Disease (MELD) scores quantify mortality risk in end-stage liver disease and organ allocation processes (Teh et al. 2005). In this study, sarcopenia independently predicted overall and recurrence-free survival following surgery (Harimoto et al. 2013). As serum albumin levels were significantly lower and indocyanine green dye retention rate at 15 min (ICGR15) values higher in sarcopenic patients than in non-sarcopenic patients (conveying less effective hepatic removal of synthetic dye from plasma, worse hepatic functional reserve and ability to regenerate), sarcopenia was significantly associated with liver dysfunction. This study strongly supported sarcopenia as a predictor of short- and long-term outcomes following hepatectomy.

Subsequent studies disagreed. A 2015 retrospective study found that while sarcopenia was independently associated with overall and disease-free survival, it was not with short-term outcomes (Voron et al. 2015). Post-operative mortality, morbidity, and major complication rates were higher in sarcopenic than non-sarcopenic subjects but not statistically significantly so.

A separate 2015 retrospective study reaffirmed initial findings from Harimoto et al. (Levolger et al. 2015). Unlike Voron et al., Levolger et al. discovered that sarcopenia was associated with short-term outcomes such as increased risk of major post-operative complications and treatment-related mortality (death within 90 days of treatment). It was also associated with some long-term outcomes, like shorter overall survival, but not disease-free survival.

Further research needs to evaluate the effectiveness of sarcopenia as a predictor of short-term outcomes following hepatectomy for hepatocellular carcinoma and clarify the extent to which it is a useful predictor of long-term outcomes.

Additionally, Voron et al. reported a wide range of BMI across sarcopenic subjects and emphasized the limited practicality of BMI in sarcopenia determination without CT analysis. Three subjects with identical BMI had varying L3mi values and sarcopenic status. Similarly, Levolger et al. noted the prevalence of sarcopenia in various body compositions and found that those overweight or obese and sarcopenic have significantly shorter median survival rates than non-sarcopenic obese or overweight. These findings highlight the necessity of using CT to separately screen for sarcopenia, which is convenient, as many hepatocellular carcinoma patients already undergo routine imaging (Voron et al. 2015).

Pancreatic adenocarcinoma and pancreatic resection

Recent literature has found that factors such as comorbidity, anemia, and sarcopenia may affect post-operative outcome as significantly as adjuvant oncological treatments (Fearon et al. 2013). Considerable variation in 30-day morbidity and mortality following cancer surgery and in long-term outcomes between countries supports the idea that factors outside traditional multidisciplinary team consideration may be important determinants of outcome (Baili et al. 2008; van Gijn et al. 2010).

A retrospective study on patients undergoing resection of pancreatic adenocarcinoma found that sarcopenia was an objective measure of patient frailty strongly predictive of long-term outcomes, independent of tumor-specific factors (Peng et al. 2012). Sarcopenia was not associated with short-term outcomes such as risk of overall morbidity or major complications, median ICU stays, or length of hospital stays. It was associated with increased risk of 3-year mortality. This relationship suggests that perhaps individual patient characteristics have a stronger impact on long-term outcomes of pancreatic resection than tumor-specific factors do.

However, more recent retrospective studies using volumetric or density psoas metrics found stronger associations between sarcopenia and short-term outcomes. In 2015, a retrospective study revealed stronger associations between total psoas volume (TPV)-sarcopenia and short-term outcomes than with TPA-sarcopenia (Amini et al. 2015). While TPA-sarcopenia was significantly related to risk of morbidity, TPV-sarcopenia was significantly associated with risk of any post-operative complication, risk of major complications, and length of hospital stay. Moreover, TPV-sarcopenia independently predicted risk of death. TPV-SO was also associated with higher risk of post-operative complications compared to non-sarcopenic obese.

The same year, Joglekar et al. investigated the Hounsfield unit average calculation (HUAC), a measure of psoas muscle density and fatty infiltration, along with TPA (Joglekar et al. 2015). Like TPV-sarcopenia, they found that HUAC-sarcopenia was associated with more short-term outcomes than TPA-sarcopenia. TPA-sarcopenia was associated with longer length of hospital stay, while HUAC-sarcopenia was associated with longer length of hospital stay, length of ICU stay, risk of any post-operative complication, and risk of major complications. One point of contrast between Joglekar et al. and Amini et al. was that unlike TPV-sarcopenia, HUAC-sarcopenia did not strongly predict long-term outcomes.

These findings reiterate the importance of identifying the most clinically significant assessment methods of sarcopenia before determining its utility as a predictor. Amini et al. determined that volumetric standards for sarcopenia like TPV might be more clinically useful as predictors of cancer surgery outcomes than cross-sectional area measures such as TPA. Similarly, a definition based on muscle density forecasted short-term outcomes better than TPA (though not long-term outcomes) (Joglekar et al. 2015).

Strategies to minimize the impact of sarcopenia and SO

While sarcopenia assessment can help identify cancer surgery patients at risk of worse outcomes, it is important to note that sarcopenia and SO themselves are modifiable. The most effective interventions to date are physical exercise and adequate nutritional protein intake (Deutz et al. 2014; Bauer et al. 2013). Pharmacological therapies for sarcopenia including inhibitors of myostatin, testosterone, selected androgen receptor modulators, ghrelin agonists, and angiotensin-converting enzyme (ACE) inhibitors have been evaluated, but preliminary trials have found that they are less effective than postulated (Molfino et al. 2016; Morley et al. 2014). In older adults vulnerable to functional decline, moderate-intensity physical activity significantly reduces risk of onset of major mobility disability compared to health education and, to a larger degree, risk of persistent mobility disability (Pahor et al. 2014). Since the primary outcome of sarcopenia is mobility disability, a proven intervention from the mobility disability literature, moderate physical activity, is a promising intervention for non-aging sarcopenic patients as well. In addition, relative sarcopenia in obese elderly was significantly ameliorated by diet regimens, exercise programs, or their combination (Villareal et al. 2011). Fat mass decreased under diet or exercise programs or their combination, but lean body mass decreased less under diet-exercise than with only diet and increased under an exercise program. A diet and exercise program yielded the greatest improvements in physical performance and the most consistent changes in strength, balance, and gait and thus may be an important therapy for SO subpopulations.

Conclusions

The impact of sarcopenia on post-operative oncologic outcomes and its usefulness as a predictor is still unclear and often conflicting, particularly in the case of hepatectomy for colorectal liver metastases and hepatectomy for hepatocellular carcinoma. However, sarcopenia is promising as a predictor of short-term outcomes following colorectal cancer surgery and long-term outcomes following hepatectomy for hepatocellular carcinoma. SO is promising as a predictor of long-term outcomes following hepatectomy for hepatocellular carcinoma and short-term outcomes following pancreatic resection. The other associations need additional clarification, as studies provided inconsistent results.

There remains considerable variation in definition, cutoffs, and assessment methods for sarcopenia and SO, which makes translation to clinical practice complicated. Recent criteria incorporating both grip strength and appendicular skeletal muscle allow more clinically meaningful associations with long-term outcomes and are preferred to definitions excluding a functional component (Studenski et al. 2014; McLean et al. 2014). Though ramifications have been explored in geriatric populations, sarcopenia assessment may be more easily assimilated into clinical practice for cancer surgery patients, as routine imaging is already completed for these populations. Semi-automated segmentation software also promises to play a major role in streamlining sarcopenia assessment integration into routine practice.

Sarcopenia and SO may predict short- and long-term outcomes, and effective identification of patients at risk of poorer outcomes from cancer surgery allows for tailored interventions. As clinicians become increasingly aware of this subtle form of malnutrition, addressing sarcopenia preoperatively can optimize outcomes for at-risk patients.

Future directions

Further research is needed to reach consensus regarding the ideal manner of assessing sarcopenia in order to predict outcomes after various cancer surgeries and across cancers in a broad clinical sense. The prevalence and impact of SO in various cancer surgeries requires further examination. Risk of mortality associated with SO for all types of patients should be further evaluated (Prado et al. 2008; Batsis et al. 2013). It remains unclear whether the added risk from SO is the sum of the individual impacts of obesity and sarcopenia or whether these conditions further interact with each other. Finally, current interventions for sarcopenia and SO have not been robustly verified, due to challenges from risk of adverse reactions when dealing with sarcopenic populations (Cesari M 2016). Furthermore, these interventions have yet to be tested specifically with regard to cancer surgery patients.

Abbreviations

ACE: Angiotensin-converting enzyme; ASA: American Society of Anesthesiologists; ASM: Appendicular skeletal muscle; BIA: Bioelectric impedance analysis; BMI: Body mass index; CT: Computerized tomography; DXA: Dual x-ray energy absorptiometry; GI: Gastrointestinal; HCC: Hepatocellular carcinoma; HUAC: Hounsfield unit average calculation; IADL: Instrumental activities of daily living; ICGR15: Indocyanine green dye retention rate at 15 min; L3mi: Total skeletal muscle cross-sectional area at the level of the third lumbar vertebrae; LSSCEP: Liver surgery-specific composite endpoint; MELD: Model for End-Stage Liver Disease; MRI: Magnetic resonance imaging; PD: Psoas density; SD: Standard deviation; SFD: Subcutaneous fat distance; SO: Sarcopenic obesity; TBF: Total body fat; TFLV: Total functional liver volume; TPA: Total psoas area; TPV: Total psoas volume; WC: Waist circumference

Acknowledgements
Not applicable.

Funding
Not applicable. There were no sources of funding for this research.

Authors' contributions
KM drafted the manuscript. JB, JM, and SH helped draft and critically review the manuscript. All authors read and approved the final version.

Competing interests
JB has received honoraria from the 2014 Merck/American Geriatrics Society New Investigator Award and is supported by the National Institute On Aging of the National Institutes of Health under Award Number K23AG051681. This content is solely the responsibility of the authors and does not necessarily represent the official views of the National Institutes of Health. SH serves on the advisory board for Emmi Solutions and Mallinckrodt Pharmaceuticals. KM and JM declare no competing interests.

Author details
[1]Dartmouth College, Hanover, NH, USA. [2]Dartmouth-Hitchcock Medical Center, Lebanon, NH, USA. [3]Geisel School of Medicine at Dartmouth, Hanover, NH, USA. [4]The Dartmouth Institute for Health Policy & Clinical Practice, Lebanon, NH, USA.

References
Amini N, Spolverato G, Gupta R, Margonis GA, Kim Y, Wagner D, Rezaee N, Weiss MJ, Wolfgang CL, Makary MM, et al. Impact total psoas volume on short- and long-term outcomes in patients undergoing curative resection for pancreatic adenocarcinoma: a new tool to assess sarcopenia. J Gastrointest Surg. 2015; 19(9):1593–602.

Baili P, Micheli A, De Angelis R, Weir HK, Francisci S, Santaquilani M, Hakulinen T, Quaresmas M, Coleman MP. Life tables for world-wide comparison of relative survival for cancer (CONCORD study). Tumori. 2008;94(5):658–68.

Batsis JA, Barre LK, Mackenzie TA, Pratt SI, Lopez-Jimenez F, Bartels SJ. Variation in the prevalence of sarcopenia and sarcopenic obesity in older adults associated with different research definitions: dual-energy X-ray absorptiometry data from the National Health and Nutrition Examination Survey 1999-2004. J Am Geriatr Soc. 2013;61(6):974–80.

Batsis JA, Mackenzie TA, Barre LK, Lopez-Jimenez F, Bartels SJ. Sarcopenia, sarcopenic obesity and mortality in older adults: results from the National Health and Nutrition Examination Survey III. Eur J Clin Nutr. 2014a;68(9):1001–7.

Batsis JA, Sahakyan KR, Rodriguez-Escudero JP, Bartels SJ, Lopez-Jimenez F. Normal weight obesity and functional outcomes in older adults. Eur J Intern Med. 2014b;25(6):517–22.

Batsis JA, Mackenzie TA, Bartels SJ, Sahakyan KR, Somers VK, Lopez-Jimenez F. Diagnostic accuracy of body mass index to identify obesity in older adults: NHANES 1999-2004. Int J Obes (2005). 2016;40(5):761–7.

Bauer JM, Sieber CC. Sarcopenia and frailty: a clinician's controversial point of view. 2008 (0531-5565 (Print)).

Bauer J, Biolo G, Cederholm T, Cesari M, Cruz-Jentoft AJ, Morley JE, Phillips S, Sieber C, Stehle P, Teta D, et al. Evidence-based recommendations for optimal dietary protein intake in older people: a position paper from the PROT-AGE Study Group. J Am Med Dir Assoc. 2013;14(8):542–59.

Baumgartner RN, Koehler KM, Gallagher D, Romero L, Heymsfield SB, Ross RR, Garry PJ, Lindeman RD. Epidemiology of sarcopenia among the elderly in New Mexico. Am J Epidemiol. 1998;147(8):755–63.

Baumgartner RN, Wayne SJ, Waters DL, Janssen I, Gallagher D, Morley JE. Sarcopenic obesity predicts instrumental activities of daily living disability in the elderly. Obes Res. 2004;12(12):1995–2004.

Bonekamp S, Ghosh P, Crawford S, Solga SF, Horska A, Brancati FL, Diehl AM, Smith S, Clark JM. Quantitative comparison and evaluation of software packages for assessment of abdominal adipose tissue distribution by magnetic resonance imaging. Int J Obes. 2008;32(1):100–11.

Buettner S, Wagner D, Kim Y, Margonis GA, Makary MA, Wilson A, Sasaki K, Amini N, Gani F, Pawlik TM. Inclusion of sarcopenia outperforms the modified frailty index in predicting 1-year mortality among 1,326 patients undergoing gastrointestinal surgery for a malignant indication. 2016 (1879-1190 (Electronic)).

Cesari M, Nobili A, Vitale G. Frailty and sarcopenia: from theory to clinical implementation and public health relevance. Eur J Intern Med. 2016. http://dx.doi.org/10.1016/j.ejim.2016.07.021

Chien MY, Huang Ty Fau - Wu Y-T, Wu YT. Prevalence of sarcopenia estimated using a bioelectrical impedance analysis prediction equation in community-dwelling elderly people in Taiwan. 2008 (1532-5415 (Electronic)).

Clavien PA, Barkun J, de Oliveira ML, Vauthey JN, Dindo D, Schulick RD, de Santibanes E, Pekolj J, Slankamenac K, Bassi C, et al. The Clavien-Dindo classification of surgical complications: five-year experience. Ann Surg. 2009;250(2):187–96.

Clegg A, Young J Fau - Iliffe S, Iliffe S Fau - Rikkert MO, Rikkert Mo Fau - Rockwood K, Rockwood K. Frailty in elderly people. 2013 (1474-547X (Electronic)).

Cruz-Jentoft AJ, Baeyens JP, Bauer JM, Boirie Y, Cederholm T, Landi F, Martin FC, Michel JP, Rolland Y, Schneider SM, et al. Sarcopenia: European consensus on definition and diagnosis: report of the European Working Group on Sarcopenia in Older People. Age Ageing. 2010;39(4):412–23.

Davison KK, Ford Es Fau - Cogswell ME, Cogswell Me Fau - Dietz WH, Dietz WH. Percentage of body fat and body mass index are associated with mobility limitations in people aged 70 and older from NHANES III. 2002 (0002-8614 (Print)).

Dello SA, Lodewick TM, van Dam RM, Reisinger KW, van den Broek MA, von Meyenfeldt MF, Bemelmans MH, Olde Damink SW, Dejong CH. Sarcopenia negatively affects preoperative total functional liver volume in patients undergoing liver resection. HPB. 2013;15(3):165–9.

Deutz NE, Bauer JM, Barazzoni R, Biolo G, Boirie Y, Bosy-Westphal A, Cederholm T, Cruz-Jentoft A, Krznaric Z, Nair KS, et al. Protein intake and exercise for optimal muscle function with aging: recommendations from the ESPEN Expert Group. Clin Nutr. 2014;33(6):929–36.

Dodson S, Baracos Ve Fau - Jatoi A, Jatoi A Fau - Evans WJ, Evans Wj Fau - Cella D, Cella D Fau - Dalton JT, Dalton Jt Fau - Steiner MS, Steiner MS. Muscle wasting in cancer cachexia: clinical implications, diagnosis, and emerging treatment strategies. 2011 (1545-326X (Electronic)).

Fearon KC, Voss Ac Fau - Hustead DS, Hustead DS. Definition of cancer cachexia: effect of weight loss, reduced food intake, and systemic inflammation on functional status and prognosis. 2006 (0002-9165 (Print)).

Fearon K, Strasser F, Anker SD, Bosaeus I, Bruera E, Fainsinger RL, Jatoi A, Loprinzi C, MacDonald N, Mantovani G, et al. Definition and classification of cancer cachexia: an international consensus. Lancet Oncol. 2011;12(5):489–95.

Fearon KC, Jenkins JT, Carli F, Lassen K. Patient optimization for gastrointestinal cancer surgery. Br J Surg. 2013;100(1):15–27.

Fielding RA, Vellas B Fau - Evans WJ, Evans Wj Fau - Bhasin S, Bhasin S Fau - Morley JE, Morley Je Fau - Newman AB, Newman Ab Fau - Abellan van Kan G, Abellan van Kan G Fau - Andrieu S, Andrieu S Fau - Bauer J, Bauer J Fau - Breuille D, Breuille D Fau - Cederholm T, et al. Sarcopenia: an undiagnosed condition in older adults. Current consensus definition: prevalence, etiology, and consequences. International Working Group on Sarcopenia. 2011 (1538-9375 (Electronic)).

Fouladiun M, Korner U Fau - Bosaeus I, Bosaeus I Fau - Daneryd P, Daneryd P Fau - Hyltander A, Hyltander A Fau - Lundholm KG, Lundholm KG. Body composition and time course changes in regional distribution of fat and lean tissue in unselected cancer patients on palliative care—correlations with food intake, metabolism, exercise capacity, and hormones. 2005 (0008-543X (Print)).

Gallagher D, Visser M, De Meersman RE, Sepulveda D, Baumgartner RN, Pierson RN, Harris T, Heymsfield SB. Appendicular skeletal muscle mass: effects of age, gender, and ethnicity. J Appl Physiol. 1997;83(1):229–39.

Gallagher D, Heymsfield SB, Heo M, Jebb SA, Murgatroyd PR, Sakamoto Y. Healthy percentage body fat ranges: an approach for developing guidelines based on body mass index. Am J Clin Nutr. 2000;72(3):694–701.

Harimoto N, Shirabe K, Yamashita YI, Ikegami T, Yoshizumi T, Soejima Y, Ikeda T, Maehara Y, Nishie A, Yamanaka T. Sarcopenia as a predictor of prognosis in patients following hepatectomy for hepatocellular carcinoma. Br J Surg. 2013; 100(11):1523–30.

Heymsfield SB, Smith R, Aulet M, Bensen B, Lichtman S, Wang J, Pierson Jr RN. Appendicular skeletal muscle mass: measurement by dual-photon absorptiometry. Am J Clin Nutr. 1990;52(2):214–8.

Irving BA, Weltman JY, Brock DW, Davis CK, Gaesser GA, Weltman A. NIH ImageJ and Slice-O-Matic computed tomography imaging software to quantify soft tissue. Obesity (Silver Spring, Md). 2007;15(2):370–6.

Joglekar S, Asghar A, Mott SL, Johnson BE, Button AM, Clark E, Mezhir JJ.

Sarcopenia is an independent predictor of complications following pancreatectomy for adenocarcinoma. J Surg Oncol. 2015;111(6):771–5.

Kyle UG, Pirlich M Fau - Lochs H, Lochs H Fau - Schuetz T, Schuetz T Fau - Pichard C, Pichard C. Increased length of hospital stay in underweight and overweight patients at hospital admission: a controlled population study. 2005 (0261-5614 (Print)).

Lentine Kl Fau - Axelrod D, Axelrod D Fau - Abbott KC, Abbott KC. Interpreting body composition in kidney transplantation: weighing candidate selection, prognostication, and interventional strategies to optimize health. 2011 (1555-905X (Electronic)).

Levolger S, van Vledder MG, Muslem R, Koek M, Niessen WJ, de Man RA, de Bruin RW, Ijzermans JN. Sarcopenia impairs survival in patients with potentially curable hepatocellular carcinoma. J Surg Oncol. 2015;112:208–13.

Lieffers JR, Bathe OF, Fassbender K, Winget M, Baracos VE. Sarcopenia is associated with postoperative infection and delayed recovery from colorectal cancer resection surgery. Br J Cancer. 2012;107(6):931–6.

Lodewick TM, van Nijnatten TJ, van Dam RM, van Mierlo K, Dello SA, Neumann UP, Olde Damink SW, Dejong CH. Are sarcopenia, obesity and sarcopenic obesity predictive of outcome in patients with colorectal liver metastases? HPB. 2015;17(5):438–46.

Makary MA, Segev DL, Pronovost PJ, Syin D, Bandeen-Roche K, Patel P, Takenaga R, Devgan L, Holzmueller CG, Tian J, et al. Frailty as a predictor of surgical outcomes in older patients. J Am Coll Surg. 2010;210(6):901–8.

Malafarina V, Uriz-Otano F Fau - Iniesta R, Iniesta R Fau - Gil-Guerrero L, Gil-Guerrero L. Sarcopenia in the elderly: diagnosis, physiopathology and treatment. 2012 (1873-4111 (Electronic)).

McLean RR, Shardell MD, Alley DE, Cawthon PM, Fragala MS, Harris TB, Kenny AM, Peters KW, Ferrucci L, Guralnik JM, et al. Criteria for clinically relevant weakness and low lean mass and their longitudinal association with incident mobility impairment and mortality: the Foundation for the National Institutes of Health (FNIH) Sarcopenia Project. J Gerontol A Biol Sci Med Sci. 2014;69(5):576–83.

Mitsiopoulos N, Baumgartner RN, Heymsfield SB, Lyons W, Gallagher D, Ross R. Cadaver validation of skeletal muscle measurement by magnetic resonance imaging and computerized tomography. J Appl Physiol. 1998;85(1):115–22.

Miyamoto Y, Baba Y, Sakamoto Y, Ohuchi M, Tokunaga R, Kurashige J, Hiyoshi Y, Iwagami S, Yoshida N, Yoshida M, et al. Sarcopenia is a negative prognostic factor after curative resection of colorectal cancer. Ann Surg Oncol. 2015; 22(8):2663–8.

Molfino A, Amabile MI, Rossi Fanelli F, Muscaritoli M. Novel therapeutic options for cachexia and sarcopenia. Expert Opin Biol Ther. 2016;16(10):1239–44.

Moon HG, Ju YT, Jeong CY, Jung EJ, Lee YJ, Hong SC, Ha WS, Park ST, Choi SK. Visceral obesity may affect oncologic outcome in patients with colorectal cancer. Ann Surg Oncol. 2008;15(7):1918–22.

Morley JE, von Haehling S, Anker SD. Are we closer to having drugs to treat muscle wasting disease? J Cachex Sarcopenia Muscle. 2014;5(2):83–7.

Mueller N, Murthy S Fau - Tainter CR, Tainter Cr Fau - Lee J, Lee J Fau - Riddell K, Riddell K Fau - Fintelmann FJ, Fintelmann Fj Fau - Grabitz SD, Grabitz Sd Fau - Timm FP, Timm Fp Fau - Levi B, Levi B Fau - Kurth T, Kurth T Fau - Eikermann M, et al. Can sarcopenia quantified by ultrasound of the rectus femoris muscle predict adverse outcome of surgical intensive care unit patients as well as frailty? A prospective, observational cohort study. 2015 (1528-1140 (Electronic)).

Pahor M, Guralnik JM, Ambrosius WT, Blair S, Bonds DE, Church TS, Espeland MA, Fielding RA, Gill TM, Groessl EJ, et al. Effect of structured physical activity on prevention of major mobility disability in older adults: the LIFE study randomized clinical trial. JAMA. 2014;311(23):2387–96.

Peng PD, van Vledder MG, Tsai S, de Jong MC, Makary M, Ng J, Edil BH, Wolfgang CL, Schulick RD, Choti MA, et al. Sarcopenia negatively impacts short-term outcomes in patients undergoing hepatic resection for colorectal liver metastasis. HPB. 2011;13(7):439–46.

Peng P, Hyder O, Firoozmand A, Kneuertz P, Schulick RD, Huang D, Makary M, Hirose K, Edil B, Choti MA, et al. Impact of sarcopenia on outcomes following resection of pancreatic adenocarcinoma. J Gastrointest Surg. 2012;16(8):1478–86.

Prado CM, Lieffers JR, McCargar LJ, Reiman T, Sawyer MB, Martin L, Baracos VE. Prevalence and clinical implications of sarcopenic obesity in patients with solid tumours of the respiratory and gastrointestinal tracts: a population-based study. Lancet Oncol. 2008;9(7):629–35.

Romero-Corral A, Somers VK, Sierra-Johnson J, Thomas RJ, Collazo-Clavell ML, Korinek J, Allison TG, Batsis JA, Sert-Kuniyoshi FH, Lopez-Jimenez F. Accuracy of body mass index in diagnosing obesity in the adult general population. Int J Obes. 2008;32(6):959–66.

Roubenoff R. Sarcopenic obesity: the confluence of two epidemics. (1071-7323 (Print)).

Sabel MS, Lee J, Cai S, Englesbe MJ, Holcombe S, Wang S. Sarcopenia as a prognostic factor among patients with stage III melanoma. Ann Surg Oncol. 2011;18(13):3579–85.

Sabel MS, Terjimanian M, Conlon AS, Griffith KA, Morris AM, Mulholland MW, Englesbe MJ, Holcombe S, Wang SC. Analytic morphometric assessment of patients undergoing colectomy for colon cancer. J Surg Oncol. 2013;108(3):169–75.

Shen W, Punyanitya M, Wang Z, Gallagher D, St-Onge MP, Albu J, Heymsfield SB, Heshka S. Total body skeletal muscle and adipose tissue volumes: estimation from a single abdominal cross-sectional image. J Appl Physiol. 2004;97(6):2333–8.

Singh M, Stewart R, White H. Importance of frailty in patients with cardiovascular disease. 2014 (1522-9645 (Electronic)).

Studenski SA, Peters KW, Alley DE, Cawthon PM, McLean RR, Harris TB, Ferrucci L, Guralnik JM, Fragala MS, Kenny AM, et al. The FNIH sarcopenia project: rationale, study description, conference recommendations, and final estimates. J Gerontol A Biol Sci Med Sci. 2014;69(5):547–58.

Teh SH, Christein J, Donohue J, Que F, Kendrick M, Farnell M, Cha S, Kamath P, Kim R, Nagorney DM. Hepatic resection of hepatocellular carcinoma in patients with cirrhosis: Model of End-Stage Liver Disease (MELD) score predicts perioperative mortality. J Gastrointest Surg. 2005;9(9):1207–15. discussion 1215.

Tsai S. Importance of lean body mass in the oncologic patient. Nutr Clin Pract. 2012;27(5):593–8.

van Gijn W, Gooiker GA, Wouters MW, Post PN, Tollenaar RA, van de Velde CJ. Volume and outcome in colorectal cancer surgery. Eur J Surg Oncol. 2010;36 Suppl 1:S55–63.

van Vledder MG, Levolger S, Ayez N, Verhoef C, Tran TC, Ijzermans JN. Body composition and outcome in patients undergoing resection of colorectal liver metastases. Br J Surg. 2012;99(4):550–7.

Villareal DT, Banks M Fau - Siener C, Siener C Fau - Sinacore DR, Sinacore Dr Fau - Klein S, Klein S. Physical frailty and body composition in obese elderly men and women. 2004 (1071-7323 (Print)).

Villareal DT, Chode S, Parimi N, Sinacore DR, Hilton T, Armamento-Villareal R, Napoli N, Qualls C, Shah K. Weight loss, exercise, or both and physical function in obese older adults. N Engl J Med. 2011;364(13):1218–29.

Visser M, Kritchevsky SB, Goodpaster BH, Newman AB, Nevitt M, Stamm E, Harris TB. Leg muscle mass and composition in relation to lower extremity performance in men and women aged 70 to 79: the health, aging and body composition study. J Am Geriatr Soc. 2002;50(5):897–904.

Voron T, Tselikas L, Pietrasz D, Pigneur F, Laurent A, Compagnon P, Salloum C, Luciani A, Azoulay D. Sarcopenia impacts on short- and long-term results of hepatectomy for hepatocellular carcinoma. Ann Surg. 2015;261(6):1173–83.

Yoshizumi T, Nakamura T, Yamane M, Islam AH, Menju M, Yamasaki K, Arai T, Kotani K, Funahashi T, Yamashita S, et al. Abdominal fat: standardized technique for measurement at CT. Radiology. 1999;211(1):283–6.

Zamboni M, Mazzali G, Fantin F, Rossi A, Di Francesco V. Sarcopenic obesity: a new category of obesity in the elderly. Nutr Metab Cardiovasc Dis. 2008; 18(5):388–95.

13

How efficient is patient discharge following lower limb arthroplasty?

Elizabeth Ashby[1*], Claire Matejowsky[2], Michael G Mythen[3], Fares S Haddad[4] and Michael PW Grocott[3,5,6]

Abstract

Background: Appropriately timed patient discharge is essential for optimal patient care and efficient hospital functioning. The post-operative morbidity survey (POMS) is the only validated prospective method of measuring short-term post-operative morbidity. It has not previously been used as a bed utilisation tool.

Methods: We collected POMS data from 529 consecutive lower-limb arthroplasty patients over a 1-year period and recorded the number of patients remaining in the hospital without morbidity, together with alternative reasons for remaining in hospital. Data was collected on post-operative days (POD) 3, 5, 8 and 15.

Results: On POD 3, 45% of hip arthroplasty patients and 52% of knee arthroplasty patients remained in hospital with no identifiable morbidity. On POD 5, 53% of hip arthroplasty patients and 47% of knee arthroplasty patients remained in hospital with no identifiable morbidity. These figures declined by POD 8 and 15. The most common reason for inappropriate bed occupancy was ongoing physiotherapy and occupational therapy.

Conclusions: We believe POMS is able to identify patients remaining in hospital with no significant morbidity and has utility as a prospective bed utilisation tool. Addition of a mobility measure to POMS may improve its utility in detecting morbidity requiring hospitalisation, particularly following lower limb arthroplasty.

Keywords: Bed utilisation, Arthroplasty, Post-operative morbidity

Background

Appropriately timed discharge of patients following surgery is essential for optimal patient care and efficient hospital functioning. A patient discharged early is at risk of under-diagnosis of medical complications with consequent adverse outcome. A patient whose discharge is delayed is at risk of developing a hospital-associated complication (for example, hospital-acquired infection) and incurs an unnecessary cost to the health-care provider. Post-operative patients should be discharged at the earliest safe opportunity to reduce the rate of hospital-associated complications and the cost of each in-patient episode. Appropriate discharge timing should increase the throughput of patients and reduce waiting times.

Historically, hospitals in the UK have been paid according to contracts with no financial incentive to treat increased numbers of patients. This changed in 2000 when the National Health Service (NHS) Plan [1] announced that hospital incomes would be directly linked to activity. Payment by results [2] began in 2003 and now every healthcare provider is paid a sum (tariff) for each procedure undertaken. In the UK, many patients remain in hospitals with no medical indication [3]. One study showed that 31% of post-operative patients remained in hospitals inappropriately [4]. Payment by results aims to reduce this figure by rewarding efficiency and encouraging increased activity.

In order to improve efficiency, hospitals must first recognise inappropriate bed occupancy. The post-operative morbidity survey (POMS) [5] is the only validated prospective method of measuring short-term post-operative morbidity in the literature. POMS was designed to identify morbidity of a type and severity that could delay hospital discharge. The survey focuses on indicators of organ system dysfunction (for example, inability to tolerate enteral diet) rather than traditional diagnostic categories (for example, deep vein thrombosis). POMS assesses nine domains of morbidity (Table 1). Data is obtained from observation charts, medication charts, patient

* Correspondence: elizabethashby@doctors.org.uk
[1]Catterall Unit, Royal National Orthopaedic Hospital, Brockley Hill, Stanmore, Middlesex HA7 4LP, UK
Full list of author information is available at the end of the article

Table 1 Criteria for a positive POMS score

Variable	Criteria for positive result
Pulmonary	Requires supplementary oxygen or ventilatory support
Infection	Currently on antibiotics or temperature >38°C in the last 24 hours
Renal	Oliguria (<500 ml/day), elevated creatinine (>30% pre-op level), catheter *in situ* (for non-surgical reason)
Gastrointestinal	Unable to tolerate enteral diet for any reason
Cardiovascular	Diagnostic tests or treatment within the last 24 h for: myocardial infarction, hypotension (requiring pharmacological therapy or fluids > 200 ml/h), atrial/ventricular arrhythmia or cardiogenic pulmonary oedema
Central nervous system	Presence of new focal deficit, coma, confusion or delirium
Wound complications	Wound dehiscence requiring surgical exploration or drainage of pus from operative wound with or without isolation of organisms
Haematological	Requirement of blood transfusion, platelets, fresh frozen plasma, or cryoprecipitate within the last 24 h
Pain	Wound pain requiring parenteral opioids or regional anaesthesia

notes, routine blood test results and direct patient questioning and observation. No additional investigations are required. The data collection process is simple to allow routine screening of large numbers of patients. POMS has been shown to be reliable, valid and acceptable to patients [6]. POMS has been used in outcomes research [7] and in effectiveness research [8].

In the US, over 98% of post-operative in-patients had morbidity defined by POMS [5]. This implies that patients with a POMS score of 0 are fit for discharge.

Therefore, as well as providing useful clinical research and audit data, POMS may have utility for assessing and improving hospital bed utilisation.

The aim of this study is to identify inappropriate bed occupancy following lower limb arthroplasty using POMS. We report the reasons for delayed discharge and suggest ways to improve bed utilisation.

Methods

Ethical approval was gained from the Joint UCLH/UCL Committee on the Ethics of Human Research (ref. number 01/0116) prior to commencement of the study. The requirement for consent was waived as collection of POMS has become a routine part of service evaluation within our institution. All patients aged 18 or over undergoing elective lower limb arthroplasty at University College Hospitals NHS Trust over a 12-month period were eligible for inclusion into this prospective cohort study. There were no exclusion criteria ensuring a consecutive sample was taken. Elective lower limb arthroplasty procedures included unicompartmental knee replacement (UKR), total knee replacement (TKR), revision total knee replacement, hip resurfacing (HR), total hip replacement (THR) and revision total hip replacement.

Data was collected by one of two study nurses. The age, sex, American Society of Anesthesiologists (ASA) physical status score and length of in-patient stay for each patient were recorded. POMS data were collected on post-operative days (POD) 3, 5, 8 and 15 if the patient remained in hospital. Presence of morbidity was defined as occurring in any patient meeting POMS criteria in one or more domains of the survey on the day of data collection. For patients remaining in hospital without morbidity on POD 8 and POD 15, the reason was recorded. The use of mobility aids on these days was also noted.

The number and percentage of patients with no identifiable morbidity according to POMS was calculated for POD 3, 5, 8 and 15. The number of days each patient remained in hospital with no morbidity was calculated by distracting the day on which the patient first had a POMS score of 0 from his or her total length of stay. An overall estimated cost saving was calculated by multiplying this figure by the average cost for one orthopaedic in-patient night.

The number of patients developing postoperative morbidity after a period free of morbidity was recorded. The number of readmissions to the same hospital in the first year following discharge was also recorded.

Results

Data collection was completed on 529 patients. Patient characteristics of the study population are shown in Table 2. The mean age of all study patients was 68.9 years, the median ASA physical status score was 2 and 62% of patients were female. The median length of stay was 7 days, and the overall in-patient mortality rate was 0.4%.

A) Hip arthroplasty patients

The location of hip arthroplasty patients on POD 3, 5, 8 and 15 is shown in Table 3. Many patients undergoing HR remained in the hospital with no identified morbidity on POD 3 (75%), 5 (78%) and 8 (16%). All HR patients had been discharged by POD 15.

Many THR patients remained in hospital with no identifiable morbidity on POD 3 (46%), 5 (54%), 8(34%) and 15 (7%). Patients undergoing revision THR patients remained in the hospital with no identifiable morbidity on POD 3 (11%), 5 (29%), 8 (31%) and 15 (3%). Discharge status and prevalence of morbidity for all hip arthroplasty patients combined are presented in Figure 1.

B) Knee arthroplasty patients

The location of knee arthroplasty patients on POD 3, 5, 8 and 15 is shown in Table 4. Many patients undergoing

Table 2 Demographics of the study population

	Number performed	Mortality rate (%)	Age (years)		ASA physical status score		% Male	Length of stay (days)	
			Mean	Range	Median	Range		Median	Range
UKR	66	1	66.1	45 to 87	2	1 to 3	45	5	2 to 52
TKR	226	0	70.3	23 to 90	2	1 to 3	36	6	3 to 37
RTKR	8	0	71.6	46 to 88	2	1 to 3	25	13	3 to 102
HR	32	0	51.6	22 to 70	1	1 to 3	50	6	4 to 13
THR	162	0	70.7	21 to 89	2	1 to 3	36	8	3 to 51
RTHR	35	3	72.2	26 to 88	2	1 to 3	36	14	6 to 93
Total	529	0.4	68.9	21 to 90	2	1 to 3	38	7	2 to 102

UKR remained in the hospital with no identified morbidity on POD 3 (63%), 5 (39%) and 8 (6%). All UKR patients had been discharged by POD 15.

Many TKR patients remained in the hospital with no identifiable morbidity on POD 3 (50%), 5 (50%), 8 (19%) and 15 (4%). Revision TKR patients remained in the hospital with no identifiable morbidity on POD 3 (52%), 5 (47%), 8 (17%) and 15 (3%). Discharge status and prevalence of morbidity for all knee arthroplasty patients combined are presented in Figure 2.

C) Overall inappropriate bed occupancy days

Table 5 shows the average number of days that postoperative patients remained in the hospital with no identifiable morbidity. HR patients stayed an average of 2.36 days with no morbidity, THR patients 4.19 days and revision THR patients 10.37 days. UKR patients stayed an average of 1.76 days with no identifiable morbidity, TKR patients 2.73 days and revision TKR patients 14.38 days.

D) Cost of inappropriate bed occupancy days

529 patients were included in this study. These patients remained in the hospital for a total of 1,965 days with no morbidity as defined by POMS. A surgical in-patient bed costs up to £400 per night [9]. If these patients had been discharged when their POMS score was 0, a saving of up to £786,000 could have been made.

E) Reasons for patients with no morbidity remaining in hospital

Of the 529 patients participating in this study, 120 remained in hospital with no morbidity defined by POMS on POD 8, and 20 patients remained with no identifiable morbidity on POD 15. The reasons for non-discharge are shown in Figure 3. The most common reason is continuing physiotherapy and occupational therapy input. Other reasons include waiting for home equipment, waiting for a rehabilitation bed, waiting for a social services package of care and patients feeling unwell with negative investigations.

Of the patients remaining in hospital with no morbidity identified by POMS, 24% were mobilising with a zimmer frame, 55% were mobilising with two crutches, 14% with a single crutch and 7% were mobilising unaided. This study did not record how far patients could mobilise or whether they could climb stairs.

Table 3 Location of patients following hip arthroplasty

			POD 3	POD 5	POD 8	POD 15
Procedure	HR	Patients discharged	0/32 (0%)	2/32 (6%)	27/32 (84%)	32/32 (100%)
		Inpatients POMS >0	8/32 (25%)	5/32 (16%)	0/32 (0%)	0/32 (0%)
		Inpatients POMS = 0	24/32 (75%)	25/32 (78%)	5/32 (16%)	0/32 (0%)
	THR	Patients discharged	0/162 (0%)	13/162 (8%)	78/162 (48%)	138/162 (85%)
		Inpatients POMS >0	87/162 (54%)	62/162 (38%)	29/162 (18%)	13/162 (8%)
		Inpatients POMS = 0	75/162 (46%)	87/162 (54%)	55/162 (34%)	11/162 (7%)
	Revision THR	Patients discharged	0/35 (0%)	0/35 (0%)	3/35 (9%)	20/35 (57%)
		Inpatients POMS >0	31/35 (89%)	25/35 (71%)	21/35 (60%)	14/35 (40%)
		Inpatients POMS = 0	4/35 (11%)	10/35 (29%)	11/35 (31%)	1/35 (3%)
	TOTAL	Patients discharged	0/230 (0%)	16/230 (7%)	109/230 (47%)	191/230 (83%)
		Inpatients POMS >0	127/230 (55%)	92/230 (40%)	50/230 (22%)	27/230 (12%)
		Inpatients POMS = 0	103/230 (45%)	122/230 (53%)	71/230 (31%)	12/230 (5%)

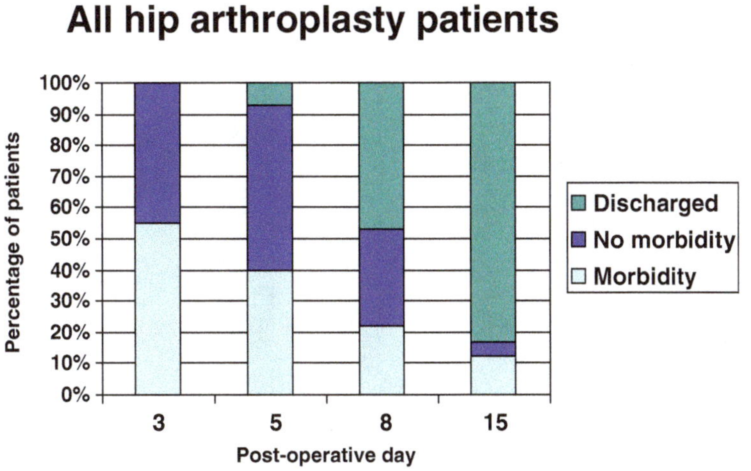

Figure 1 Discharge status and prevalence of morbidity following all types of hip arthroplasty.

F) New morbidity and readmission

Thirty-eight out of 529 patients developed morbidity as an in-patient following a period without morbidity. Five of these patients underwent a second surgical procedure and developed morbidity in the second post-operative period. Thirty patients (6.2%) developed morbidity following a period without morbidity. Twenty-five of these patients developed wound morbidity: 24 patients had no morbidity on POD 3 but developed wound morbidity by POD 5, and 1 revision arthroplasty patient had no morbidity on POD 5 but developed wound morbidity by POD 8. Six patients developed cardiovascular morbidity after a period with no morbidity: 5 patients were prescribed anticoagulation (2 for pulmonary embolus and 3 for deep vein thrombosis) and 1 patient had a myocardial infarction. One patient developed neurological morbidity (a cerebro-vascular accident) after a period without morbidity, and 1 patient developed infectious morbidity (an infected peripheral cannula site) after a period without morbidity.

No patient in this study was readmitted to the same hospital in the first year following discharge for any reason relating to their surgery.

Discussion

This study identifies many patients remaining in hospital with no identifiable morbidity following lower-limb arthroplasty in a UK teaching hospital. The rate of inappropriate bed occupancy varies with time after surgery and type of arthroplasty.

The most common reason for patients remaining in hospital with no identifiable morbidity was ongoing physiotherapy and occupational therapy. This suggests that improving pre- and post-operative planning could improve appropriate bed occupancy. Patients could be taught post-operative physiotherapy exercises in group classes prior to surgery. Occupational therapists could assess each patient's home environment and ensure necessary modifications are made. In the post-operative

Table 4 Location of patients following knee arthroplasty

			Day 3 post-op	Day 5 post-op	Day 8 post-op	Day 15 post-op
Procedure	UKR	Patients discharged	7/66 (11%)	33/66 (50%)	59/66 (89%)	65/66 (98%)
		Inpatients POMS >0	17/66 (26%)	7/66 (11%)	3/66 (5%)	1/66 (2%)
		Inpatients POMS = 0	42/66 (63%)	26/66 (39%)	4/66 (6%)	0/66 (0%)
	TKR	Patients discharged	0/226 (0%)	22/226 (10%)	145/226 (64%)	211/226 (93%)
		Inpatients POMS >0	114/226 (50%)	90/226 (40%)	38/226 (17%)	7/22 (3%)
		Inpatients POMS = 0	112/226 (50%)	114/226 (50%)	43/226 (19%)	8/226 (4%)
	Revision TKR	Patients discharged	0/8 (0%)	1/8 (13%)	1/8 (13%)	6/8 (75%)
		Inpatients POMS >0	6/8 (75%)	4/8 (50%)	5/8 (62%)	1/8 (12.5%)
		Inpatients POMS = 0	2/8 (25%)	3/8 (37%)	2/8 (25%)	1/8 (12.5%)
	TOTAL	Patients discharged	7/300 (2%)	56/300 (19%)	205/300 (68%)	282/300 (94%)
		Inpatients POMS >0	137/300 (46%)	101/300 (34%)	46/300 (15%)	9/300 (3%)
		Inpatients POMS = 0	156/300 (52%)	143/300 (47%)	49/300 (17%)	9/300 (3%)

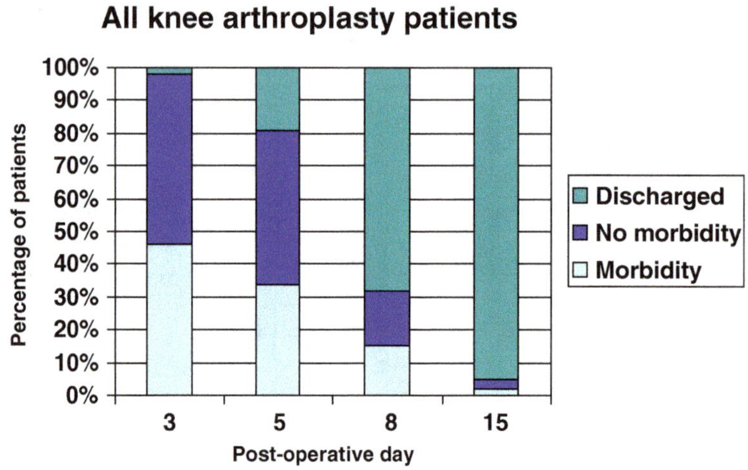

Figure 2 Discharge status and prevalence of morbidity following all types of knee arthroplasty.

period 'fast-track' pathways could be used to ensure maximum therapy input at the earliest possible opportunity. Some physiotherapy and occupational therapy could be provided post-operatively in a rehabilitation unit or at the patient's home rather than in hospital. This would require safety and cost evaluation prior to implementation.

Three of the top five reasons for patients remaining in hospital with no identifiable morbidity relate to 'social' issues (awaiting home equipment, awaiting a rehabilitation bed, awaiting a package of care from social services). Pre-operative clinics could identify and address these problems prior to admission. Such clinics could also be used to manage patient expectation so they are aware of the difficulties they may encounter in the post-operative period and the expected timing of discharge.

This study has several strengths. A large consecutive dataset was collected prospectively using a validated methodology for measuring post-operative morbidity. This is the first published study to prospectively evaluate the appropriateness of discharge following lower limb joint replacement surgery.

Table 5 Number of inappropriate inpatient days classified by type of arthroplasty

	Total number of patients	Total number of inappropriate in-patient days	Average number of inappropriate in-patient days per patient
HR	33	78	2.36
THR	162	678	4.19
Revision THR	35	363	10.37
UKR	63	111	1.76
TKR	227	620	2.73
Revision TKR	8	115	14.38
Total	528	1965	3.72

The weaknesses of this study are that it was conducted in a single centre, POMS is not validated as a bed utilisation tool, there was not daily recording of data so the calculation of excess days are an approximation, and patient mobility was not fully assessed. Data was collected regarding mobility aids, but the distance each patient could mobilise was not recorded.

This is the first time that POMS has been used as a bed utilisation tool. It has not been validated for this purpose but has previously been used to identify patients in hospitals without morbidity [5,6]. In the US, over 98% of in-patients had morbidity defined by POMS [5] suggesting that patients with POMS score of 0 were rapidly discharged. In a previous UK study, 63% of orthopaedic patients remained in hospital with no morbidity on POD 3 and 42% on POD 5 suggesting that discharge efficiency was lower in the UK institution. In the US, many post-operative arthroplasty patients are discharged to a rehabilitation unit. This practice is far less common in the UK and may partially account for the discrepancy in discharge efficiency.

Use of POMS as a bed utilisation tool relies on the assumption that it captures all reasons for remaining in hospital. In this study, the main reason for remaining in hospital with no identifiable morbidity was 'ongoing physiotherapy and occupational therapy input'. A specific concern in this patient group, who are often elderly and frail, is that they may not have adequate mobility to be discharged safely. Including a specific domain for mobility may improve the sensitivity of POMS for morbidity requiring hospitalisation following orthopaedic surgery. The domain should assess the ability to walk short distances, ability to climb a flight of stairs and a balance and falls assessment. Whilst this domain could be

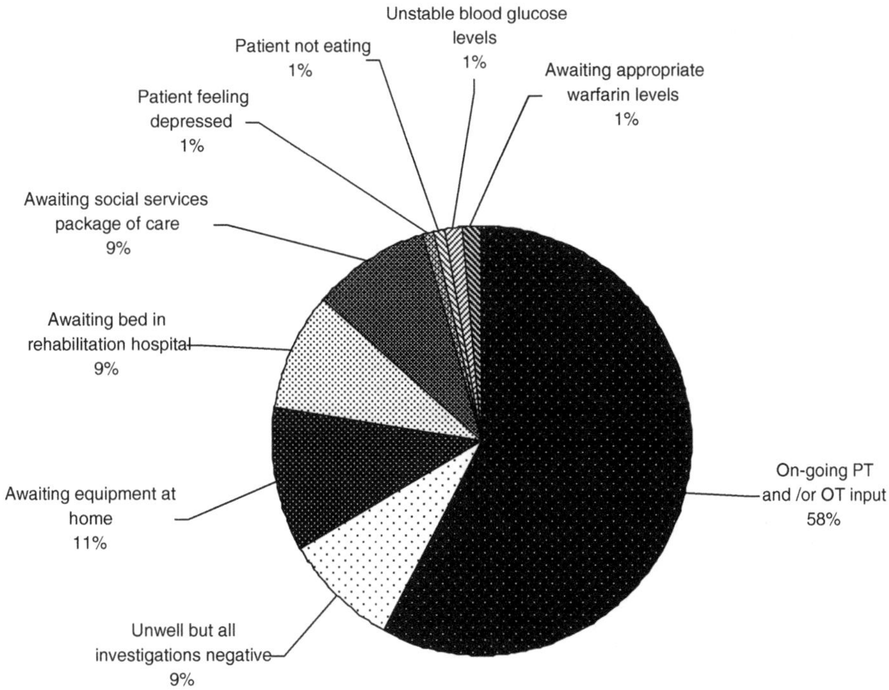

Figure 3 Reasons lower-limb arthroplasty patients with no morbidity remained in the hospital on post-operative days 8 and 15.

especially relevant for orthopaedic patients, this requires further investigation.

Use of POMS as a 'fitness for discharge' tool rests on the assumption that patients do not develop new morbidity after they have become free from morbidity, either in hospital or following discharge. No patients were readmitted to the study hospital in the first post-operative year for complications linked to surgery. However, 33 patients (6.2%) developed 'new' morbidity following a period without morbidity whilst in hospital. This highlights a limitation of prospectively using POMS as a 'fitness for discharge' tool. 25 of 33 (76%) of these patients developed wound morbidity after a period with no morbidity. To overcome this potential problem, primary arthroplasty patients should have regular wound reviews until POD 5 and revision arthroplasty patients until POD 8. This could be performed in an outpatient or primary care setting by a doctor or nurse. Extra capacity would be needed to ensure no negative impact on existing services. This would add cost to each patient episode but would be more cost effective than patients remaining in hospital. Patients should be aware of the risk of deep vein thrombosis, pulmonary embolus, myocardial infarction and cerebro-vascular accident following discharge and receive clear written instructions regarding symptoms and management. As long as these precautionary measures are in place, POMS has potential as a bed utilisation tool.

The most commonly used tool to assess appropriate bed utilisation in the literature is the Appropriateness Evaluation Protocol (AEP) [10]. AEP is a retrospective tool that relies on data from the inpatient record. It has been shown to be valid and reliable in some studies [10] but not in others [11]. POMS is a prospective tool that could be used in real time to assist with appropriate patient discharge. AEP is a retrospective tool that can only be used to evaluate past events. Data for POMS is collected directly from contemporary data sources whilst the patient is in hospital; AEP relies solely on past patient records and is therefore dependent on completeness and accuracy of record keeping for reliable functioning.

AEP has been used in several European countries to examine bed utilisation. In Portugal, 50% of inpatient days were deemed inappropriate [12], in Italy 37.3% [3], in Germany 28% [13], in Switzerland 8% to 15% [14] and in France 7% [15]. This study indicates bed utilisation in the UK is comparable to that seen in Portugal and Italy but such a direct comparison may have limited validity since different bed utilisation tools have been used.

The finding that many fewer patients remain in the hospital with no morbidity (as defined by POMS) in the US when compared with the UK suggests that bed utilisation in the US is superior to that seen in the UK. The implementation of 'payment by results' in the UK aims to improve appropriate bed occupancy to optimise patient care and improve efficiency. If the patients in this study had been discharged when they first had no morbidity defined by POMS, a saving of over £750,000 could have been made in 1 year (based on a cost of £400 per bed-day). This money could be reinvested in rehabilitation services with a strong emphasis on therapies rather than being spent on unnecessary inpatient medical care.

Conclusions

We believe that POMS is able to identify patients remaining in hospital without clinically significant morbidity and may be used prospectively as a bed utilisation tool. To use the survey for this purpose, it may be useful to add an additional measure to assess mobility.

Abbreviations

AEP: appropriateness evaluation protocol; ASA: American Society of Anesthesiologists; HR: hip resurfacing; POD: post-operative day; POMS: post-operative morbidity survey; THR: total hip replacement; TKR: total knee replacement; UK: United Kingdom; UKR: unicondylar knee replacement; US: United States (of America).

Competing interests

The authors declare that they have no competing interests.

Authors' contributions

EA participated in the design of the study, analysed the data and wrote the manuscript. CM collected data and helped with data analysis. MGM and FSH participated in the design and coordination of the study as well as interpretation of the data. MPWG participated in the study design, data analysis and helped to write the manuscript. All authors read and approved the final manuscript.

Authors' information

EA is an orthopaedic registrar at the Royal National Orthopaedic Hospital, Middlesex. CM is affiliated to the Surgical Outcomes Research Centre, University College London Hospitals. MGM is a medical professor of anaesthesia at the UCL Institute of Child Health; Surgical Outcomes Research Centre, Joint UCH/UCL Comprehensive Biomedical Research Centre. FSH is a professor of orthopaedic surgery at the University College London Hospital. MPWG is a professor of Anaesthesia and Critical Care Medicine, Integrative Physiology and Critical Illness Group, Clinical and Experimental Sciences at the University of Southampton; University Hospital Southampton/University of Southampton NIHR Respiratory Biomedical Research Unit; senior lecturer at the UCL Institute of Child Health and at the Surgical Outcomes Research Centre, Joint UCH/UCL Comprehensive Biomedical Research Centre.

Acknowledgements

We would like to acknowledge Maj Mutch for collecting much of the data and Ramani Moonesinghe for managing the data.

Funding

Funding was received from the Special Trustees of the Middlesex Hospital and University College Hospital/UCL NIHR Biomedical Research Centre.

Author details

[1]Catterall Unit, Royal National Orthopaedic Hospital, Brockley Hill, Stanmore, Middlesex HA7 4LP, UK. [2]Surgical Outcomes Research Centre, University College London Hospital, 235 Euston Road, Fitzrovia, London NW1 2BU, UK. [3]UCL Institute of Child Health, Surgical Outcomes Research Centre, Joint UCLH/UCL Comprehensive Biomedical Research Centre, Gower Street, London WC1E 6BT, UK. [4]University College London Hospital, 235 Euston Road, Fitzrovia, London NW1 2BU, UK. [5]Integrative Physiology and Critical Illness Group, Clinical and Experimental Sciences, University of Southampton, University Road, Southampton SO17 1BJ, UK. [6]NIHR Respiratory Biomedical Research Unit, University Hospital Southampton/University of Southampton, University Road, Southampton SO17 1BJ, UK.

References

1. UK Department of Health. The NHS Plan. http://www.dh.gov.uk/prod_consum_dh/groups/dh_digitalassets/@dh/@en/@ps/documents/digitalasset/dh_118522.pdf. Accessed 1 July 2000.
2. UK Department of Health. Response to reforming NHS financial flows: introducing payment by results. http://www.dh.gov.uk/prod_consum_dh/groups/dh_digitalassets/@dh/@en/documents/digitalasset/dh_4018704.pdf. Accessed October 2002.
3. Angelillo IF, Ricciardi G, Nante N, Boccia A, Bianco A, La Torre G, et al. Appropriateness of hospital utilisation in Italy. Public Health. 2000;114:9–14.
4. Alijani A, Hanna GB, Ziyaie D, Burns SL, Campbell KL, McMurdo ME, et al. Instrument for objective assessment of appropriateness of surgical bed occupancy: validation study. BMJ. 2003;326:1243–4.
5. Bennett-Guerrero E, Welsby I, Dunn TJ, Young LR, Wahl TA, Diers TL, et al. The use of a postoperative morbidity survey to evaluate patients with prolonged hospitalization after routine, moderate-risk, elective surgery. Anesth Analg. 1999;89:514–9.
6. Grocott MPW, Browne JP, Van der Meulen J, Matejowsky C, Mutch M, Hamilton MA, et al. The Post-Operative Morbidity Survey was validated and used to describe morbidity following major surgery. J Clin Epidemiol. 2007;60:919–28.
7. Bennett-Guerrero E, Feierman DE, Barclay GR, Parides MK, Sheiner PA, Mythen MG, et al. Preoperative and intraoperative predictors of postoperative morbidity, poor graft function, and early rejection in 190 patients undergoing liver transplantation. Arch Surg. 2001;136:1177–83.
8. Wakeling HG, McFall MR, Jenkins CS, Woods WG, Miles WF, Barclay GR, et al. Intraoperative oesophageal Doppler guided fluid management shortens postoperative hospital stay after major bowel surgery. Br J Anaesth. 2005;95:634–42.
9. Webb A. Solutions for reducing length of stay. Health Service Journal. http://www.hsj.co.uk/resource-centre/solutions-for-reducing-length-of-stay/373020.article. Accessed 14 January 2008.
10. Gertman PM, Restuccia JD. The appropriateness evaluation protocol: a technique for assessing unnecessary days of hospital care. Med Care. 1981;19:855–71.
11. Kalant N, Berlinquet M, Diodati JG, Dragatakis L, Marcotte F. How valid are utilization review tools in assessing appropriate use of acute care beds? Can Med Assoc J. 2000;162:1809–13.
12. Bentes M, Gonsalves ML, Santos M, Pina E. Design and development of a utilization review program in Portugal. Int J Qual Health Care. 1995;7:201–12.
13. Sangha O, Schneeweiss S, Wildner M, Cook EF, Brennan TA, Witte J, et al. Metric properties of the appropriateness evaluation protocol and predictors of inappropriate hospital use in Germany: an approach using longitudinal patient data. Int J Qual Health Care. 2002;14:483–92.
14. Santos-Eggimann B, Paccaud F, Blanc T. Medical appropriateness of hospital utilization: an overview of the Swiss experience. Int J Qual Health Care. 1995;7:227–32.
15. D'Alche-Gautier M, Maiza D, Chastang F. Assessing the appropriateness of hospitalisation days in a French university hospital. Int J of Health Care Qual Assurance. 2004;17:87–91.

14

The impact of complications following open colectomy on hospital finances

David N Flynn[1], Rebecca M Speck[1,2], Najjia N Mahmoud[3], Guy David[4,5] and Lee A Fleisher[1,2,5*]

Abstract

Background: When hospitals suffer financial losses when postoperative complications occur, they may have a direct financial incentive to initiate quality improvement programs. The purpose of this research was to determine the relationship between complications following open colectomy and hospital finances.

Methods: After obtaining Institutional Review Board approval, we conducted a retrospective chart review of 276 open colectomies performed at the Hospital of the University of Pennsylvania. The medical records were manually reviewed for complications that occurred within 30 days after surgery. Financial information, including total, fixed and variable costs, was obtained from the hospital's cost accounting database. Reimbursement assuming payment by Medicare was calculated. Differences in costs, reimbursements and total margins were analyzed.

Results: Of 276 patient records reviewed, 61 (22%) of the patients experienced postoperative complications. When complications occurred, mean total costs increased from \$23,101 to \$48,180, fixed costs increased from \$14,516 to \$30,339 and variable costs increased from \$8,535 to \$17,848 ($P < 0.001$ for each comparison); the mean reimbursement increased from \$23,231 to \$35,651 ($P < 0.001$); and the total margin decreased from \$131 to – \$12,528 ($P < 0.001$). Complications were associated with a more than twofold increase in length of stay in the hospital. Multiple regression modeling indicated similar increases in each of the financial variables and length of stay as a result of postoperative complications. The impact of these complications on each outcome measure was similar in effect for patients in the matched subset of 100 patients.

Conclusion: Our results demonstrate a financial incentive for hospitals to investigate quality improvement measures to prevent postoperative complications and avoid the associated financial losses.

Keywords: Cost, Complications, Colectomy

Background

Value is the new focus of the American health-care system [1], with payers, providers and policy makers searching for ways to improve outcomes and contain costs [2]. Complications following surgery are value-destroying events because they contribute to poor outcomes while increasing the costs borne by hospitals and health-care payers [3]. As a result, initiatives designed to prevent surgical complications, such as the National Surgical Quality Improvement Program (NSQIP), have gained increasing importance at both the individual hospital and nationwide levels [4].

The impact of improved health-care quality on hospital finances is of great importance to hospital financial managers and administrators. Launching an initiative to reduce surgical complications requires allocation of scarce hospital resources, potentially at the expense of alternative quality improvement programs [5,6]. Quantifying the impact of postoperative complications on hospital resources is therefore a useful exercise that can help financial managers optimally allocate these resources to benefit both patients and hospitals.

* Correspondence: lee.fleisher@uphs.upenn.edu
[1]Department of Anesthesiology and Critical Care, Perelman School of Medicine, University of Pennsylvania, 3400 Spruce Street, Philadelphia, PA 19104, USA
[2]Center for Pharmacoepidemiology Research and Training, Center for Clinical Epidemiology and Biostatistics, Perelman School of Medicine, University of Pennsylvania, 423 Guardian Drive, Philadelphia, PA 19104, USA
Full list of author information is available at the end of the article

Colectomy has become a focus of quality improvement initiatives because of the large number of these operations performed each year and the high incidence of associated complications. The procedure, performed on nearly 275,000 patients annually [7], has been shown in several studies to have 30-day complication rates exceeding 25% [8-10]. A 2008 study of 36 general surgical procedures involving more than 129,000 patients found that colectomy, though it represented less than 10% of all cases, was responsible for 24.3% of all adverse events and the greatest share of morbidity, mortality and increased length of stay (LOS) of the procedures studied [9]. Furthermore, a majority of adverse events involving colon resection are considered preventable [11], suggesting that quality improvement applied to colon surgery could be a particularly fruitful undertaking.

Although numerous studies have demonstrated that surgical complications significantly increase hospital costs, data regarding the overall financial impact of postoperative complications on hospitals are scarce. Although some of these additional costs may be offset by higher reimbursement from payers [3,12], little is known about the sources of increased hospital costs or the extent to which payers compensate hospitals for increased expenses for postoperative complications.

We hypothesized that surgical complications would be financially detrimental to hospitals, resulting in increased costs and decreased profit margins. In this study, we examined the increment in hospital costs and reimbursements associated with complications following open colectomies at a large academic medical center. We modeled reimbursement under the simplifying assumption that all patients were insured by Medicare. Using cost and reimbursement data, we calculated total margins (that is, profitability) and compared the results between patients who experienced complications and patients who did not. Finally, we discussed the implications of our results on the financial case for complication prevention from the perspective of hospital financial managers and administrators.

Methods

Study design and setting

We conducted a retrospective review of all medical records of patients who underwent open partial colectomy with anastomosis during a 4-year period (2007 through 2010) at the Hospital of the University of Pennsylvania, a large, urban academic medical center. This study was conducted after we received approval from the Institutional Review Board of the University of Pennsylvania. Approval included a waiver of documentation of informed consent, given the retrospective, minimal risk nature of the research. The study was conducted and reported in accordance with the Strengthening the Reporting of Observational Studies in Epidemiology statement for observational studies [13].

Data sources

Patient data and dates of admissions were obtained from the hospital's administrative database. Complications were identified by manual review of the hospital's electronic medical records. Financial data were obtained from the hospital's internal cost accounting database (Horizon Performance Manager Cost Accounting System; McKesson, San Francisco, CA, USA). The accounting system assigns a unit cost to each charge item or service provided (excluding physicians' professional fees) using either the relative value unit (RVU) or ratio of cost to charge (RCC) cost accounting methods. The RCC method is used to determine the costs of medications and supplies, and the RVU method is used to assign costs to particular services, from both service centers (for example, nursing or radiology) and support centers (for example, information technology or housekeeping) [7]. The costs for each item or service provided during an encounter are then mapped to charge categories (fixed costs, variable labor costs and variable supply costs), which are then added to determine the total cost of resources consumed during each encounter.

Participants

Study patients were located by searching the hospital's administrative database for Current Procedural Terminology (CPT) code 41440 (open partial colectomy with anastomosis). Study exclusion criteria included (1) age younger than 18 years, (2) concomitant surgery involving an organ outside the lower gastrointestinal (GI) tract, (3) failure to perform surgery within 48 hours after hospital admission and/or (4) incomplete medical or financial records. Demographic data collected for each patient included age, gender, American Society of Anesthesiologists (ASA) physical status score and body mass index (BMI).

Complications

Each patient's electronic medical record was manually reviewed for major complications occurring within 30 days after surgery. Complications abstracted included deep wound surgical site infection (SSI), organ/space infection SSI, sepsis, *Clostridium difficile* colitis, pneumonia, myocardial infarction, new-onset arrhythmia, cardiac arrest, pulmonary embolism, acute renal failure and/or acute kidney injury, cerebrovascular accident, hemorrhage requiring transfusion of more than 4 U of packed red blood cells (RBCs), bowel obstruction, reoperation, death and other complications. *Other complications* included any condition not present upon admission that could potentially be harmful to the patient's health that was documented in the medical record by an attending physician. We used standard American College of Surgeons NSQIP definitions when available. *C. difficile* colitis and bowel obstruction were recorded on the basis of the attending physician's diagnosis.

Financial outcomes and lengths of stay

Clinical data were merged with financial data to determine the costs associated with each patient's care. Costs examined included total costs, fixed costs and variable costs. For patients who were readmitted to the hospital within 30 days after the initial surgery, the cost of each inpatient encounter was added to determine the total cost for all hospital admissions. All costs were adjusted to 2010 US dollars (USD) using the hospital inpatient services subcategory of the Consumer Price Index (CPI) obtained from the US Bureau of Labor Statistics [12].

The patients in this study were insured by various payers, including Medicare, Medicaid and commercial insurers, so, in addition to obtaining the actual payments, we calculated expected reimbursements under the simplifying assumption that all study patients were insured by Medicare only. This step was included to eliminate the impact of payer mix on financial outcomes, which may vary substantially between hospitals and have a significant impact on reimbursement and overall profitability. We calculated the expected Medicare reimbursement for each patient using the Medicare Severity Diagnosis-Related Group (MS-DRG) payment rate at our hospital during each year of services. (A brief overview of the Medicare system is provided in the Appendix). A unique MS-DRG was assigned for each admission using an automated MS-DRG grouper based on International Classification of Disease, Ninth Revision (ICD-9) discharge and procedure codes (3M Co, St Paul, MN, USA). Payment rates for 2007 were not available, so the corresponding 2008 rates were used for patients treated during 2007 and 2008. Payments were adjusted to 2010 USD using the general CPI. LOS was also calculated for each patient. For patients who were readmitted within 30 days after surgery, LOS from the index visit and subsequent readmissions occurring within the study period were added to determine the total LOS associated with the procedure.

Statistical methods

Bivariate comparisons of continuous data were made using Student's *t*-test. The impact of complications on financial variables was analyzed using multiple linear regression analysis. Additional explanatory variables used in the regression analysis included age, age-squared (to allow for nonlinear effects of age on the rate of complications), gender, ASA classification and BMI.

To control for potential confounding effects resulting from underlying differences between groups, we used the Coarsened Exact Matching (CEM) algorithm [14] to match patients who experienced complications on a one-to-one basis to patients without complications. Patients were matched for age, gender, ASA classification and BMI. CEM is relatively a new nonparametric matching method developed to address limitations of more widely used methods such as propensity score matching. CEM has been described in detail elsewhere, so we will discuss it here only briefly. When performing CEM, the original values of the covariates are first coarsened, or divided into two or more user-defined ranges or categories. The CEM algorithm is then used to create a set of strata, each of which contains variables that share identical coarsened values for every covariate. Strata that contain patients in both the treatment and control groups are retained, and patients from the treatment group and control group paired within each stratum. After matching has been performed, the coarsened values are replaced by their original values, allowing subsequent analysis of the uncoarsened values of each covariate to proceed.

We used CEM because it offers several advantages over existing methods, such as Propensity Score Matching (PSM). First, CEM is a member of the Monotonic Imbalance Bounding (MIB) class of matching methods, which generalizes the Equal Percent Bias Reducing (EPBR) class (comprising PSM and many other popular matching methods, such as Mahalanobis matching, Genetic Matching and others), eliminating key assumptions required to generate unbiased estimates of treatment effects. Second, with CEM, the process used to create matches is reversed. With CEM (and MIB methods in general), the user chooses the maximum level of imbalance *ex ante* (determined by the level of coarsening), with the number of matches produced as a result. With EPBR methods, the number of matched observations is chosen *ex ante*, with an unknown amount of imbalance produced as a result. Thus, with CEM, the need for repeated postmatch balance-checking, model modification and rematching required by other methods is eliminated, although the level of coarsening may need to be altered to produce a satisfactory sample size. Third, with CEM, the imbalance on one covariate can be changed in isolation without affecting the imbalance on any other covariates. This contrasts with EPBR methods, in which altering the imbalance on one covariate changes the imbalance on all other covariates, sometimes in unpredictable ways. Fourth, CEM has been shown through simulation on multiple data sets to be superior to alternative matching methods by producing matches with reduced imbalance, bias, variance, model dependence, estimation error and mean square error [15,16].

All statistical analyses were conducted using Stata version 11.0 software (StataCorp, Austin, TX, USA). For all calculations, statistical significance was defined by *P*-values less than 0.05.

Results

A total of 380 patients were identified, 276 of whom met our inclusion criteria. Reasons for exclusion included concomitant surgery outside the lower GI tract (47 patients), surgery more than 48 hours after admission (48 patients) and incomplete medical or financial records (3 patients). An additional six patients met two exclusion criteria because they had concomitant surgery outside the GI tract more than 48 hours after admission.

Among the 276 included patients, 61 patients (22% of the total) experienced one or more major complications (Table 1). The most common complication was organ/space SSI (5.1% of patients), followed by new-onset arrhythmia (4.7%), reoperation (4.7%) and bowel obstruction (4.0%). All other complications were relatively uncommon, occurring in fewer than 3.0% of patients. Only one patient death occurred, which followed the only recorded cardiac arrest (believed to be precipitated by a massive pulmonary embolism). Postoperative complications were often related. For example, 9 of the 13 reoperations were performed as a result of either deep SSI or organ and/or surgical space infections.

Unmatched sample

There were no statistically significant differences between patient groups with respect to age, gender, BMI or ASA classification in the unmatched samples (Table 2). However, patients in the complications group tended to be older, more often male and had higher ASA scores than those in the uncomplicated group. Mean LOS was more than twice as long for patients who experienced complications (15.6 days) than for those who had no complications (7.3 days).

Table 1 Number and incidence of complications[a]

Complications	Number of patients	%
Deep SSI	5	1.8%
Organ/space SSI	14	5.1%
Sepsis	5	1.8%
Clostridium difficile colitis	4	1.4%
Pneumonia	8	2.9%
Bowel obstruction	11	4.0%
Acute kidney injury	6	2.2%
Cerebrovascular accident	2	0.7%
Pulmonary embolism	4	1.4%
New-onset arrhythmia	13	4.7%
Myocardial infarction	5	1.8%
Cardiac arrest	1	0.4%
Unplanned intubation	6	2.2%
Reoperation	13	4.7%
Death	1	0.4%
Other infections	7	2.5%

[a]SSI: Surgical site infection. The category "Other infections" included readmission for unexplained severe gastritis, hypotension of unknown cause prompting transfer to the surgical intensive care unit (SICU), upper-extremity ischemia presumed to be caused by vasospasm, respiratory depression from opiate overdose requiring SICU transfer, readmission for biliary colic requiring surgical intervention, readmission for chylous ascites requiring paracentesis and postdural puncture headache requiring epidural blood patch ($n = 1$ for each complication).

Complications were associated with dramatic increases in total, fixed and variable costs; increased reimbursements; and decreased total margins (Table 2). The mean total cost was $23,101 for patients in the uncomplicated group compared to $48,180 for those in the complications group, a difference of $24,079. Fixed and variable costs were more than doubled when complications occurred. Mean reimbursement was $12,420 higher for patients in the complications group ($35,651) than for patients in the uncomplicated group ($23,231). Patients in the uncomplicated group generated a small but positive total margin (that is, gain) of $131 per patient, whereas patients in the complications group generated a large negative total margin (that is, loss) of $12,528 per patient.

Table 3 displays the results of the multiple linear regression analysis for each outcome variable, adjusted for the effects of age, age-squared, gender, ASA classification and BMI. The results of this analysis were similar to the unadjusted differences between the two groups with regard to the mean values (Table 2). Complications were associated with an increase in total cost of $24,889, an increase in reimbursement of $12,326 and a decrease in total margin of $12,563.

Matched sample

The 50 patients in who experienced complications were matched to 50 similar patients who without complications. Suitable matches were not found for the remaining 11 patients who had complications. Differences in age, gender, BMI and ASA classification were minimal between complication groups in the matched sample (Table 2).

Complications were associated an increase in total costs of $26,351, an increase in reimbursement of $12,108 and a decrease in total margin of $14,244. Complications were associated with an increase in LOS of 8.5 days.

The results of the multivariate regression analysis (Table 3) were nearly identical to the unadjusted results. After adjustment, complications were associated with an increase in total cost of $26,269, an increase in reimbursement of $12,138 and a decrease in total margin of $14,131.

Discussion

The purpose of this study was to evaluate the financial impact of surgical complications following open colectomy from the perspective of hospital financial managers and administrators. To eliminate the impact of payer mix on our

Table 2 Patient demographic data, length of stay and financial data by complication group for matched and unmatched samples[a]

	Entire cohort ($N = 276$)				Matched sample ($n = 100$)			
Variable	Uncomplicated	Complications	*P*-value	Difference	Uncomplicated	Complications	*P*-value	Difference
Patients, *n* (%)	215 (78%)	61 (22%)	–	–	50	50	–	–
Mean age, years (SD)	60.2 (14.8)	62.9 (13.3)	0.20	2.7	63.6 (12.9)	63.7 (12.3)	0.97	0.1
Females, *n* (%)	113 (53%)	27 (44%)	0.25	–	24 (48%)	24 (48%)	1.0	–
ASA class, mean (SD)	2.5 (0.5)	2.6 (0.5)	0.21	0.1	2.6 (0.50)	2.6 (0.50)	1.0	0
BMI, mean (SD)	28.4 (7.3)	28.7 (6.3)	0.74	0.3	28.1 (6.4)	28.2 (5.7)	0.93	0.1
LOS (days), mean (SD)	7.3 (2.4)	15.6 (7.8)	<0.001	8.3	7.4 (2.1)	15.9 (7.5)	<0.001	8.5
Total cost, mean (SD)	$23,101 (6,914)	$48,180 (26,596)	<0.001	$25,079	$23,381 (6,712)	$49,733 (28,279)	<0.001	$26,351
Fixed cost, mean (SD)	$14,516 (4,252)	$30,229 (16,340)	<0.001	$15,713	$14,807 (4,509)	$31,233 (17,333)	<0.001	$16,426
Variable cost, mean (SD)	$8,535 (2,904)	$17,848 (10,356)	<0.001	$9,313	$8,526 (2,656)	$18,397 (11,066)	<0.001	$9,871
Reimbursement, mean (SD)	$23,231 (6,761)	$35,651 (13,445)	<0.001	$12,420	$23,632 (7,110)	$35,739 (13,327)	<0.001	$12,108
Total margin, mean (SD)	$131 (8,309)	−$12,528 (26,113)	0.001	−$12,659	$250 (7,781)	−$13,993 (27,144)	<0.001	−$14,244

[a]ASA: American Society of Anesthesiology; BMI: Body mass index. Total margin = Reimbursement – Total cost. Financial data are US dollars.

results, we used the simplifying assumption that all patients included in the study were insured by Medicare. We found that major surgical complications were associated with higher total hospital cost and reimbursement, but decreased profitability, under Medicare payment. When complications occurred, cost increased from $23,101 to $48,180, reimbursement increased from $23,231 to $35,651 and profitability fell from a gain of $131 to a loss of $12,528.

There were no statistically significant differences in demographics or health-related attributes between study groups. This suggests that patient baseline health status cannot explain the cause or risk of complications observed. However, there were minor, non–statistically significant differences between our study groups. Patients who experienced major complications tended to be older, were assigned a higher preoperative ASA classification and were more likely to be male. Each of these factors could independently impact cost and profitability. We used a powerful matching algorithm to generate nearly perfectly matched study groups to control for these effects. Interestingly, the financial impact of major complications was even greater between the matched study groups than the original unmatched groups. This provides strong support for the assertion that the observed differences in financial outcomes were driven by the occurrence of complications rather than by variability between groups.

We used multivariate linear regression to evaluate the impact of complication status, age/age-squared, ASA classification, BMI and gender on cost, reimbursement, profitability and LOS. Only complication status had a statistically significant impact on outcomes, increasing total cost by $24,889, increasing reimbursement by $12,326 and decreasing profitability by $12,563. The results of multivariate analyses performed on the matched sample were nearly identical. This further supports the argument that complication status, rather than other factors, independently drives financial performance and strongly suggests that hospitals could benefit financially by preventing complications.

LOS has an important but underappreciated impact on hospital finances. Any event that prolongs LOS generates an opportunity cost for hospitals, especially as the health care environment is moving toward bundled payment [17,18]. Whenever a patient's LOS is prolonged, the hospital's available bed capacity is decreased, thus limiting the hospital's ability to admit additional revenue-generating patients. The cost of a missed admission is equal to the expected revenue minus the expected variable cost (that is, the contribution margin). Because variable costs make up a small component of a hospital's total costs, the contribution margin will nearly always be large and positive. We found that complications more than doubled the LOS, indicating that the hospital could treat two uncomplicated patients in the same time required to treat single patients who experienced a major complication. Thus, our data indicate that hospitals suffer financially in at least two ways when complications occur: first, through lower expected profit margins due to treating patients who experience complications, and second, via the opportunity cost generated when capacity is consumed by prolonged hospital LOS.

Medicare has recently started to deny payment for selected diagnoses when readmissions occur within 30 days of discharge, including congestive heart failure, myocardial infarction and pneumonia [19]. This policy will eventually be extended to include other conditions, including readmissions related to surgical complications. For the purposes of this study, we assumed that all

Table 3 Relationships between major surgical complications and cost, reimbursement, total margin and length of stay, controlling for effects of age, gender, American Society of Anesthesiology score and body mass index[a]

	Entire patient cohort ($N = 276$)						Matched sample ($n = 100$)					
Dependent variable	Total cost	Fixed cost	Variable costs	Reimbursement	Total margin	Length of stay (days)	Total cost	Fixed cost	Variable costs	Reimbursement	Total margin	LOS (days)
Complication	$24,889[b]	$15,610[b]	$9,228[b]	$12,326[b]	–$12,563[b]	8.29[b]	$26,269[b]	$16,368[b]	$9,846[b]	$12,138[b]	–$14,131[b]	8.456[b]
	(2,024)	(1,246)	(799)	(1,272)	(2,083)	(0.607)	(4,168)	(2,566)	(1,634)	(2,175)	(4,022)	(1.116)
Age	-$118	–$54	–$63	–$153	–$35	–0.135	$854	$572	$281	$16	–$838	0.256
	(393)	(242)	(155)	(247)	(404)	(0.118)	(1,498)	(922)	(587)	(782)	(1,445)	(401)
Age-squared	$1	$1	$1	$1	$0	0.001	–$8	–$6	–$3	$0	$8	–0.002
	(3)	(2)	(1)	(2)	(3)	(0.001)	(12)	(7)	(5)	(6)	(12)	(0.003)
Female gender	$2,047	$1,258	$796	–$578	–$2,625	0.493	$4,442	$2,698	$1,759	–$991	–$5,432	1.093
	(1,680)	(1,034)	(663)	(1,056)	(1,729)	(0.504)	(4,313)	(2,655)	(1,691)	(2,251)	(4,161)	(1.154)
ASA score	$2,598	$1,397	$1,200	$1,391	–$1,207	0.611	$2,272	$1,194	$1,074	–$159	–$2,430	0.411
	(1,758)	(1,082)	(694)	(1,104)	(1,809)	(0.528)	(4,755)	(2,927)	(1,864)	(2,482)	(4,588)	(1.272)
BMI	$53	$38	$16	–$110	–$163	0.006	–$51	–$17	–$34	–$208	–$158	–0.024
	(121)	(75)	(48)	(76)	(125)	(0.036)	(375)	(231)	(147)	(196)	(362)	(0.100)
Constant	$15,636	$9,791	$5,797	$27,531[b]	$11,895	8.011[c]	–$2,900	–$2,330	–$584	$31,214	$34,114	0.494
	(11,860)	(7,298)	(4,682)	(7,450)	(12,202)	(3.559)	(45,162)	(27,804)	(17,704)	(23,573)	(43,578)	(12,090)[c]
Observations	276	276	276	276	276	276	100	100	100	100	100	100
R^2	0.3764	0.3835	0.3509	0.2733	0.1391	0.4290	0.3137	0.3197	0.2945	0.2600	0.1496	0.3928

[a]ASA: American Society of Anesthesiology; BMI: Body mass index; LOS: Length of stay. [b]$P < 0.001$. [c]$P < 0.05$. All values were obtained using multiple linear regression techniques as described in the Methods section. Values in parentheses are standard errors.

readmissions were reimbursed fully by Medicare. Denial of payment for readmissions would result in losses greater than those calculated in this study, thus providing additional incentives for hospitals to prevent complications and the readmissions that frequently accompany them.

Eappen and coauthors [17] found that surgical complications were associated with increased total margin for commercially insured patients but decreased total margin for patients who were self-insured or covered by Medicare or Medicaid. Owing to the relatively small sample size in our study, we assumed that all patients were insured by Medicare, thus eliminating the impact of payer mix on our results. In contrast to the findings of Eappen *et al.*, however, when we used actual payment received in the analysis, regardless of payer type, patients who experienced complications generated negative margins (losses averaging nearly $8,000/patient), whereas uncomplicated patients generated positive margins (gains of nearly $1,200/patient). This suggests that the financial incentive to prevent complications is preserved when actual payment is considered at our institution.

In this study, we did not evaluate the impact of individual types of complications on financial performance or the preventability of different complications. Previous studies have demonstrated that certain complications are far more expensive to treat than others [20,21]. Additionally, certain complications may be far more difficult to prevent than others, whereas some complications may simply be inevitable because of the underlying disease burden of surgical patients. From a strictly financial standpoint, treatment of patients with complications that are both preventable and associated with the highest cost should be prioritized.

This study has several limitations that warrant discussion. First, physicians' professional fees and payments were not included in the analyses, so our results may understate both the increase in cost and reimbursement associated with complications. Second, because our chart review was limited to a single hospital, patients whose readmissions occurred at other hospitals were not included in our analysis. Although it may have been feasible for us to contact all study patients and inquire about readmissions elsewhere, we used retrospective data in this study. The only potentially link of patients to this study would have been direct contact for a research telephone call, which they did not consent to at the time of procedure. Third, although we modeled reimbursement by assuming all patients were insured through Medicare, our study population might not be representative of the Medicare population. The average age of patients in each complication group, for example, was slightly less than the minimum age of 65 years at which patients become eligible for Medicare benefits. The fourth limitation concerns the generalizability of this study to other settings. All of the data in this study derived from a single US institution, with its own unique cost structure and patient population. Thus, it is difficult to predict how accurately the cost increases found in this study would predict changes in cost associated with complications at other hospitals. Moreover, hospitals operating outside of the United States generate revenue based on the financing systems of their home countries, which may differ significantly from the MS-DRG rates used in this study to determine reimbursement and calculate margins. In many countries, however (for example, England, France and Germany) the methods used to derive rates (or tariffs) share many similarities to Medicare's MS-DRGs, including adjustment for patients' comorbidities, complications and local market forces [22]. Therefore, we can predict that both costs and payments in these settings would increase when complications occur, but additional research is required to determine the extent to which payment increases offset increased expenditures.

Conclusions

Our results provide a strong argument for financial investment in quality improvement from the perspective of the hospital administrator. Increases in Medicare reimbursement resulting from postoperative complications are not large enough to compensate the hospital for the increase in total costs associated with complications. Prevention of surgical complications therefore can help to improve care quality while improving cost-effectiveness.

Appendix: the US Medicare system

Medicare is a social health insurance program administered by the US Department of Health and Human Services. Eligible beneficiaries include Americans ages 65 or older as well as Americans of any age with certain chronic diseases. Medicare is a large source of payment for inpatient hospital care in the United States, comprising 27% of all acute care hospital revenue in 2012 [23].

Medicare payment is broken into different components, each of which pays for different aspects of medical care. Medicare Part A (hospital insurance) pays for inpatient hospital care, home health care, skilled nursing facilities and hospice care. Medicare Part B (supplementary medical insurance) pays for outpatient physician and nursing services, diagnostic imaging and testing, and outpatient hospital procedures. Medicare Part D (prescription drug plan) is a voluntary, premium-based program that helps to subsidize the cost of prescription drugs for Medicare beneficiaries.

Inpatient hospital care (Medicare Part A) is financed by the Medicare inpatient prospective payment system. Each hospital is paid a predetermined amount per discharge based on the beneficiary's clinical condition and treatment strategy, which are captured through MS-DRGs. The payment rates for each MS-DRG are updated each year in an attempt to account for the average cost of resources required to treatment patients in that MS-DRG. Payments for individual hospitals are further adjusted on the basis of geographic differences with regard to labor prices, costs of providing graduate medical education and compensation of hospitals that provide care to a disproportionate share of low-income patients.

The MS-DRG system consists of 335 base DRGs, which are split into two or three MS-DRGs on the basis of the presence of one or more complications or comorbidities (CCs) or major CCs. For example, a healthy patient who undergoes a colectomy with no resulting complications may be assigned MS-DRG 331 (major small- or large-bowel procedures without CCs), whereas a patient with multiple comorbidities may be assigned MS-DRG 330 (major small- or large-bowel procedures with CCs) and a patient who experiences a serious complication may be assigned MS-DRG 329 (major small- or large-bowel procedure with major CCs). Accordingly, the hospital would receive the highest payment for MS-DRG 329, less for MS-DRG 330 and the least for MS-DRG 331.

Abbreviations

ASA: American Society of Anesthesiologists; BMI: Body mass index; CEM: Coarsened Exact Matching; CPI: Consumer Price Index; CPT: Current Procedural Terminology; EPBR: Equal Percent Bias Reducing; ICD-9: International Classification of Diseases Ninth Revision; LOS: Length of stay; MIB: Monotonic Imbalance Bounding; MS-DRG: Medicare Severity Diagnosis-Related Group; NSQIP: National Surgical Quality Improvement Program; PSM: Propensity score matching; RBC: Red blood cell; RCC: Ratio of cost to charge; RVU: Relative value unit; SSI: Surgical site infection; USD: US dollars.

Competing interests

The authors declare that they have no competing interests.

Authors' contributions

DF participated in the study design, completed data collection and drafted the manuscript. RS participated in study design and coordination and performed the statistical analysis. NM participated in the study design and helped to draft the manuscript. GD participated in the study design and performed the statistical analysis. LF conceived the study, participated in its design and coordination, and helped to draft the manuscript. All authors read and approved the final manuscript.

Acknowledgements

The authors would like to acknowledge the assistance of Marc A LaPergola, Director of Operational Reimbursement and Managed Care Analysis, University of Pennsylvania Health System, for his assistance with gathering the financial data. No financial compensation was provided for his contribution to this study.

Author details

[1]Department of Anesthesiology and Critical Care, Perelman School of Medicine, University of Pennsylvania, 3400 Spruce Street, Philadelphia, PA 19104, USA. [2]Center for Pharmacoepidemiology Research and Training, Center for Clinical Epidemiology and Biostatistics, Perelman School of Medicine, University of Pennsylvania, 423 Guardian Drive, Philadelphia, PA 19104, USA. [3]Department of Surgery, Hospital of the University of Pennsylvania, 3400 Spruce Street, Philadelphia, PA 19104, USA. [4]Department of Health Care Management, The Wharton School, University of Pennsylvania, Colonial Penn Center, 3641 Locust Walk, Philadelphia, PA 19104, USA. [5]Senior Fellow, Leonard Davis Institute of Health Economics, University of Pennsylvania, Colonial Penn Center, 3641 Locust Walk, Philadelphia, PA 19104, USA.

References

1. Porter ME: **What is value in health care?** *N Engl J Med* 2010, **363:**2477–2481.
2. Lee TH: **Putting the value framework to work.** *N Engl J Med* 2010, **363:**2481–2483.
3. Dimick JB, Weeks WB, Karia RJ, Das S, Campbell DA Jr: **Who pays for poor surgical quality? Building a business case for quality improvement.** *J Am Coll Surg* 2006, **202:**933–937.
4. Ingraham AM, Richards KE, Hall BL, Ko CY: **Quality improvement in surgery: the American College of Surgeons National Surgical Quality Improvement Program approach.** *Adv Surg* 2010, **44:**251–267.
5. Dunagan WC, Murphy DM, Hollenbeak CS, Miller SB: **Making the business case for infection control: pitfalls and opportunities.** *Am J Infect Control* 2002, **30:**86–92.
6. Weeks WB, Bagian JP: **Making the business case for patient safety.** *Jt Comm J Qual Saf* 2003, **29:**51–54.
7. Agency for Healthcare Research and Quality (AHRQ): **HCUPnet: healthcare cost and utilization project.** In . Rockville, MD: AHRQ. [http://hcupnet.ahrq.gov/]. Accessed 2 March 2014.
8. Obeid NM, Azuh O, Reddy S, Webb S, Reickert C, Velanovich V, Horst HM, Rubinfeld I: **Predictors of critical care-related complications in colectomy patients using the National Surgical Quality Improvement Program: exploring frailty and aggressive laparoscopic approaches.** *J Trauma Acute Care Surg* 2012, **72:**878–883.
9. Schilling PL, Dimick JB, Birkmeyer JD: **Prioritizing quality improvement in general surgery.** *J Am Coll Surg* 2008, **207:**698–704.
10. Singh PP, Srinivasa S, Lemanu DP, Kahokehr AA, Hill AG: **The Surgical Recovery Score correlates with the development of complications following elective colectomy.** *J Surg Res* 2013, **184:**138–144.
11. Gawande AA, Thomas EJ, Zinner MJ, Brennan TA: **The incidence and nature of surgical adverse events in Colorado and Utah in 1992.** *Surgery* 1999, **126:**66–75.
12. Hemmila MR, Jakubus JL, Maggio PM, Wahl WL, Dimick JB, Campbell DA Jr, Taheri PA: **Real money: complications and hospital costs in trauma patients.** *Surgery* 2008, **144:**307–316.
13. von Elm E, Altman DG, Egger M, Pocock SJ, Gøtzsche PC, Vandenbroucke JP, STROBE Initiative: **The Strengthening the Reporting of Observational Studies in Epidemiology (STROBE) statement: guidelines for reporting observational studies.** *Lancet* 2007, **370:**1453–1457.
14. Blackwell M, Iacus S, King G, Porro G: **cem: Coarsened Exact Matching in Stata.** *Stata J* 2009, **9:**524–546.
15. Iacus SM, King G, Porro G: **Multivariate matching methods that are Monotonic Imbalance Bounding.** *J Am Stat Assoc* 2011, **106:**345–361.
16. Wells AR, Hamar B, Bradley C, Gandy WM, Harrison PL, Sidney JA, Coberley CR, Rula EY, Pope JE: **Exploring robust methods for evaluating treatment and comparison groups in chronic care management programs.** *Popul Health Manag* 2013, **16:**35–45.
17. Eappen S, Lane BH, Rosenberg B, Lipsitz SA, Sadoff D, Matheson D, Berry WR, Lester M, Gawande AA: **Relationship between occurrence of surgical complications and hospital finances.** *JAMA* 2013, **309:**1599–1606.
18. Gawande A: **Testing, testing: the health-care bill has no master plan for curbing costs. Is that a bad thing?** *New Yorker* 2009:34–41. 14 December.
19. Joynt KE, Jha AK: **A path forward on Medicare readmissions.** *N Engl J Med* 2013, **368:**1175–1177.
20. Speir AM, Kasirajan V, Barnett SD, Fonner E Jr: **Additive costs of postoperative complications for isolated coronary artery bypass grafting patients in Virginia.** *Ann Thorac Surg* 2009, **88:**40–46.

21. Carey K, Stefos T, Zhao S, Borzecki AM, Rosen AK: **Excess costs attributable to postoperative complications.** *Med Care Res Rev* 2011, **68:**490–503.
22. Quentin W, Scheller-Kreinsen D, Blümel M, Geissler A, Busse R: **Hospital payment based on diagnosis-related groups differs in Europe and holds lessons for the United States.** *Health Aff (Millwood)* 2013, **32:**713–723.
23. Martin AB, Hartman M, Whittle L, Catlin A, National Health Expenditure Accounts Team: **National health spending in 2012: rate of health spending growth remained low for the fourth consecutive year.** *Health Aff (Millwood)* 2014, **33:**67–77.

15

Predicting, preventing, and identifying delirium after cardiac surgery

Jason B. O'Neal* and Andrew D. Shaw

Abstract

Delirium after cardiac surgery is a major problem. The exact mechanisms behind delirium are not understood. Potential pathways of delirium include neurotransmitter interference, global cognitive disorder, and neuroinflammation. Several predisposing and precipitating risk factors have been identified for postoperative delirium. The development of delirium following cardiac surgery is associated with worse outcomes in the perioperative period. Multiple interventions are being explored for the prevention and treatment of delirium. Studies investigating the potential roles of biomarkers in delirium as well as pharmacological interventions to reduce the incidence and duration of delirium are necessary to mitigate this negative outcome.

Keywords: Postoperative delirium, Cardiac surgery, Neuroinflammation

Background

Delirium is a syndrome defined as an acute state of confusion and inattention which may be accompanied by an altered level of consciousness and disorganized thinking (Cole 2004). The American Psychiatric Association's Diagnostic and Statistical Manual, 5th edition (DSM-V), provides five key components of delirium (Association AP 2013): a disturbance in attention and awareness; the disturbance is acute and develops over a short period of time while fluctuating during the course of the day; a disturbance in cognition occurs; these disturbances are not explained by another neurocognitive disorder and do not occur during a state of reduced level of arousal including coma; and there is evidence to suggest that the disturbance is caused by a medical condition, substance intoxication or withdrawal, or side effect of a medication. Other features of delirium may include psychomotor disturbances and variable emotional states. Delirium can be categorized into three subgroups: hypoactive, hyperactive, or mixed. The most common type of delirium is hypoactive. When making the diagnosis of delirium, agitation must not be misinterpreted as hyperactive delirium.

Given the range of symptoms and sub-types, the diagnosis of delirium may be difficult and under-recognized by healthcare professionals (Boustani et al. 2010). Several scales are available to assist in making the correct diagnosis. A comparison of methods in the intensive care unit (ICU) found the confusion assessment method for the ICU (CAM-ICU) to be the most valid and reliable delirium assessment tool when compared with the Nursing Delirium Screening Scale (Nu-DESC) and Delirium Detection Score (DDS) (Luetz et al. 2010). Using these tests is time-consuming, especially for providers not formally trained to complete the assessment. The optimal method(s) for assessing postoperative delirium following surgery has yet to reach a generalized consensus although the CAM-ICU is the most commonly used method by clinicians.

Postoperative delirium has been studied in various surgical patient populations. The most extensively studied groups are patients undergoing orthopedic procedures such as total hip arthroplasty or total knee arthroplasty and cardiovascular surgery patients (van Meenen et al. 2014). Delirium is associated with negative hospital outcomes including a tenfold increased risk of death, a fivefold increased risk of nosocomial complications (Inouye 2006), poor 1-year functional recovery, and postoperative cognitive decline (Saczynski et al. 2012). The long-term cognitive decline seen in some patients after the development of delirium is similar to that of Alzheimer's patients (Pandharipande et al. 2013). With reports of up to 50 % of patients over 60 years old developing postoperative delirium following cardiac surgery

* Correspondence: jason.b.oneal@vanderbilt.edu
Department of Anesthesiology, Vanderbilt University Medical Center, Nashville, TN, USA

(Rudolph et al. 2009), this patient population poses a major burden for healthcare.

This review article discusses the pathophysiology, risk factors, and complications of postoperative delirium following cardiac surgery. Pharmacological interventions which may reduce postoperative delirium and the potential role of biomarkers in this patient population are presented. In addition, we discuss several considerations for future studies in the field.

Review

Pathophysiology

The underlying mechanisms behind delirium are not fully understood. Several hypotheses exist for the pathophysiology of delirium such as neuroinflammation (Fig. 1). The stress associated with cardiac surgery, especially when cardiopulmonary bypass (CPB) is utilized, leads to a systemic inflammatory response. Elevated levels of chemokines, cytokines, and other inflammatory markers may contribute to endothelial dysfunction and disruption of the blood brain barrier (BBB) (Rudolph et al. 2008). When this occurs, the brain is susceptible to neuronal injury via neuroinflammation and the activation of microglia ensues which may be a key component to the development of delirium (Cerejeira et al. 2010).

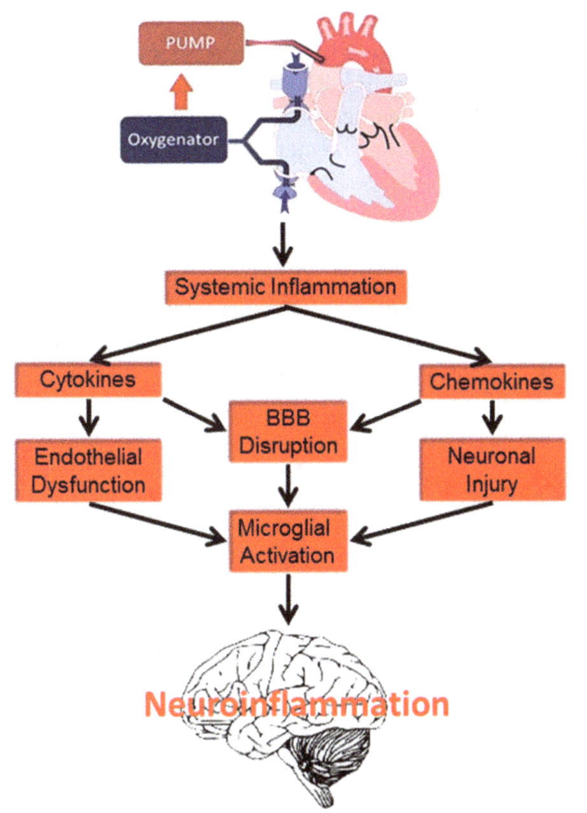

Fig. 1 Cardiopulmonary bypass and neuroinflammation

Neurotransmitter interference may lead to delirium. Reduced levels of plasma cholinesterase activity have a correlation with delirium (Cerejeira et al. 2012; Trzepacz 1996), while increased levels of dopamine may also play a part (Gaudreau & Gagnon 2005). This theory is further supported by evidence which suggests anticholinergic medications and dopaminergic medications instigate delirium (Gaudreau & Gagnon 2005; Trzepacz & van der Mast 2002).

Other theories focus on a more global cognitive disorder in which a single molecule cannot be implicated in delirium, but rather communication in the brain as a whole is impaired. This may include disturbances in the prefrontal and parietal networks, or subcortical structures including the basal ganglia, reticular activating system, thalamic nuclei, and cerebellum (Trzepacz & van der Mast 2002).

In cardiac surgery, the exposure to CPB and the stress endured by the patient produces significant inflammation, and the processes of neuroinflammation provide a logical pathway. This may also hold true in various ICU patients with a diagnosis of sepsis, severe burn injury, or polytrauma. Yet the evidence for an imbalance of certain neurotransmitters and delirium is supported and has been known for years (Cerejeira et al. 2012; Trzepacz 1996). Therefore, delirium is likely multifactorial in nature and components from each theory may be involved.

Biomarkers

A direction to expand our understanding of the mechanisms behind delirium and to identify patients at increased risk for delirium after cardiac surgery is through targeting biomarkers. Several studies have investigated biomarkers in heart disease, dementia, heart failure, and various settings of delirium, mostly in critically ill patients (Wiltfang 2014; Gaggin & Januzzi 2013; van den Boogaard et al. 2011; Khan et al. 2011). Multiple biomarkers have associations with delirium and may offer support when assessing risk, establishing diagnosis, and quantifying severity of delirium (Khan et al. 2011; Marcantonio et al. 2006).

A focused approach when evaluating biomarkers is necessary, and one that aims to quantify the probable components of neuroinflammation—endothelial dysfunction, BBB compromise, and neuronal injury—as they relate to cardiac surgery and postoperative delirium may be a promising direction. Previous studies have included pro-inflammatory, anti-inflammatory, and also neuron-specific biomarkers. A study investigating both IL-2 and TNF-α in coronary artery bypass grafting (CABG) patients with CPB not only found a correlation between each biomarker and delirium but also provided cutoff levels for increased risk of 907.5 U/ml and 10.95 pg/ml, respectively (Kazmierski et al. 2014). High levels of IL-2 were associated with a higher risk of delirium following cardiac surgery in another study (Baranyi & Rothenhausler 2014). A prospective cohort looking at pterins in postoperative delirium found that the preoperative neopterin level predicted delirium and postoperative neopterin and homovanillic acid levels were associated with delirium after cardiac surgery (Osse et al. 2012). Even with several studies showing associations of specific biomarkers and delirium, a review concluded that not enough evidence existed to support the clinical use of any biomarker for the diagnosis of delirium (Khan et al. 2011). The review did however state that S100B, insulin-like growth factor-1 (IGF-1), and some inflammatory markers demonstrated promising results.

The biomarker S100B has been associated with delirium and acute brain dysfunction in previous studies and is considered a validated measure of BBB disruption (Blyth et al. 2009). BBB disruption and neuron injury via neuroinflammation may contribute to delirium, and therefore, S100B provides support for this theory. Ubiquitin C-terminal hydrolase L1 (UCHL1) is a neuron-specific enzyme recognized in traumatic brain injury patients as a marker for direct neuron injury (Blyth et al. 2011; Brophy et al. 2011). In addition, a link between this enzyme and neurodegeneration has been suggested (Figueiredo-Pereira et al. 2014; Jara et al. 2013). The biomarker UCHL1 has yet to be investigated in delirium and could provide a novel way to predict and screen patients at risk for delirium following cardiac surgery by directly detecting injury to neurons. Another pathway to consider is impaired endothelial vascular reactivity as an association with endothelial vascular injury and brain dysfunction has been demonstrated (Hughes et al. 2013).

Risk factors

Many risk factors are associated with postoperative delirium. While some may predispose patients to delirium, other risk factors precipitate delirium such as medications given during the perioperative period. Predisposing risk factors are typically long-standing with the patient and should be recognized preoperatively in order to screen patients for increased risk. Precipitating risk factors must be considered by clinicians when treating any patient, especially patients already at high risk for postoperative delirium. Each type of risk factor can be modifiable or non-modifiable, and if possible, those that are modifiable should be optimized in the perioperative period.

Advanced age is a well-recognized risk factor for postoperative delirium. Age has been shown to be an independent risk factor in numerous studies (Chung et al. 2015; Trabold & Metterlein 2014). And with the average age of patients undergoing open-heart surgery in the mid-1960s (O'Neal et al. 2013), many patients automatically fall into a higher risk stratification.

Patients with cognitive impairment are also at risk for postoperative delirium. The incidence of dementia is estimated at 9.8 per 1000 person-years (Ruitenberg et al. 2001), and with humans living longer in a world of steadily increasing population, the prevalence of dementia will continue to rise over the foreseeable future. Impaired cognition may be unrecognized in some patients as people suffering from mild cognitive impairment may present for surgery undiagnosed as symptoms can be subtle at this stage of the disease (Robinson et al. 2012). Thus, these patients are at a greater risk for delirium without healthcare workers being aware. Clinicians should consider screening patients for cognitive impairment prior to surgery and then attempt to avoid and/or mitigate any potential precipitating risk factors in this population.

Other preoperative conditions found to have associations with postoperative delirium include anemia, dehydration, electrolyte abnormalities, and signs of malnutrition (Trabold & Metterlein 2014). A small prospective study of hospitalized patients over the age of 70 years found anemia and dehydration to be risk factors for delirium (Joosten et al. 2006). The finding of anemia as a risk factor was also demonstrated in patients after lumbar spine surgery (Fineberg et al. 2013). This finding has not been reproduced after cardiac surgery; however, whether or not addressing these risk factors prior to surgery can influence the outcome of delirium has yet to be elucidated. Studies which investigate the incidence of delirium after the correction of anemia, dehydration, or other conditions prior to undergoing cardiac surgery should be conducted.

Another consideration is pharmacotherapy before, during, and after surgery. A review of medications taken by patients in the perioperative period of cardiac surgery identified preoperative antipsychotics as an independent risk factor for delirium (Tse et al. 2012). Other preoperative medications that may contribute to delirium include statins, antihypertensives, anticholinergics, antidepressants, benzodiazepines, and opioids which are common home medications for patients undergoing cardiac surgery (Tse et al. 2012). Intraoperative medications associated with delirium include both fentanyl and ketamine while diazepam has inconclusive results (Tse et al. 2012). As for postoperative medications, risperidone was shown to reduce the incidence of delirium by almost one third when taken by patients after cardiac surgery as a preventive strategy (Prakanrattana & Prapaitrakool 2007). However, the large effect size in reducing delirium in patients receiving risperidone (11.1 vs. 31.7 %; RR, 0.35 (95 % CI 0.16 to 0.77); $P = 0.009$) has yet to be reproduced.

Oxygen delivery to the brain is critical for optimal performance of the brain's activities. Cerebral oximetry continuously measures cerebral oxygenation in both hemispheres of the brain and is sometimes used in cardiac surgery as a monitor to stratify risk in patients throughout the perioperative period (Vretzakis et al. 2014). Previous studies have found a correlation between low preoperative cerebral oxygenation and postoperative delirium (Schoen et al. 2011). Desaturations in cerebral oximetry readings while on bypass are associated with several adverse outcomes (Vohra et al. 2009), but whether or not this may contribute to delirium is unknown.

Outcomes

Delirium is a condition that may affect a patient for several days or weeks. It is associated with many significant adverse effects and poor outcomes. The progression of dementia after suffering from an episode of delirium may lead to a significant decline in both physical and cognitive functioning (Morandi et al. 2014). This is also evident in patients without an underlying dementia as delirium is associated with declines in both condition and functional level in older patients (Inouye 2006). After cardiac surgery, patients diagnosed with delirium have a higher risk for falls, increased length of stay in the hospital, higher likelihood of discharge to a nursing home or home with assisted care, and prolonged inpatient physical therapy duration (Mangusan et al. 2015). Delirium after CABG surgery is also associated with increased mortality up to 10 years postoperatively (Gottesman et al. 2010).

The outcomes for patients developing delirium are clearly worse than patients who do not. Whether the poor outcomes are a direct effect of delirium or a marker of disease severity is unclear. Either way, these negative outcomes lead to increased costs in not only the healthcare field but also social costs as families incur the increased burdens of time and money to care for relatives diagnosed with delirium. Strategies to reduce healthcare costs are becoming a major focus within the field of medicine. Interventions to effectively treat delirium and its complications are being explored, and strategies to reduce healthcare costs are on the rise (Zaubler et al. 2013). The treatment of delirium is important, but discovering ways to prevent delirium is ideal and would likely equate to the greatest decrease in overall healthcare costs and improved outcomes.

Pharmacological interventions

The identification and correction of risk factors including dehydration, electrolyte imbalance, and anemia are important and should be emphasized in every patient. And while these non-pharmacological interventions and others such as reorientation, effective communication, and maintenance of consistent sleep-wake cycles are considered first-line interventions for delirium (Young et al. 2010), the discovery of pharmacological agents which decrease the incidence or duration of delirium has great potential. With the current lack of understanding behind the exact pathophysiology of delirium, the present prevention and treatment strategies are inadequate. As previously mentioned, second-generation antipsychotics were shown to decrease the incidence of postoperative delirium when administered prophylactically (Hirota & Kishi 2013); however, only one study in this review was specific to cardiac surgery patients (Prakanrattana & Prapaitrakool 2007). Also, a total of six studies were included in this meta-analysis. Other studies have suggested patients taking preoperative antipsychotics are actually at a greater risk for delirium (Tse et al. 2012). The use of antipsychotics is a potential treatment option as they may alter and subsequently correct neurotransmitter imbalances in delirious patients (Hirota & Kishi 2013; Schotte et al. 1996), but the majority of interventions for delirium after cardiac surgery aim to optimize analgesia and sedation regimens in the ICU and preemptively treat delirium.

Postoperative pain may contribute to the condition of delirium (Fong et al. 2006). Pain after cardiac surgery can be moderate to severe with incisions to the lower extremities and sternum and also the placement of chest tubes. With the potential for bleeding and increased risk of kidney injury, nonsteroidal anti-inflammatory drugs (NSAIDs) are not ideal in this patient population. Ketamine is one option for pain postoperatively, but it may increase the risk of delirium (Tse et al. 2012), and the potential side effect of hallucinations should also be considered. The usual analgesic regimen after cardiac surgery includes an opiate. Opiates, such as morphine and hydromorphone, have many deleterious side effects including nausea/vomiting, ileus, bladder dysfunction, and respiratory depression (Memis et al. 2010). Opioids also increase the risk of postoperative delirium, especially in elderly patients (Tse et al. 2012). The use of intravenous acetaminophen (IVA) has been shown in multiple studies to reduce the amount of opiates consumed by surgical patients (O'Neal 2013). IVA possesses no psychoactive properties, and it has both rapid and effective analgesic properties while considered to be a safe and well-tolerated medication (Candiotti et al. 2010). Given the reduction in opiate consumption, reliable analgesic properties, and safety profile, IVA may be an alternative for patients undergoing cardiac surgery.

In addition to optimizing pain control after cardiac surgery, choosing the most appropriate sedation regimen is important when trying to reduce the chance for postoperative delirium. The importance of periodically weaning sedation should not be overlooked. Overly sedating patients is associated with delayed extubation and higher mortality in the ICU (Shehabi et al. 2013; Shehabi et al. 2012). Finding the appropriate balance of sedation and adequate analgesia should be targeted in cardiac surgery patients.

An ideal choice for sedation in the ICU is a medication that provides both sedation and pain relief. Dexmedetomidine is a selective α-2 receptor agonist which provides sedation and also has an analgesic component. Some clinicians use caution before administering this medication given the side effect profile which includes bradycardia, hypotension, and hypertension with loading doses. Cardiac surgery patients have the advantage of pacer wire implants to avoid the side effect of bradycardia, and since these patients are in the ICU, hypotension can be treated with vasopressors when appropriate. A study comparing sedation with propofol to dexmedetomidine in the ICU found no difference between the two with regard to bradycardia and hypotension; however, dexmedetomidine was associated with an increased risk of hypertension in patients receiving a loading dose initially (Xia et al. 2013). This undesired side effect might be avoided by foregoing the loading dose. Given its sedative and analgesic properties with limited side effects, dexmedetomidine could be the ideal medication for cardiac surgery patients, and multiple studies have investigated the role of dexmedetomidine in reducing delirium.

A typical sedation regimen in the ICU includes benzodiazepines and/or propofol. The link between benzodiazepines and delirium has been demonstrated (Zaal et al. 2015; Taipale et al. 2012), and therefore, many trials have aimed to compare these agents to dexmedetomidine. The MENDS trial was a double-blind randomized, controlled trial that found the use of dexmedetomidine to result in fewer days of delirium in medical and surgical ICU patients when compared to lorazepam (Pandharipande et al. 2007). Achieving the goal sedation level was also superior in the dexmedetomidine group, but mortality and cost did not differ when compared to the lorazepam group. A larger randomized, controlled trial SEDCOM suggested that medical and surgical ICU patients sedated with dexmedetomidine spent less time on the ventilator, experienced fewer episodes of delirium, and developed less tachycardia and hypertension than patients sedated with midazolam (Riker et al. 2009). Researchers have used these findings in medical and surgical ICUs to study the effects of dexmedetomidine specifically in cardiac surgery ICU patients.

A meta-analysis including 11 randomized, controlled or cohort studies found the use of dexmedetomidine for sedation in cardiac surgery patients' shortened ventilator time, reduced the incidence of postoperative arrhythmias, and reduced the incidence of delirium (Lin et al. 2012). An issue with this analysis is that some of the main studies included in the analysis had poor designs and variable methods to assess for delirium. The DEXCOM study was a randomized, controlled trial which showed a decreased duration of delirium (5 vs. 2 days, (95 % CI 1.09 to 6.67); $P = 0.0317$) in patients sedated with dexmedetomidine versus morphine (Shehabi et al. 2009). The study found no difference in incidence of delirium, although the baseline delirium rate was only 15 %. Propofol was used in both study groups, and when assessing delirium, the CAM-ICU scale was used on both intubated and extubated patients. A prospective, randomized, open-label trial comparing dexmedetomidine to propofol to midazolam for sedation after cardiac surgery found an incidence of only 3 % in the dexmedetomidine group versus 50 % in both the propofol and midazolam groups (Maldonado et al. 2009). The large reduction in incidence of delirium is unprecedented as no other study has shown such a drastic reduction. A retrospective cohort consisting of data collected from 250 hospitals found that patients receiving dexmedetomidine/propofol/midazolam had a decreased incidence of delirium compared to the propofol/midazolam group, but the method for assessing delirium was not described (Dasta et al. 2006). Also, the primary endpoint of this study was cost, which was also reduced in the dexmedetomidine/propofol/midazolam group.

More recent studies continue to support the use of dexmedetomidine after cardiac surgery for reduction of delirium. When comparing dexmedetomidine to remifentanil for sedation after cardiac surgery, a reduction in the incidence of delirium was shown in the dexmedetomidine group (8.96 vs. 22.67 %; $P < 0.05$) (Park et al. 2014). The study found no differences between the two groups with respect to length of stay in the ICU, time to extubation, hospital length of stay, and other postoperative complications. Another recent single-blinded, prospective randomized trial found that when compared to propofol, the use of dexmedetomidine for sedation after cardiac surgery resulted in reduced incidence (odds ratio (OR) 0.46 (95 % CI 0.23 to 0.92); $P = 0.028$), delayed onset, and also shorter duration of delirium (Djaiani et al. 2015). A retrospective cohort investigating outcomes after CABG found a decreased mortality in patients receiving dexmedetomidine perioperatively (Ji et al. 2014). A reduction in the risk of delirium in patients receiving dexmedetomidine (adjusted OR, 0.431 (95 % CI 0.265 to 0.701); $P = 0.0007$) was also reported when compared to patients who did not receive dexmedetomidine. A larger retrospective study including CABG and CABG plus valve surgery patients also found a reduction in delirium (5.46 vs. 7.42 %; adjusted OR, 0.53 (95 % CI 0.37 to 0.75); $P = 0.003$) and decreased 1-year mortality (3.17 vs. 7.95 %; adjusted OR, 0.47 (95 % CI 0.312 to

0.701); $P = 0.0002$) in patients receiving dexmedetomidine (Ji et al. 2013).

Other interventions are also being studied. The use of high-dose dexamethasone (1 mg/kg) in cardiac surgery patients failed to show a difference in the incidence or duration of delirium (Sauer et al. 2014). The theory that the inflammatory response from surgery and cardiopulmonary bypass contributes to delirium drove the hypothesis of this study. The use of intraoperative Bispectral Index (BIS)-guided and end-tidal anesthetic concentration-guided depth of anesthesia protocols is another direction investigators have taken (Whitlock et al. 2014). No difference was shown with either of these monitors; however, low average volatile anesthetic dose was found to be a predictor of delirium. This may be reflective of patients with poorer health and could potentially assist with screening for patients at higher risk for delirium.

A systematic review and meta-analysis supported the use of dexmedetomidine, antipsychotics, and multicomponent interventions for strategies to reduce postoperative delirium based on the review of 38 randomized controlled trials but did state that one of the greatest obstacles in evaluating delirium studies is the lack of continuity in evaluation of delirium (Zhang et al. 2013). This is a major issue when clinicians are trying to extrapolate these findings and utilize them in clinical practice. When the majority of the randomized clinical trials on postoperative delirium show vast inconsistencies in the method chosen to evaluate delirium, the evidence may seem insufficient and unreliable by intensivists. And even though evidence suggests benefits of using certain interventions to reduce postoperative delirium after cardiac surgery, more studies are necessary which aim to universalize the assessment of delirium.

Future studies

Studies on this topic are not lacking in quantity but more so in quality. Establishing a reliable, convenient, and consistent method for diagnosing delirium is a must for researchers in this field. More recent studies utilize multiple assessment tools, but until a universal screening method for delirium is accepted, it will be difficult for studies to change clinical practice with their results.

Projects involving biomarkers and their role in delirium after cardiac surgery are limitless. Aiming to target biomarkers shown to have a correlation with delirium in non-cardiac surgery patients should be investigated in cardiac surgery. Biomarkers linked to the mechanisms of delirium should also be characterized potentially through targeting biomarkers of the neuroinflammatory pathway of endothelial dysfunction, BBB disruption, and neuronal injury. This may lead to identifying patients at higher risk, preemptively treating those patients, and further defining the severity of disease in patients with delirium. Finding ways to effectively treat cerebral oxygen desaturations during CPB may also reduce postoperative delirium.

Modifications to medications administered before, during, and after surgery should continue to be investigated. The avoidance of medications such as benzodiazepines and opiates by using other sedatives and analgesics has proven to decrease delirium. Considering the flaws in studies using dexmedetomidine in the ICU, more research is necessary with this medication to determine the optimal dosing and timing of its use and solidify the evidence that it decreases delirium after cardiac surgery. The use of IVA may limit opiate consumption and play a role in decreasing delirium in these patients. An ongoing trial investigating the effects of both dexmedetomidine and IVA on delirium following cardiac surgery may provide sufficient evidence to support the use of these medications in the prevention of postoperative delirium (NCT02546765). Other analgesics such as gabapentin and pregabalin given preoperatively should also be considered.

Conclusions

Delirium is an ongoing issue in cardiac surgery patients. Many risk factors are known, and some can be modified perioperatively. The complications associated with postoperative delirium lead to increased morbidity and mortality as well as higher healthcare costs. Several interventions in the ICU after cardiac surgery have been investigated, but the results have yet to significantly change clinical practice. The role of biomarkers in postoperative delirium after cardiac surgery is promising but not yet fully elucidated. More research and randomized clinical trials in this field is both warranted and necessary given the negative outcomes associated with delirium.

Abbreviations

BBB: blood brain barrier; BIS: Bispectral Index; CABG: coronary artery bypass grafting; CAM-ICU: confusion assessment method for the ICU; CPB: cardiopulmonary bypass; DDS: Delirium Detection Score; DSM-V: Diagnostic and Statistical Manual, 5th edition; ICU: intensive care unit; IGF-1: insulin-like growth factor-1; IV: intravenous; IVA: intravenous acetaminophen; MMSE: Mini-Mental State Examination; NSAIDs: nonsteroidal anti-inflammatory drugs; Nu-DESC: Nursing Delirium Screening Scale; UCHL1: ubiquitin C-terminal hydrolase L1.

Competing interests

The authors declare that they have no competing interests.

Authors' contributions

JBO and ADS were both involved in the preparation of the article. Both authors read and approved the final manuscript.

Acknowledgements

The research reported in this publication was supported by the National Institutes of Health under award number 5T32 GM108554. The content is solely the responsibility of the authors and does not necessarily represent the official views of the National Institutes of Health.

References

Association AP. Diagnostic and statistical manual of mental disorders. 5th ed. Washington, DC: Elsevier Inc.; 2013.

Baranyi A, Rothenhausler HB. The impact of soluble interleukin-2 receptor as a biomarker of delirium. Psychosomatics. 2014;55(1):51–60.

Blyth BJ et al. Validation of serum markers for blood–brain barrier disruption in traumatic brain injury. J Neurotrauma. 2009;26(9):1497–507.

Blyth BJ et al. Elevated serum ubiquitin carboxy-terminal hydrolase L1 is associated with abnormal blood–brain barrier function after traumatic brain injury. J Neurotrauma. 2011;28(12):2453–62.

Boustani M et al. Impact and recognition of cognitive impairment among hospitalized elders. J Hosp Med. 2010;5(2):69–75.

Brophy GM et al. Biokinetic analysis of ubiquitin C-terminal hydrolase-L1 (UCH-L1) in severe traumatic brain injury patient biofluids. J Neurotrauma. 2011;28(6):861–70.

Candiotti KA et al. Safety of multiple-dose intravenous acetaminophen in adult inpatients. Pain Med. 2010;11(12):1841–8.

Cerejeira J et al. The neuroinflammatory hypothesis of delirium. Acta Neuropathol. 2010;119(6):737–54.

Cerejeira J et al. The cholinergic system and inflammation: common pathways in delirium pathophysiology. J Am Geriatr Soc. 2012;60(4):669–75.

Chung KS et al. Risk factors of delirium in patients undergoing total knee arthroplasty. Arch Gerontol Geriatr. 2015;60(3):443–7.

Cole MG. Delirium in elderly patients. Am J Geriatr Psychiatry. 2004;12(1):7–21.

Dasta JF et al. Addition of dexmedetomidine to standard sedation regimens after cardiac surgery: an outcomes analysis. Pharmacotherapy. 2006;26(6):798–805.

Djaiani G, et al. Dexmedetomidine versus propofol sedation reduces delirium after cardiac surgery: a randomized controlled trial. Anesthesiology, 2015.

Figueiredo-Pereira ME et al. Neuroinflammation and J2 prostaglandins: linking impairment of the ubiquitin-proteasome pathway and mitochondria to neurodegeneration. Front Mol Neurosci. 2014;7:104.

Fineberg SJ et al. Incidence and risk factors for postoperative delirium after lumbar spine surgery. Spine (Phila Pa 1976). 2013;38(20):1790–6.

Fong HK, Sands LP, Leung JM. The role of postoperative analgesia in delirium and cognitive decline in elderly patients: a systematic review. Anesth Analg. 2006;102(4):1255–66.

Gaggin HK, Januzzi Jr JL. Biomarkers and diagnostics in heart failure. Biochim Biophys Acta. 2013;1832(12):2442–50.

Gaudreau JD, Gagnon P. Psychotogenic drugs and delirium pathogenesis: the central role of the thalamus. Med Hypotheses. 2005;64(3):471–5.

Gottesman RF et al. Delirium after coronary artery bypass graft surgery and late mortality. Ann Neurol. 2010;67(3):338–44.

Hirota T, Kishi T. Prophylactic antipsychotic use for postoperative delirium: a systematic review and meta-analysis. J Clin Psychiatry. 2013;74(12):e1136–44.

Hughes CG et al. Association between endothelial dysfunction and acute brain dysfunction during critical illness. Anesthesiology. 2013;118(3):631–9.

Inouye SK. Delirium in older persons. N Engl J Med. 2006;354(11):1157–65.

Jara JH, Frank DD, Ozdinler PH. Could dysregulation of UPS be a common underlying mechanism for cancer and neurodegeneration? Lessons from UCHL1. Cell Biochem Biophys. 2013;67(1):45–53.

Ji F et al. Perioperative dexmedetomidine improves outcomes of cardiac surgery. Circulation. 2013;127(15):1576–84.

Ji F et al. Perioperative dexmedetomidine improves mortality in patients undergoing coronary artery bypass surgery. J Cardiothorac Vasc Anesth. 2014;28(2):267–73.

Joosten E et al. Is anaemia a risk factor for delirium in an acute geriatric population? Gerontology. 2006;52(6):382–5.

Kazmierski J et al. Raised IL-2 and TNF-alpha concentrations are associated with postoperative delirium in patients undergoing coronary-artery bypass graft surgery. Int Psychogeriatr. 2014;26(5):845–55.

Khan BA et al. Biomarkers for delirium—a review. J Am Geriatr Soc. 2011;59 Suppl 2:S256–61.

Lin YY et al. Can dexmedetomidine be a safe and efficacious sedative agent in post-cardiac surgery patients? A meta-analysis. Crit Care. 2012;16(5):R169.

Luetz A et al. Different assessment tools for intensive care unit delirium: which score to use? Crit Care Med. 2010;38(2):409–18.

Maldonado JR et al. Dexmedetomidine and the reduction of postoperative delirium after cardiac surgery. Psychosomatics. 2009;50(3):206–17.

Mangusan RF et al. Outcomes associated with postoperative delirium after cardiac surgery. Am J Crit Care. 2015;24(2):156–63.

Marcantonio ER et al. Serum biomarkers for delirium. J Gerontol A Biol Sci Med Sci. 2006;61(12):1281–6.

Memis D et al. Intravenous paracetamol reduced the use of opioids, extubation time, and opioid-related adverse effects after major surgery in intensive care unit. J Crit Care. 2010;25(3):458–62.

Morandi A et al. Delirium superimposed on dementia strongly predicts worse outcomes in older rehabilitation inpatients. J Am Med Dir Assoc. 2014;15(5):349–54.

O'Neal JB. The utility of intravenous acetaminophen in the perioperative period. Front Public Health. 2013;1:25.

O'Neal WT et al. Preoperative atrial fibrillation and long-term survival after open heart surgery in a rural tertiary heart institute. Heart Lung. 2013;42(6):442–7.

Osse RJ et al. High preoperative plasma neopterin predicts delirium after cardiac surgery in older adults. J Am Geriatr Soc. 2012;60(4):661–8.

Pandharipande PP et al. Effect of sedation with dexmedetomidine vs lorazepam on acute brain dysfunction in mechanically ventilated patients: the MENDS randomized controlled trial. JAMA. 2007;298(22):2644–53.

Pandharipande PP et al. Long-term cognitive impairment after critical illness. N Engl J Med. 2013;369(14):1306–16.

Park JB et al. Efficacy and safety of dexmedetomidine for postoperative delirium in adult cardiac surgery on cardiopulmonary bypass. Korean J Thorac Cardiovasc Surg. 2014;47(3):249–54.

Prakanrattana U, Prapaitrakool S. Efficacy of risperidone for prevention of postoperative delirium in cardiac surgery. Anaesth Intensive Care. 2007;35(5):714–9.

Riker RR et al. Dexmedetomidine vs midazolam for sedation of critically ill patients: a randomized trial. JAMA. 2009;301(5):489–99.

Robinson TN et al. Preoperative cognitive dysfunction is related to adverse postoperative outcomes in the elderly. J Am Coll Surg. 2012;215(1):12–7. discussion 17–8.

Rudolph JL et al. Chemokines are associated with delirium after cardiac surgery. J Gerontol A Biol Sci Med Sci. 2008;63(2):184–9.

Rudolph JL et al. Derivation and validation of a preoperative prediction rule for delirium after cardiac surgery. Circulation. 2009;119(2):229–36.

Ruitenberg A et al. Incidence of dementia: does gender make a difference? Neurobiol Aging. 2001;22(4):575–80.

Saczynski JS et al. Cognitive trajectories after postoperative delirium. N Engl J Med. 2012;367(1):30–9.

Sauer AM et al. Intraoperative dexamethasone and delirium after cardiac surgery: a randomized clinical trial. Anesth Analg. 2014;119(5):1046–52.

Schoen J et al. Preoperative regional cerebral oxygen saturation is a predictor of postoperative delirium in on-pump cardiac surgery patients: a prospective observational trial. Crit Care. 2011;15(5):R218.

Schotte A et al. Risperidone compared with new and reference antipsychotic drugs: in vitro and in vivo receptor binding. Psychopharmacology (Berl). 1996;124(1–2):57–73.

Shehabi Y et al. Prevalence of delirium with dexmedetomidine compared with morphine based therapy after cardiac surgery: a randomized controlled trial (DEXmedetomidine COmpared to Morphine-DEXCOM study). Anesthesiology. 2009;111(5):1075–84.

Shehabi Y et al. Early intensive care sedation predicts long-term mortality in ventilated critically ill patients. Am J Respir Crit Care Med. 2012;186(8):724–31.

Shehabi Y et al. Sedation depth and long-term mortality in mechanically ventilated critically ill adults: a prospective longitudinal multicentre cohort study. Intensive Care Med. 2013;39(5):910–8.

Taipale PG et al. The association between nurse-administered midazolam following cardiac surgery and incident delirium: an observational study. Int J Nurs Stud. 2012;49(9):1064–73.

Trabold B, Metterlein T. Postoperative delirium: risk factors, prevention, and treatment. J Cardiothorac Vasc Anesth. 2014;28(5):1352–60.

Trzepacz PT. Anticholinergic model for delirium. Semin Clin Neuropsychiatry. 1996;1(4):294–303.

Trzepacz PT, van der Mast R. The neuropathophysiology of delirium. Oxford: Oxford University Press; 2002.

Tse L et al. Pharmacological risk factors for delirium after cardiac surgery: a review. Curr Neuropharmacol. 2012;10(3):181–96.

van den Boogaard M et al. Biomarkers associated with delirium in critically ill patients and their relation with long-term subjective cognitive dysfunction; indications for different pathways governing delirium in inflamed and noninflamed patients. Crit Care. 2011;15(6):R297.

van Meenen LC et al. Risk prediction models for postoperative delirium: a systematic review and meta-analysis. J Am Geriatr Soc. 2014;62(12):2383–90.

Vohra HA, Modi A, Ohri SK. Does use of intra-operative cerebral regional oxygen saturation monitoring during cardiac surgery lead to improved clinical outcomes? Interact Cardiovasc Thorac Surg. 2009;9(2):318–22.
Vretzakis G et al. Cerebral oximetry in cardiac anesthesia. J Thorac Dis. 2014;6 Suppl 1:S60–9.
Whitlock EL et al. Postoperative delirium in a substudy of cardiothoracic surgical patients in the BAG-RECALL clinical trial. Anesth Analg. 2014;118(4):809–17.
Wiltfang J. Clinically validated molecular biomarkers of neurodegenerative dementia. Nervenarzt. 2014;85(11):1372–81.
Xia ZQ et al. Clinical benefits of dexmedetomidine versus propofol in adult intensive care unit patients: a meta-analysis of randomized clinical trials. J Surg Res. 2013;185(2):833–43.
Young J et al. Diagnosis, prevention, and management of delirium: summary of NICE guidance. BMJ. 2010;341:c3704.
Zaal IJ et al. Benzodiazepine-associated delirium in critically ill adults. Intensive Care Med. 2015;41(12):2130–7.
Zaubler TS et al. Quality improvement and cost savings with multicomponent delirium interventions: replication of the Hospital Elder Life Program in a community hospital. Psychosomatics. 2013;54(3):219–26.
Zhang H et al. Strategies for prevention of postoperative delirium: a systematic review and meta-analysis of randomized trials. Crit Care. 2013;17(2):R47.

16

Hemodynamics and tissue oxygenation during balanced anesthesia with a high antinociceptive contribution

Jaap Jan Vos[1*], Marieke Poterman[1], Laura N Hannivoort[1], Victor W Renardel De Lavalette[2], Michel MRF Struys[1], Thomas WL Scheeren[1] and Alain F Kalmar[1,3]

Abstract

Background: In particular surgical conditions, a balanced anesthesia with a high-antinociceptive contribution is required. This may induce cardiovascular impairment and thus compromise tissue oxygenation. In this prospective observational study, we investigated the hemodynamic stability and tissue oxygen saturation (StO_2) in 40 patients with a high-antinociceptive general anesthesia, goal-directed fluid therapy, and norepinephrine. In addition, optimal surgical conditions and safe and fast emergence are pivotal parts of anesthetic management.

Methods: In high-antinociceptive propofol/remifentanil anesthesia with bispectral index (BIS) between 40 and 60, norepinephrine was administered to maintain mean arterial pressure (MAP) above 80% of individual baseline. Fluid was administered if the Δ plethysmographic waveform amplitude exceeded 10%. Surgical and recovery conditions, hemodynamic responses, and tissue oxygenation were investigated.

Results: Mean (SD) StO_2 at the left thenar eminence increased from 83 (6)% before to 86 (4)% 20 min after induction of anesthesia (p <0.05). Cardiac index dropped from 3.0 (0.7) to 2.1 (0.4) L min^{-1} (p <0.05), MAP from 109 (16) to 83 (14) mm Hg, and heart rate from 73 (12) to 54 (8) bpm (p <0.05). Thirteen out of 40 patients received a fluid bolus. The median (range) norepinephrine administration rate was 0.05 (0.0–0.10) μg kg^{-1} min^{-1}. After complete akinesia in all patients during surgery, a median (IQR) extubation time of 311 (253–386) s was observed.

Conclusions: This high-antinociceptive balanced anesthesia with goal-directed fluid and vasopressor therapy adequately preserved StO_2 and hemodynamic homeostasis.

Keywords: Propofol, Remifentanil, Cardiac output, Fluid therapy, Balanced anesthesia, Tissue oxygenation, Norepinephrine

Background

Induction to a level of anesthesia adequate to tolerate laryngoscopy requires a combination of hypnotics and analgesics that may induce significant hemodynamic suppression attributed to peripheral vasodilatation, loss of venous tone causing reduction in preload and venous return, and to a lesser extent, a decreased myocardial contractility. After intubation, the sudden decrease in nociceptive stimuli often results in hypotension and frequently requires administration of vasoactive medication if surgical stimulation remains absent for a significant time. These agents may however jeopardize hemodynamic stability and tissue oxygenation [1]. Yet, particular surgical interventions require a sustained high level of analgesia, although only occasional but intense nociceptive stimuli occur in between long periods of low stimulation. In these fluctuating surgical conditions, maintaining a stable anesthesia (which can, among other variables, be reflected by a BIS-value between 40 and 60) may be challenging in view of the fluctuating noxious stimuli. A reliable method to assess the quality

* Correspondence: j.j.vos@umcg.nl
[1]Department of Anesthesiology, University of Groningen, University Medical Center Groningen, Groningen, The Netherlands
Full list of author information is available at the end of the article

of analgesia level is complete tolerance to laryngoscopy, which reflects an equal tolerance to typical surgical stimuli [2].

In addition, many of these surgical interventions have only limited analgesic needs once the procedure is finished making the pharmacological profile of remifentanil suitable for this purpose.

In most surgical conditions, a sound approach to compensate for alternating stimuli would be decreasing the level of analgesia. However, in many procedures where continuous muscle relaxants are undesirable and complete akinesia is nonetheless required, an alternative strategy must be pursued while addressing obvious concerns regarding hemodynamic disturbances and awareness [3].

Furthermore, a safe and fast emergence from anesthesia with avoidance of sudden increases in intra-ocular or middle-ear pressure during extubation [4,5], a full cooperative patient soon after surgery and a concise recovery period is often a pivotal part of the anesthetic management.

Whilst all these desired anesthetic requirements are being addressed, adequate tissue perfusion and oxygenation must be preserved. Only relying on the arterial blood pressure to maintain adequate tissue oxygenation is insufficient, yet most advanced hemodynamic monitoring devices are moderately to highly invasive and are associated with rare but serious complications limiting their value in many patients [6-8]. In the surgical settings described above (with a substantial percentage of day-case surgery), non-invasive monitoring (i.e., providing sufficient information without the risk of inducing complications) is mandatory. The Inspectra® device (Hutchinson Technology, Hutchinson, KS, USA) can be used to continuously monitor the tissue oxygen saturation (StO_2) non-invasively on the thenar muscle using near-infrared spectroscopy (NIRS) [9] while the Nexfin® monitor (Edwards Lifesciences, Irvine, CA, USA) permits non-invasive measurement of various hemodynamic variables in a beat-to-beat fashion [9-14]. The aim of this observational study was to describe the adequacy of tissue oxygenation and hemodynamic stability together with the quality of the surgical conditions and emergence from anesthesia in a tightly-specified balanced anesthesia with a high-antinociceptive contribution combined with a goal-directed fluid and vasopressor therapy.

Methods

After the Institutional Ethics Committee approval (Ref: 2012.052, Ethics Committee, University Medical Center Groningen, Groningen, The Netherlands), 40 consecutive adult patients scheduled for a day-case surgery under general anesthesia were recorded and written informed consent was asked for data-analysis. The study was registered at Current Controlled Clinical Trials (ISRCTN20153044).

Anesthetic management

One gram of Paracetamol was administered orally prior to admission to the OR. Intravenous access was secured using an 18G IV catheter in a left large forearm vein, and a continuous background infusion of crystalloids was started at 90 ml hr^{-1}. Anesthesia was induced with remifentanil (1 μg kg^{-1}), propofol (1–3 mg kg^{-1}), and cisatracurium (0.1 mg kg^{-1}).

In patients with preexisting cardiovascular comorbidities such as hypertension, reported peripheral or coronary artery disease in whom post-induction hypotension—defined as a 20% decrease [15,16] in baseline mean arterial pressure (MAP)—can be expected, a norepinephrine (10 μg) single bolus was co-administered prophylactically.

After tracheal intubation, the lungs were ventilated in a volume controlled mode with a tidal volume of 8 ml kg^{-1} lean body weight with a mixture of O_2/air (F_iO_2 0.4) and 5 cm H_2O PEEP. The respiratory rate was adjusted to keep an end-tidal CO_2 pressure between 4.5 and 5.5 kPa.

Anesthesia was maintained with propofol (4 mg kg^{-1} hr^{-1}) and remifentanil (0.25 μg kg^{-1} min^{-1}) and adequate doses of hypnotics and analgesics to tolerate laryngoscopy [2,17] and to keep BIS between 40 and 60. If necessary, these doses could be increased in 30% steps. In addition, norepinephrine was infused as required to keep MAP above 80% of individual baseline (preoperative ambulatory pressure) [15,16].

The level of respiratory induced variation in the pulse oximetry plethysmographic waveform amplitude (ΔPOP) [18] was assessed 2 min after intubation; if it was found to be above 10%, hypovolemia was assumed and a fluid bolus of 500 ml colloid solution (Voluven®, Fresenius, Bad Homburg, Germany) was administered.

Administration of propofol, remifentanil, and norepinephrine was stopped simultaneously when the surgical procedure was finished. The trachea was extubated under continuous suction only after the patients were consciously responding and after they deeply inhaled upon verbal command. The extubation time, defined as the time between cessation of the syringe pumps and the moment of extubation, was recorded together with the incidence of any coughing reflex upon extubation. Any patient movement during the procedure was recorded. Two hours after recovery from anesthesia, patients were explicitly asked for any (adverse) experience in the peri-anesthetic period.

Monitoring

In addition to standard monitoring, a bispectral index (BIS) sensor (Aspect Medical Systems, Norwood, MA, USA) was placed on the forehead [19,20]. The non-invasive Inspectra® device (Model 650, Hutchinson Technology, Hutchinson, KA, USA) measures the peripheral StO_2

based on near-infrared spectrometry [9]. This device emits near-infrared light (600–800 nm) to the tissue, which then undergoes changes in its spectrum, mostly depending on the degree of microvascular hemoglobin saturation. The probe can be placed on different anatomical locations; but it was placed on the left thenar eminence because of the limited fat-layer with little inter-individual variation [9]. The anesthetist was blinded for StO_2 readings. The Nexfin® monitor (model 1) is a non-invasive advanced hemodynamic monitoring device with a working principle that is based on the volume clamp method using a photoplethysmograph and an inflatable cuff placed around the intermediate phalanx [21]. This device provides continuous calculation of arterial blood pressure, systemic vascular resistance, stroke volume, cardiac output (CO), and heart rate in a beat-to-beat fashion [10-14].

Data registration and analysis

The Philips MP70 anesthesia monitor (Philips, Eindhoven, Netherlands) was connected to a PC, and all patient data were recorded at a 1-s interval using Rugloop II data-manager software (Demed, Temse, Belgium). The time and dose of all administered drugs were recorded in the Rugloop system, together with any noteworthy events or patient responses. The following variables were recorded: SpO_2, StO_2, heart rate (HR), MAP, CO, Cardiac Index (CI), and BIS. The electronic data were imported into Microsoft Excel 2010® (Microsoft, Redmond, WA, USA). After a graphical representation, a visual inspection of the data plots was performed to correct obvious atypical values caused by artifacts.

Statistics

All statistics were performed using Microsoft Excel 2010® and PASW Statistics 18 (SPSS Inc, Chicago, IL, USA). Data were expressed as mean (SD), median (range), or number of patients (%). Normality of continuous variables was assessed using the Kolmogorov-Smirnov test. Continuous repetitive data before induction, and at 20 and 60 min thereafter were compared using the paired *t* test. Statistical significance level was set at $p < 0.05$.

Results

A total of 40 consecutive patients were screened for eligibility and subsequently enrolled.

Forty consecutive patients scheduled for ophthalmic surgery under general anesthesia were recorded. Mean (SD) age was 64 (13) years, weight was 82 (14) kg, and height was 176 (10) cm. There were 11, 23, and 6 patients of ASA classifications I, II, and III respectively. The median (range) duration of surgery was 73 (30–184) min. No use of neuromuscular reversal agents was necessary. In two patients (5%), an increase in the dosage of both propofol and remifentanil was required, whereas in one patient (2.5%), only the dosage of propofol was increased.

Overall, the median (range) administration rate of norepinephrine was 0.05 (0.00–0.10) $\mu g\ kg^{-1}\ min^{-1}$. Thirty-two patients were given a prophylactic dose of 10 µg norepinephrine at induction of anesthesia. Twenty-one patients were administered 0.05 $\mu g\ kg^{-1}\ min^{-1}$ norepinephrine continuously, while in eight patients, this administration rate could be either reduced to 0.025 $\mu g\ kg^{-1}\ min^{-1}$ or stopped. In two patients, the administration rate was increased to 0.075 $\mu g\ kg^{-1}\ min^{-1}$ and in one patient to 0.1 $\mu g\ kg^{-1}\ min^{-1}$. Eight patients did not receive norepinephrine at all. Thirteen of the forty patients showed a ΔPOP above 10% and were subsequently administered 500 ml fluid.

Evolution of hemodynamic variables and bispectral index

Figure 1A,B,C,D,E shows the time course of both the individual and mean values (in bold) of the investigated variables for the first 90 min. All data were synchronized at the start of induction of anesthesia. Figure 2 shows the mean values of all the investigated variables with a time interval of 1 min.

MAP decreased significantly from 109 (16) to 83 (14) mmHg ($p < 0.05$) after induction and remained stable afterwards. No inadvertent severe hypertension following prophylactic norepinephrine administration was observed at induction (Figure 1A). Heart rate also decreased upon induction of anesthesia from 73 (12) to 54 (8) bpm ($p < 0.05$) but remained stable afterwards (56 (9) bpm at 60 min; non-significant vs. 20 min). After an initial drop in cardiac index from 3.0 (0.7) L $min^{-1}\ m^{-2}$ at induction to 2.1 (0.4) L $min^{-1}\ m^{-2}$ at 20 min thereafter ($p < 0.05$), it gradually increased again to 2.4 (0.4) L min m^{-2} ($p < 0.05$) at 60 min. StO_2 increased significantly within minutes after induction of anesthesia from 83 (6)% before induction to 86 (4)% at 20 min after induction of anesthesia ($p < 0.05$) to remain stable thereafter (87 (4)% at 60 min after induction of anesthesia). The mean (SD) BIS value dropped from 95 (4) before induction to 44 (9) after 20 min ($p < 0.05$) and remained stable afterwards (mean BIS 44 (10) at 60 min).

Figure 3 shows the changes in CI and StO_2 from pre-anesthesia level to 20 min after induction in a scatterplot. Accordingly, a majority of patients have an increased StO_2 despite decreased CI. There was no significant correlation between CI and StO_2 values.

Quality of surgical conditions

Complete akinesia was realized in all patients in the period between induction of anesthesia and the end of surgery, while no additional relaxant was administered after intubation and 90% of the cases lasted longer than 45 min. No neuromuscular reversal agents were needed.

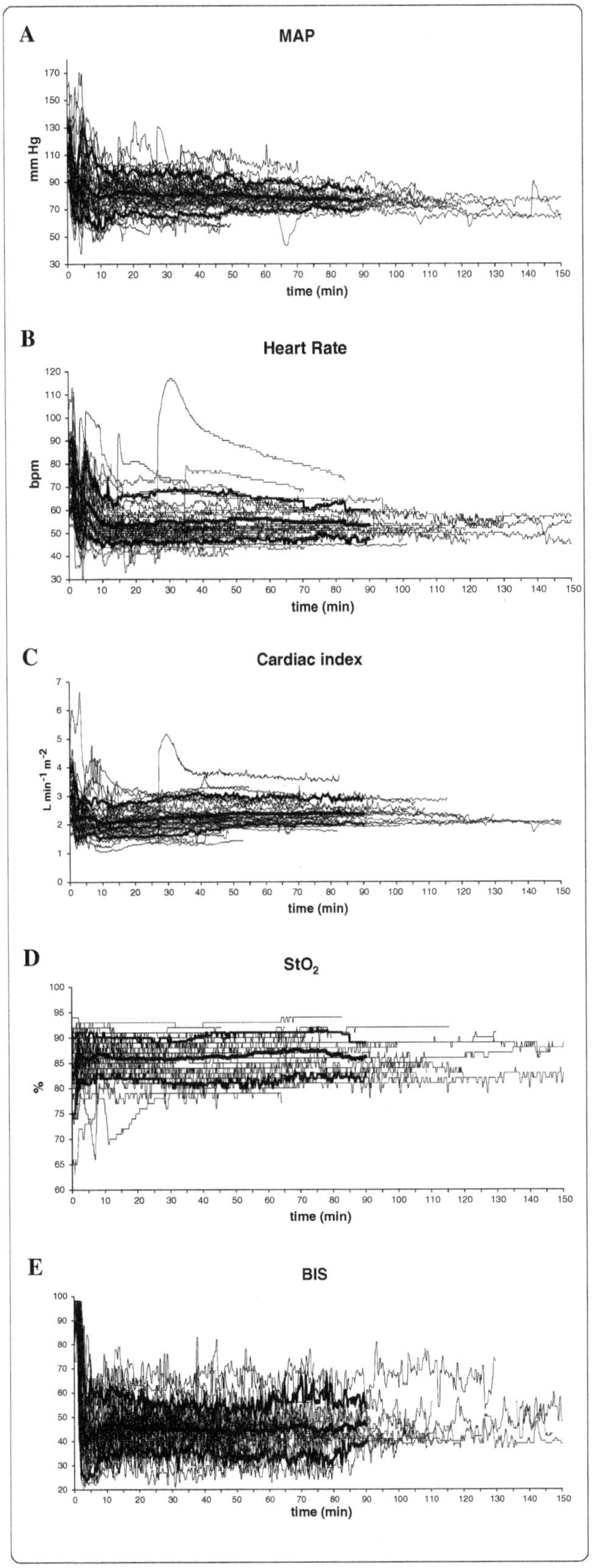

Figure 1 Evolution of individual values (grey), mean value (black), and 10th and 90th percentile (blue). (A) Mean arterial pressure. **(B)** Heart rate. **(C)** Cardiac index. **(D)** Tissue oxygen saturation. **(E)** Bispectral index. Values are shown from the moment of induction of anesthesia up to the end of the procedure. Mean and percentiles are shown for the first 90 minutes.

The median (range) extubation time was 311 (72–600) s with an interquartile range of 253–386 s. None of the patients exhibited a coughing reflex upon extubation and none of the patients reported awareness or unpleasant experiences in the peri-anesthetic period upon explicit questioning 2 h after extubation.

Discussion

In this prospective study in 40 patients, we have shown that during a high-antinociceptive balanced general anesthesia with propofol and remifentanil, goal-directed fluid administration and vasopressor support with norepinephrine results in a hemodynamically stable procedure with preservation of tissue oxygen saturation. This study performed in patients undergoing surgery with minimal noxious stimuli most of the time allows optimal quantification of the diverse effects of the anesthetic management with minimal interference of the surgical procedure. The combination of propofol/remifentanil, reported to provide an optimal depth of anesthesia, was also selected to produce a level of analgesia providing tolerance to laryngoscopy in >80% of cases (ED80) [2]. However, administration of analgesics to reach this high probability of tolerance to laryngoscopy requires a corresponding decrease in hypnotics in order to prevent excessive depth of anesthesia. Low BIS values (less than 30–40) are indicative of burst suppression [22], which is not considered a physiological EEG pattern, and has been correlated with poor outcome [16,23]. An appropriate decrease in propofol level is adequately reflected in a fitting mean (SD) BIS value of 44. This high level of antinociception proved to provide excellent analgesic and hypnotic conditions during surgery while also preventing intra- or postoperative events that might lead to increases in intra-ocular pressure or pharyngeal reflexes albeit allowing quick extubation with eventless recovery.

Critique of the methods

Firstly, the current study was neither designed as a randomized controlled trial nor has there been a control group. The study was nonetheless aimed to elucidate the effects of a balanced high-antinociceptive general anesthesia on tissue oxygen saturation in a clinical setting, for which an observational study would be the most appropriate.

Secondly, the current study was performed solely in patients undergoing ophthalmic surgery and therefore

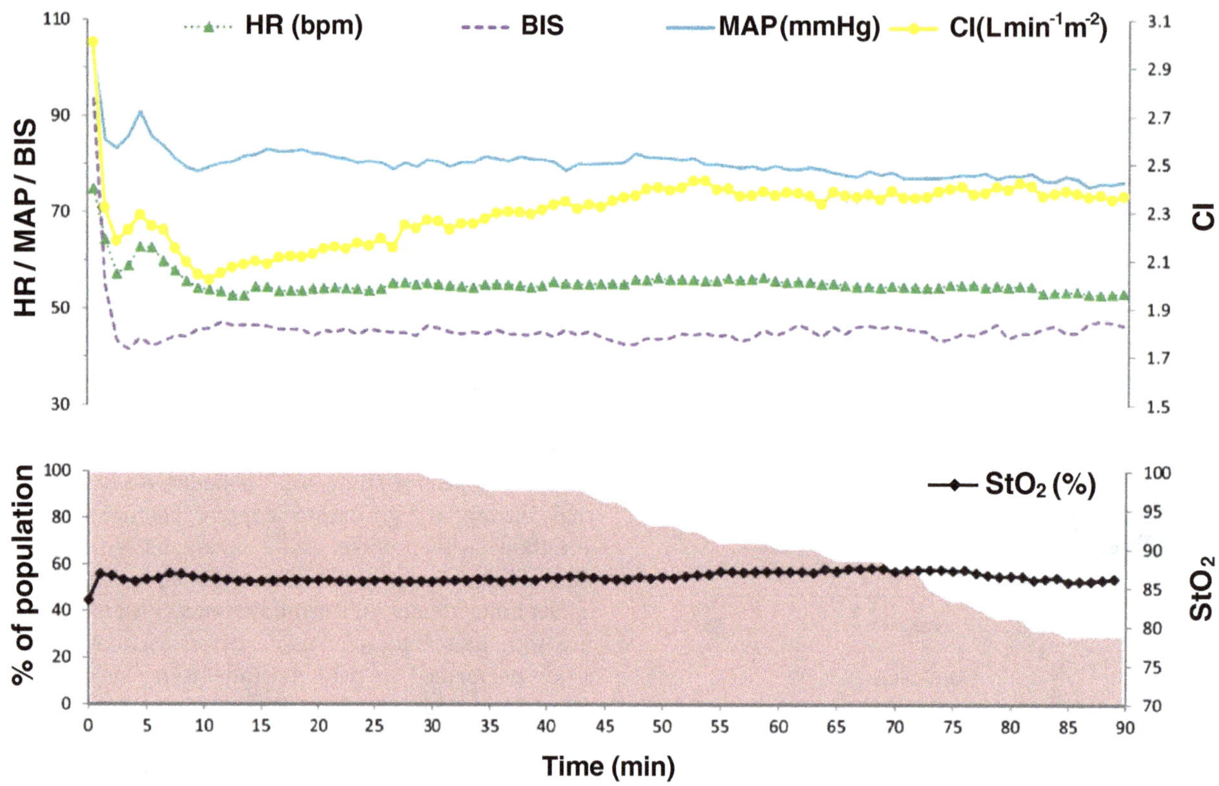

Figure 2 Time course of HR (bpm), BIS, MAP (mmHg), CI (L min^{-1} m^{-2}), and StO_2 (%). The variables are shown as mean values from induction of anesthesia up to 90 minutes thereafter. Furthermore, the percentage of the population at each time point that is still included is shown.

we cannot draw firm conclusions on the question whether this anesthetic regimen would be applicable during other types of surgery. Nevertheless, we speculate that in other surgical procedures associated with intermittent painful stimuli but requiring absolute akinesia (e.g., rigid laryngoscopy) and subsequently requiring rapid recovery with a fully responsive and cooperative patient, the investigated high-antinociceptive balanced anesthesia might be of particular use. Further studies should address this issue.

While invasive measurements are conventionally preferred to continuously assess hemodynamic variables, we used the non-invasive Nexfin® device, for which accuracy and precision of MAP measurements were recently shown, to meet the Association for the Advancement of Medical Instrumentation criteria in patients undergoing thoracic surgery [24] and also, were shown to be not inferior to noninvasive cuff manometric measurement of MAP in hemodynamically stable patients under general anesthesia [10]. This device also measures CO with a percentage error (PE) between 23% and 26% compared to thermodilution derived CO measurements as reported for patients who are awake before and after coronary artery bypass surgery [25]. Another study [14], investigating the influence of phenylephrine infusion on Nexfin® CO measurements, found a high concordance (94%) between phenylephrine-induced changes in CO measured by Nexfin® and by esophageal Doppler. The PE found in this study was however relatively high with a PE of 33% before and 42.5% after phenylephrine infusion, suggesting a reduced accuracy after vasopressor administration. Yet, Nexfin® CO accuracy still requires further investigation in patients under general anesthesia and in situations such as hemodynamic instability or during infusion of (other) vasoactive drugs, e.g., norepinephrine. Nevertheless, this device allows continuous and non-invasive monitoring of blood pressure and flow without adding additional risk to the patient. Additionally, recent technologic advances have also allowed the ability to calculate dynamic preload variables, such as pulse pressure and stroke volume variation, in an automated continuous noninvasive fashion [18], yet with a reported [26] higher accuracy in assessing fluid responsiveness than clinical ΔPOP assessment, as was performed in the current study.

Finally, the site and technology to determine tissue oxygenation may have some limitations. In particular, myoglobin can have relatively high oxygen saturation even in case of tissue hypoperfusion and decreased oxygenation, and it could be a major contributor to the readings obtained. As a consequence, there is a debate on which site should be preferred to accurately measure

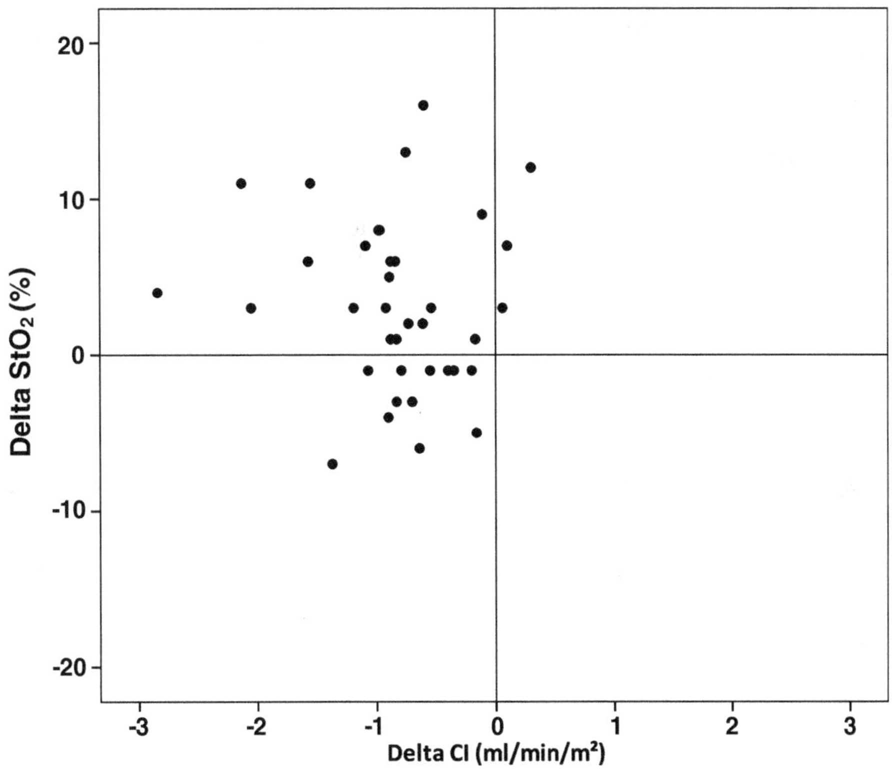

Figure 3 The change in CI and StO_2 between pre-anesthesia level and 20 min after induction.

StO_2 [27]. However, the systematic increase in StO_2 relative to baseline we observed in the current study convincingly demonstrates a favorable mixed effect of the anesthesia on global StO_2.

Quality of surgical conditions and emergence from anesthesia

In many surgical situations, a balanced high-antinociceptive general anesthesia is indicated, and a combination of propofol/remifentanil is appreciated. Based on the pharmacodynamic principle of equivalent anesthetic depth at different ratios of hypnotic/opiate, the chosen combination of propofol/remifentanil induced a sufficient level of anesthesia—reflected in normal BIS values between 40–60—although with a relatively higher contribution of remifentanil [2], resulting in a higher tolerance for sudden noxious stimuli. The favorable pharmacokinetic profile of this remifentanil/propofol combination resulted in a short median time to extubation—defined as the time interval between stopping the syringe pumps and the moment of extubation—of 311 s with low variability, together with optimal recurrence conditions: the fast elimination of propofol with still adequate analgesia at extubation results at the moment of endotracheal extubation in a complete suppression of potentially deleterious coughing reflexes and appropriate cooperation in all patients.

Hemodynamics and tissue oxygenation

Anesthesia was induced with propofol, 1–3 mg kg^{-1}, and remifentanil, 1 μg kg^{-1}: a combination that can acutely decrease vascular tonus, heart rate, and cardiac output with resulting *relative* hypotension [28], which was also observed in the current study (Figure 2).

Firstly, in order to preserve cardiac preload, 13/40 patients were administered fluid as the ΔPOP value was >10%, indicating fluid responsiveness, i.e., cardiac preload dependency.

Secondly, the decrease in CI following anesthesia induction is largely attributable to the (remifentanil-induced) decrease in heart rate (Figure 2), while stroke volume itself was relatively maintained probably because of both increased cardiac filling time and anesthesia-induced peripheral vasodilation and reduced cardiac afterload. The decrease in blood pressure after induction of anesthesia was anticipated with a single bolus of 10 μg norepinephrine at induction and a concomitantly started background infusion of norepinephrine. Most importantly, the administration of norepinephrine at the reported dose, in combination with goal-directed fluid optimization, was able to preserve a MAP at 80% of individual baseline values with a benign decrease in CO and without exerting adverse effects on StO_2.

A major concern of combining potent hypnotics/analgetics with a vasopressor is a negative end-effect on cardiac output and ultimately on tissue oxygenation. Therefore, a rational dosing is essential to obtain the desired intubation conditions and surgical stability, with optimal preservation of hemodynamic homeostasis. The stable BIS value within the recommended range reflects an adequate and reliable depth of hypnosis and demonstrates that a strong antinociceptive effect can be safely obtained if combined with an adequately adapted administration of propofol. Secondary, while the slight increase in tissue oxygenation is reassuring, a significant decrease in CI between awake and post-induction state demonstrates the potent hemodynamic effects of induction of even a balanced anesthesia. This decrease in CI is mainly based on a decrease in systemic resistance and heart rate and a preserved stroke volume. The resulting decrease in cardiac oxygen consumption, combined with a preserved peripheral tissue oxygenation, suggests that a CI decrease to this extent can be considered acceptable for induction of anesthesia. The subsequent increase in CI and stable MAP and StO_2 demonstrates that the moderate continuous doses of vasopressor are sufficient and appropriate to sustain hemodynamic stability during guaranteed optimal surgical conditions. However, the potent effects of the vasopressors must be reckoned with and must be considered in respect to other cardiovascular comorbidities. In addition, a more subtle administration of hypnotics/analgetics, such as based on TCI models, may be more appropriate in vulnerable patients.

While this desired MAP may appear relatively high for some clinicians, several reports [15,16] acknowledge the utmost importance of a preserved MAP up this value to prevent adverse outcome. Importantly, care must be taken that potent vasopressors like norepinephrine are administered with respect to appropriate safety measures, such as the preferable use of a dedicated line and avoidance of inadvertent boluses.

For patients under general anesthesia, StO_2 values around 80% are considered within the normal range [29]. The increase in StO_2 to 86(4)% in our study was most probably caused by peripheral vasodilation due to the combination of propofol and remifentanil. This finding is in contrast to a previous study in which no differences in StO_2 were found before and after induction of anesthesia [29]. The use of sufentanil in this previous study may account for this difference. Nevertheless, StO_2 is believed to be a flow-dependent variable [9]. Furthermore, it has been shown to be independent of MAP and remained almost constant at different levels of MAP [30]. It has however not yet been investigated whether thenar StO_2 values also correlate with oxygen saturation of tissues of vital importance (e.g., heart, brain, kidney, liver). Subsequently, although the data show favorable values of thenar StO_2, indicating adequate peripheral tissue oxygenation (at least in the range of MAP and CI values observed), 'macro' hemodynamic values such as CI, heart rate, and MAP are of great importance for assuring patient safety.

Conclusions

A high-antinociceptive balanced anesthesia with goal-directed fluid and norepinephrine administration preserved tissue oxygen saturation while other hemodynamic variables remained within a clinically acceptable range. Furthermore, this approach provided reliable surgical conditions, complete akinesia, and swift postoperative recovery.

Competing interests

The authors declare that they have no competing interests.

Authors' contributions

JJV was involved in the patient inclusion, data recording, data analysis and interpretation, and manuscript writing. MP participated in the data analysis and manuscript writing. LNH participated in the data analysis, pharmacologic modeling, data interpretation, and manuscript writing. WRDL was involved in the patient inclusion and manuscript writing. MMRFS and TWLS participated in the data interpretation and manuscript writing. AFK was involved in the patient inclusion and patient care, data recording, data analysis and interpretation, and manuscript writing. All authors read and approved the final manuscript.

Acknowledgements

Support for this study was solely provided by departmental and institutional funding.

Author details

[1]Department of Anesthesiology, University of Groningen, University Medical Center Groningen, Groningen, The Netherlands. [2]Department of Ophthalmology, University of Groningen, University Medical Center Groningen, Groningen, The Netherlands. [3]Department of Anaesthesiology and Intensive care medicine, Maria Middelares hospital, Ghent, Belgium.

References

1. Meng L, Cannesson M, Alexander BS, Yu Z, Kain ZN, Cerussi AE, Tromberg BJ, Mantulin WW: **Effect of phenylephrine and ephedrine bolus treatment on cerebral oxygenation in anaesthetized patients.** *Br J Anaesth* 2011, **107**:209–217.
2. Bouillon TW, Bruhn J, Radulescu L, Andresen C, Shafer TJ, Cohane C, Shafer SL: **Pharmacodynamic interaction between propofol and remifentanil regarding hypnosis, tolerance of laryngoscopy, bispectral index, and electroencephalographic approximate entropy.** *Anesthesiology* 2004, **100**:1353–1372.
3. Sandin RH, Enlund G, Samuelsson P, Lennmarken C: **Awareness during anaesthesia: a prospective case study.** *Lancet* 2000, **355**:707–711.
4. Cunningham AJ, Barry P: **Intraocular pressure–physiology and implications for anaesthetic management.** *Can Anaesth Soc J* 1986, **33**:195–208.
5. Murphy DF: **Anesthesia and intraocular pressure.** *Anesth Analg* 1985, **64**:520–530.
6. Leone M, Blidi S, Antonini F, Meyssignac B, Bordon S, Garcin F, Charvet A, Blasco V, Albanese J, Martin C: **Oxygen tissue saturation is lower in nonsurvivors than in survivors after early resuscitation of septic shock.** *Anesthesiology* 2009, **111**:366–371.
7. Brzezinski M, Luisetti T, London MJ: **Radial artery cannulation: a comprehensive review of recent anatomic and physiologic investigations.** *Anesth Analg* 2009, **109**:1763–1781.
8. Cohn SM: **Near-infrared spectroscopy: potential clinical benefits in surgery.** *J Am Coll Surg* 2007, **205**:322–332.
9. Scheeren TW, Schober P, Schwarte LA: **Monitoring tissue oxygenation by near infrared spectroscopy (NIRS): background and current applications.** *J Clin Monit Comput* 2012, **26**:279–287.

10. Vos JJ, Poterman M, Mooyaart EAQ, Weening M, Struys MMRF, Scheeren TWL, Kalmar AF: **Comparison of continuous non-invasive finger arterial pressure monitoring with conventional intermittent automated arm arterial pressure measurement in patients under general anaesthesia.** *Br J Anaesth* 2014, **113:**67–74.
11. Eeftinck Schattenkerk DW, van Lieshout JJ, van den Meiracker AH, Wesseling KR, Blanc S, Wieling W, van Montfrans GA, Settels JJ, Wesseling KH, Westerhof BE: **Nexfin noninvasive continuous blood pressure validated against riva-Rocci/Korotkoff.** *Am J Hypertens* 2009, **22:**378–383.
12. Hofhuizen CM, Lemson J, Hemelaar AE, Settels JJ, Schraa O, Singh SK, van der Hoeven JG, Scheffer GJ: **Continuous non-invasive finger arterial pressure monitoring reflects intra-arterial pressure changes in children undergoing cardiac surgery.** *Br J Anaesth* 2010, **105:**493–500.
13. Nowak RM, Sen A, Garcia AJ, Wilkie H, Yang JJ, Nowak MR, Moyer ML: **Noninvasive continuous or intermittent blood pressure and heart rate patient monitoring in the ED.** *Am J Emerg Med* 2011, **29:**782–789.
14. Chen G, Meng L, Alexander B, Tran NP, Kain ZN, Cannesson M: **Comparison of noninvasive cardiac output measurements using the nexfin monitoring device and the esophageal doppler.** *J Clin Anesth* 2012, **24:**275–283.
15. Sessler DI, Sigl JC, Kelley SD, Chamoun NG, Manberg PJ, Saager L, Kurz A, Greenwald S: **Hospital stay and mortality are increased in patients having a "triple low" of low blood pressure, low bispectral index, and low minimum alveolar concentration of volatile anesthesia.** *Anesthesiology* 2012, **116:**1195–1203.
16. Monk TG, Saini V, Weldon BC, Sigl JC: **Anesthetic management and one-year mortality after noncardiac surgery.** *Anesth Analg* 2005, **100:**4–10.
17. Bouillon TW: **Hypnotic and opioid anesthetic drug interactions on the CNS, focus on response surface modeling.** *Handb Exp Pharmacol* 2008, **182:**471–487.
18. Vos JJ, Kalmar AF, Struys MMRF, Wietasch JKG, Hendriks HGD, Scheeren TWL: **Comparison of arterial pressure and plethysmographic waveform based dynamic preload variables in assessing fluid responsiveness and dynamic arterial tone in patients undergoing major hepatic resection.** *Br J Anaesth* 2013, **110:**940–946.
19. Gan TJ, Glass PS, Windsor A, Payne F, Rosow C, Sebel P, Manberg P: **Bispectral index monitoring allows faster emergence and improved recovery from propofol, alfentanil, and nitrous oxide anesthesia. BIS utility study group.** *Anesthesiology* 1997, **87:**808–815.
20. Kearse LA Jr, Manberg P, Chamoun N, Chamoun N, de Bros F, Zaslavsky A: **Bispectral analysis of the electroencephalogram correlates with patient movement to skin incision during propofol/nitrous oxide anesthesia.** *Anesthesiology* 1994, **81:**1365–1370.
21. Imholz BP, Wieling W, van Montfrans GA, Wesseling KH: **Fifteen years experience with finger arterial pressure monitoring: assessment of the technology.** *Cardiovasc Res* 1998, **38:**605–616.
22. Besch G, Liu N, Samain E, Pericard C, Boichut N, Mercier M, Chazot T, Pili FS: **Occurrence of and risk factors for electroencephalogram burst suppression during propofol-remifentanil anaesthesia.** *Br J Anaesth* 2011, **107:**749–756.
23. Leslie K, Myles PS, Forbes A, Chan MT: **The effect of bispectral index monitoring on long-term survival in the B-aware trial.** *Anesth Analg* 2010, **110:**816–822.
24. Martina JR, Westerhof BE, van Goudoever J, de Beaumont EM, Truijen J, Kim YS, Immink RV, Jobsis DA, Hollmann MW, Lahpor JR, de Mol BA, van Lieshout JJ: **Noninvasive continuous arterial blood pressure monitoring with nexfin(R).** *Anesthesiology* 2012, **116:**1092–1103.
25. Broch O, Renner J, Gruenewald M, Meybohm P, Schottler J, Caliebe A, Steinfath M, Malbrain M, Bein B: **A comparison of the nexfin(R) and transcardiopulmonary thermodilution to estimate cardiac output during coronary artery surgery.** *Anaesthesia* 2012, **67:**377–383.
26. Rinehart J, Islam T, Boud R, Nguyen A, Alexander B, Canales C, Cannesson M: **Visual estimation of pulse pressure variation is not reliable: a randomized simulation study.** *J Clin Monit Comput* 2012, **26:**191–196.
27. Van Beest PA, Scheeren TW: **Tissue oxygen saturation as a goal, but when and where should we measure it?** *J Clin Monit Comput* 2013, **27:**211–213.
28. Habib AS, Parker JL, Maguire AM, Rowbotham DJ, Thompson JP: **Effects of remifentanil and alfentanil on the cardiovascular responses to induction of anaesthesia and tracheal intubation in the elderly.** *Br J Anaesth* 2002, **88:**430–433.
29. Bernet C, Desebbe O, Bordon S, Lacroix C, Rosamel P, Farhat F, Lehot JJ, Cannesson M: **The impact of induction of general anesthesia and a vascular occlusion test on tissue oxygen saturation derived parameters in high-risk surgical patients.** *J Clin Monit Comput* 2011, **25:**237–244.
30. Spruit RJ, Schwarte LA, Hakenberg OW, Scheeren TW: **Association of intraoperative tissue oxygenation with suspected risk factors for tissue hypoxia.** *J Clin Monit Comput* 2013, **27:**541–550.

17

The prevalence of pulmonary complications after thoracic and abdominal surgery and associated risk factors in patients admitted at a government hospital in Harare, Zimbabwe-a retrospective study

Cathrine Tadyanemhandu[1*], Rufaro Mukombachoto[1], Clement Nhunzvi[1], Farayi Kaseke[1], Vasco Chikwasha[2], Samson Chengetanai[3] and Shamila Manie[4]

Abstract

Background: The burden of HIV/AIDS in Sub-Saharan Africa has presented unusual and challenging acute surgical problems across all specialties. Thoraco-abdominal surgery cuts through muscle and thereby disrupts the normal anatomy and activity of the respiratory muscles leading to reduced lung volumes and putting the patients at greater risk of developing post-operative pulmonary complications (PPCs). PPCs remain an important cause of post-operative morbidity, mortality, and impacts on the long-term outcomes of patients post hospital discharge. The objective of the study was to determine the pulmonary complications developing after abdominal and thoracic surgery and the associated risks factors.

Methods: A retrospective records review of all abdominal and thoracic surgery patients admitted at a central hospital from January 2014 to October 2014 was done. Data collected included demographic data, surgical history, comorbidities and the PPCs present.

Results: Out of the 92 patients whose records were reviewed, 55 (59.8%) were males and 84 (91.3%) had abdominal surgery. The mean age of the patients was 42.6 years (SD = 18.4). The common comorbidities were HIV infection noted in 14(15.2%) of the patients and hypertension in 10 (13.0%). Thirty nine (42.4%) developed PPCs and the most common complications were nosocomial pneumonia in 21 (22.8%) patients, ventilator associated pneumonia in 11 (12.0%), and atelectasis in 6 (6.5%) patients. Logistic regression showed that a history of alcohol consumption, prolonged surgery, prolonged stay in hospital or critical care unit, incision type, and comorbidities were significant risk factors for PPCs ($p < 0.05$). The mortality rate was 10.9%.

Conclusion: PPCs like nosocomial and ventilator associated pneumonia were common and were associated with increased morbidity and adversely affected clinical outcomes of patients. HIV and hypertension presented significant comorbidities which the health team needed to recognize and address. Strategies to reduce the occurrence of PPCs have to be implemented through coordinated efforts by the health practitioners as a team during the entire perioperative period.

Keywords: Abdominal surgery, Thoracic surgery, Post-operative complications, Pulmonary complications, HIV infection, Comorbidities

* Correspondence: cathytadya@gmail.com
[1]Department of Rehabilitation, College of Health Sciences, University Of Zimbabwe, PO Box AV 178, Avondale, Harare, Zimbabwe
Full list of author information is available at the end of the article

Background

It is estimated that surgical conditions account for 11% of the total global burden of disease and 25 million disability-adjusted life years (DALYs) in Africa, the region with the highest concentration of surgical DALYs (38/1000 population) (Ozgediaz and Riviello 2008; Ärnlöv 2016). According to the World Health Organization (WHO), DALY is a measure of overall disease burden, expressed as the number of years lost due to ill-health, disability or early death. Human Immunodeficiency Virus (HIV) infection complicates surgical practice by increasing the occurrence of surgery related disease conditions, presenting challenges in the surgical management of HIV infected patients and necessitating the introduction of appropriate methods to improve surgical outcomes (Odimba 2010). Furthermore, these patients also present with other comorbidities such as hypertension, diabetes, and tuberculosis which further complicate their post-operative management (Hanekom, Coetzee and Faure 2006).

Surgical and trauma patients invariably experience a sudden and profound systemic insult that often leads to decompensation of subclinical conditions and sets the stage for new and potentially life-threatening complications (Sawyer and Leon 2010). In Nigeria, the majority of post-surgical complications were related either to surgery or anesthetic care, leading to a very high mortality rate in surgical units (Okafor 2009). Post-operative complications, involving the respiratory tract remain the most frequent cause of morbidity contributing to significant increases in patient discomfort, increased length of hospital stay (LOS), increased use of resources and overall hospital costs as well as mortality (Brooks-Brunn 1995; Arozullah et al., 2001; Hulzebos et al., 2003; Reeve 2008). A post-operative pulmonary complication (PPC) is defined as "any pulmonary abnormality occurring during the postoperative period and resulting in clinically significant disease or dysfunction, adversely affecting the clinical course of the primary condition" (Sharafkhaneh et al. 2008) and the specific complications were defined by Jammer et al., (2015).

Patients undergoing abdominal and thoracic surgery are most prone to PPCs since the incidence of PPCs is inversely related to the distance of the surgical incision from the diaphragm (Rudra and Das 2006). Besides the type of surgery, increased number, and complexity of thoraco-abdominal surgical procedures, increasing severity of illness and age of patients undergoing surgery are all directly related to the patients' post-surgical outcomes (Hulzebos et al., 2003) and to the incidence of PPCs. It is therefore important to understand the most common PPCs in our population so that preoperative assessment can partly focus on the risk factors for the PPCs. The main aim of this study was to determine the pulmonary complications developing after abdominal and thoracic surgery and the associated risk factors. It is envisaged that knowledge of such will help put strategies in place to minimize the occurrence of the complications as well as effectively manage them thus reducing morbidity and mortality rates.

Methods

Study setting

A retrospective records review was carried out at Parirenyatwa Group of Hospitals, the largest referral public hospital in Zimbabwe with a bed capacity of 1800. The records were accessed through the Medical Records Department, which stores the patients' records in both electronic and hard-copy formats. Patients referred to this hospital are usually from the low to middle socioeconomic classes.

Participants

Participants were selected from patients aged 16 years and older who had undergone abdominal and cardiothoracic surgery between January and October 2014 inclusive. Ethical approval was granted by the Joint Research Ethics Committee for the University of Zimbabwe and Parirenyatwa Group of Hospitals (JREC: 270/14) and the Medical Research Council of Zimbabwe (MRCZ/B/738). Permission to access patients' records from the medical records department was also sought from the Institutional Review Board.

Sample size

The sample size required to establish the prevalence of PPCs which were anticipated to be present in 10% of the patients (Kelkar 2015), with a precision of 5% was 87, at 90% confidence level (Epi Info Version 7.1.5.0). This was based on a population of 800, the estimated number of surgical admissions over a 10-month period.

Data collection

Qualifying patient records were identified from the admission and ward order books of the cardiothoracic and general surgery wards. Patient hospital numbers were used to access their electronic files from the Medical Records Department. The checklist used to document data during the record review comprised of the following variables which were selected based on a review of studies on risk factors for PPCs: demographic data (age, gender, marital status, smoking and alcohol consumption history), (up to one drink per day for women and up to two drinks per day for men) medical/surgical information (specific diagnosis, cause, surgery done, category of surgery, type of procedure, length of surgery, type of incision), clinical information (ICU admission, duration of period on mechanical ventilation, length of stay in ICU, length of hospital stay, complications, comorbidities, medication, chest X-rays results, FBC results, temperature, sputum analysis, number of pre and post-operative physiotherapy sessions received) and post-operative pulmonary complications present. The incision type was divided into three groups which included upper, midline (vertical incisions) and lower incision (transverse incisions). An upper incision was described as consisting of thoracic and other incisions above the umbilicus such as thoracoabdominal incision, median sternotomy, posterolateral, anterolateral, axillary, anterior, and posterior thoracotomies. Midline/vertical incisions included the midline and paramedian incisions and the Mayo-Robson extension of the paramedian incision. Lower or transverse incisions included the Kocher, Transverse, Rockey-Davis, Maylard, and Pfannenstiel incisions.

Data analysis

Data was analyzed using Stata (Version 13). Continuous data was summarized using means and standard deviations whereas categorical data was reported as frequencies and percentages. Chi-square test and Fisher's exact were used to test for association. Logistic regression was used to determine the risk factors for development of the PPCs in the patients. For multivariate analysis, variables were selected for inclusion into multiple logistic regression model based on $p < 0.25$ in the univariate analysis. The level of significance was set at $\alpha < 0.05$.

Table 1 Demographics and clinical information for the patients ($n = 92$)

Characteristics	PPCs present	PPCs absent
Sample size, *n* (%)	39 (42.4)	53 (57.6)
Age, mean(SD)	45.8 (17.2)	40.0 (19.1)
Gender-males, *n* (%)	26 (66.7)	29 (54.7)
Duration of surgery/min, mean(SD)	148.8 (75.0)	82.7 (35.7)
Length of CCU stay/days, mean(SD)	6.4 (7.3)	0.6 (1.3)
Hospital stay/days, mean(SD)	14 (7.6)	6.3 (7.7)
Cause of surgery, *n* (%)		
Disease	35 (89.7)	47 (88.7)
Accidents	4 (10.3)	6 (11.3)
Type of surgery, *n* (%)		
Abdominal	34 (87.2)	50 (94.3)
Cardiothoracic	5 (12.8)	3 (5.7)
Types of comorbidities, *n* (%)		
None	18 (46.1)	41 (77.4)
HIV	9 (23.1)	5 (7.5)
Hypertension	8 (20.5)	4 (7.5)
Diabetics	2 (5.1)	2 (3.7)
Previous pulmonary disease (COPD)	1 (2.6)	0
Renal disease	1 (2.6)	1 (1.9)
Post-op physiotherapy, *n* (%)		
Yes	38 (97.4)	14 (26.4)
No	1 (2.6)	39 (73.6)

Results

Demographics of the participants

A total of 92 patient records were accessed from Parirenyatwa Hospital Medical Records Department, 84 (91.3%) of whom had undergone abdominal surgery and 8 (8.7%) thoracic. Fifty-five (59.8%) patients were male and the overall mean age of all participants was 42.6 ± 18.4 years. Table 1 shows the demographic characteristics of the patients.

Clinical information and surgical history

The majority of surgeries done, 70 (76.1%) were emergency while 22 (23.9%) were elective. Surgery was due to disease conditions in 82 (89.1%) patients and trauma following an accident in 10 (10.9%) patients. Comorbidities were present in 33 (35.9%) patients, with HIV infection being the most common cormobidity in 14 (15.2%) followed by hypertension in 12 (13.0%) patients. The mean duration of surgery was 110.0 ± 64.0 min and patients had a mean duration stay in the critical care unit of 3.1 ± 5.6 days. The mean hospital stay for the cohort was 9.7 ± 7.3 days and the mortality rate was 10.9%. Midline incisions were the most common incisions having been done in 60 (65.2%) participants, lower incisions in 20 (21.7%) and upper incisions in 12 (13.1%).

Postoperative pulmonary complications and associated risk factors

Out of the 92 patients, 39 (42.4%) developed PPCs. The most common PPCs in the cohort included nosocomial pneumonia in 21 (22.8%), ventilator associated pneumonia in 11 (12.0%) and atelectasis in 6 (6.5%) patients. Post-operative physiotherapy was administered to 52 (56.5%) patients, with the median number of physiotherapy sessions being 2 (IQR = 0–9.0). The majority of the patients who developed PPCs were male, 26 (66.7%) but there was no significant association between development of PPCs and gender (X^2 (1) = 1.3343, p = .25). History of alcohol consumption was found to be a risk factor for PPC development (p = 0.038) (Table 2).

Patients who developed a PPC had longer duration of surgery, critical care stay as well length of hospital stay compared to those who did not and this was statistically significant for all variables (p < .001). The following were found to be the risk factors for developing PPCs; duration period of surgery, length of critical care stay, length of hospital stay, having a disease due to tumors and presence of comorbidities (Table 3).

Table 2 Demographic risk factors for postoperative pulmonary complications

Characteristic	Postoperative pulmonary complication		OR (95% CI)	*p* value
	Yes	No		
Age, mean ± sd	45.8 ± 17.2	40.2 ± 19.1	1.02 (0.99–1.04)	0.156
Gender				
Female	13	24	1	0.250
Male	26	29	1.66 (0.70–3.90)	
Smoking history				
No	29	45	1	0.212
Yes	10	8	1.94 (0.69–5.49)	
Alcohol consumption history				
No	23	42	1	0.038
Yes	16	11	2.66 (1.06–6.67)	

Table 4 Univariate analysis of surgical related risks factors for postoperative pulmonary complications

Characteristic	Postoperative pulmonary complication		OR (95% CI)	*p* value
	Yes	No		
Cause of surgery				
Disease	35	47	1.12 (0.29–4.26)	0.871
Trauma	4	6	1	
Category of surgery				
Emergency	31	39	1.39 (0.52–3.74)	0.513
Elective	8	14	1	
Incision type				
Lower	2	18	1	0.005[a]
Middle	30	30	9 (1.92–42.23)	
Upper	7	5	12.6 (1.97–80.76)	0.008[a]

[a]Denotes statistically significant

Under surgery related risk factors, the type of the incision was found to be a major risk factor, especially if it was either a middle or an upper incision (Table 4).

Multivariate analysis was done to determine the risk factors and to control for possible confounding variables. The only factors which were statistically significant in the development of PPCs in the patients were duration of surgery and length of hospital stay (Table 5).

Discussion

Studies conducted in low-income countries showed that 10–15% of hospital admissions were due to diseases amenable to surgical treatment, of which diseases were more prevalent in the young population compared to high income countries (Hanekom, Coetzee and Faure 2006, Frankel et al., 2007, Semer, Sullivan and Meara 2010, Chalya et al., 2011, Pearse et al., 2012, Kodra, Shpata and Ohri 2016) and the same pattern was noted in the current study. The affected age group in African countries of between 15 and 44 years is the predominant economically active segment of the population. Previous reports indicated that in this age group traumatic injuries from road traffic crashes or assault were the second most common cause of morbidity and mortality after HIV infection, particularly in males (Hanekom, Coetzee and Faure 2006, Ntumba and Juma 2011). However, our study sample showed lower prevalence of

Table 3 Univariate analysis of clinical risk factors for postoperative pulmonary complications

Characteristic	Postoperative pulmonary complication		OR (95% CI)	*p* value
	Yes	No		
Duration period of surgery (min), mean ± sd	148.8 ± 75.0	82.7 ± 35.7	1.02 (1.01–1.03)	<0.001[a]
Length of critical care stay (days), mean ± sd	6.4 ± 7.3	0.6 ± 1.3	1.73 (1.32–2.26)	<0.001[a]
Length of hospital stay (days), mean ± sd	14 ± 7.6	6.3 ± 7.7	1.36 (1.17–1.57)	<0.001[a]
Category of diagnosis				
Inflammations	17	34	1	0.634
Infective	7	10	1.33 (0.41–4.36)	
Trauma	5	3	2.00 (.36–10.97)	0.425
Tumors	10	6	3.60 (1.04–12.42)	0.043[a]
Comorbidities				
None	17	42	1	0.001[a]
Present	22	11	4.94 (1.97–12.36)	
Outcome				
Deceased	5	5	1	0.607
Discharged	34	48	0.71 (0.19–2.64)	

[a]Denotes statistically significant

Table 5 Multiple logistic regression for risk factors for developing pulmonary complications after surgery

Characteristic	Postoperative pulmonary complication		OR (95% CI)	*p* value
	Yes	No		
Age, mean ± sd	45.8 ± 17.2	40.2 ± 19.1	0.99 (0.93–1.06)	0.826
Gender				
Female	13	24	1	0.857
Male	26	29	0.85 (0.15–4.89)	
Smoking history				
No	29	45	1	0.069
Yes	10	8	0.06 (0.00–1.24)	
Alcohol consumption history				
No	23	42	1	0.060
Yes	16	11	7.02 (0.92–53.46)	
Duration period of surgery (min), mean ± sd	148.8 ± 75.0	82.7 ± 35.7	1.03 (1.01–1.05)	0.003[a]
Length of hospital stay (days), mean ± sd	14 ± 7.6	6.3 ± 7.7	1.21 (1.03–1.42)	0.019[a]
Incision type				
Lower	2	18	1	0.313
Middle	30	30	5.06 (0.22–118.10)	
Upper	7	5	2.89 (0.04–194.32)	0.621
Category of diagnosis				
Inflammations	17	34	1	0.476
Infective	7	10	0.50 (0.07–3.41)	
Trauma	5	3	0.43 (0.03–6.73)	0.550
Masses	10	6	2.68 (0.28–26.03)	0.394
Comorbidities				
None	17	42	1	0.066
Present	22	11	6.01 (0.89–40.66)	

[a]Denotes statitically significant

HIV in both elective and traumatic surgery patients when compared to reports from other African countries (Hanekom, Coetzee and Faure 2006, Odimba 2010, Pandie et al., 2012).

The majority of patients had abdominal surgery mainly due to infection or the presence of tumors. This compared well with reports from other countries like India, Malawi, and Ethiopia where abdominal surgery was the most common surgery performed especially in the central hospitals (Bhat, Shinde and Chaudhari 2006, Lavy et al., 2007, Denu et al., 2015). The commonest causes for laparotomies in African countries have been listed as injuries, infections and neoplasms (Grimes et al., 2012, Tadyanemhandu and Manie 2015). In Zimbabwe, the prevalence of violent or injury related surgeries have been reported to be higher in the Southern part of the country, in the Matebeleland Region as compared to the Northern part (Tadyanemhandu and Manie 2015). The current study was done in the Northern part of the country, hence the small number of injury related surgeries.

Post-operative pulmonary complications were very high indicating the burden of morbidity experienced by patients undergoing thoracic and abdominal surgery in a low income country hospital. The final outcome of critically ill surgical and trauma patients depends, to a large extent, on events that take place after the original injury, surgical emergency or elective procedure (Sawyer and Leon 2010). A significant proportion of patients in our study developed various PPCs which further impacted on the duration of stay in either critical care or general hospital stay potentially worsening final outcomes.

The prevalence of PPCs in our study was found to be 42.4%. The prevalence rate for development of PPCs in our study falls in the range of 5–80% which was reported for non-thoracic surgeries by Fisher, Majumdar and McAlister (2002). The reason for this wide variation was attributed to the set-up, pre-operative and intraoperative risk factors (Rock and Rich 2003), use of different diagnostic criteria or definitions for PPCs, the type of surgery category and the type of patients recruited (Smetana 2009). The reason why our prevalence rate was relatively high might be due to the surgical specialties under consideration, since it has been reported that the prevalence of PPCs is high in abdominal and cardiothoracic surgery patients. Nosocomial pneumonia was the most common PPC identified in our study. This was similar to other studies which highlighted that pneumonia was the most common PPC as it ranked third after urinary tract infection and wound infection (Inoue et al., 2013; Denu et al. 2015). The other complications included atelectasis, respiratory failure, and pleural effusion which were also reported in other studies (Jensen and Yang 2007, Okafor 2009).

To reduce the incidence or prevalence of PPCs, there must be an understanding of patient conditions that increase the risk of developing PPCs and of effective interventions available to reduce the impact of pre-existing patient's conditions on the subsequent development of PPCs (Rudra and Das 2006, Denu et al., 2015, Kodra, Shpata and Ohri 2016). The risk factors for development of PPCs from our study were found to be incision type, presence of comorbidities, duration of surgery, length of critical care stay, and hospital stay. These findings were also reported in other studies which looked at predictors of PPCs in patients (Rudra and Das 2006; Jensen and Yang 2007; Denu et al. 2015, Kodra, Shpata and Ohri 2016). Gender, age over 65 years and category of surgery were not found to be associated with development of PPCs in our study contrary to other studies (Jensen and Yang 2007, Denu et al., 2015, Kodra, Shpata and Ohri 2016). This may be due to a small number of patients over the age of 60 in our study as majority was below the age of 45. However, there is evidence that advanced age is an important predictor of postoperative pulmonary complications, even after adjustment for comorbid conditions (Qaseem et al. 2006). Moreover, following any type of surgery, patients are reluctant to move because of fear of damaging the incision site and the pain associated with any movement. This predisposes the patients to the complications of immobility. Development of PPCs will further result in prolongation of mechanical ventilation, CCU stay or hospital stay, and this was evident in our study during comparisons between the group which developed PPCs and the one which did not. It is assumed that this resulted in substantial economic burden on the hospital resources. Surgical patients from 28 European countries have been reported to have a median critical care stay of 1.2 days (IQR = 0.9–3.6) and a median duration of hospital stay of 3.0 days (IQR = 1.0–70), far lower than what is reported in most African countries (Hanekom et al., 2006, Chalya et al. 2011, Tadyanemhandu and Manie 2015). The mortality rate for our study was comparable to the 12.3% reported in South Africa (Hanekom et al., 2006) but lower than 32.7% reported in Tanzania. A plausible reason for the high mortality in Tanzania was the fact that the study was focused on trauma admissions only and not any other cause. Furthermore, high income countries reported very low mortality rates as exemplified by the 4% obtained in the study of 28 European nations (Pearse et al., 2012). After controlling for other variables in our cohort, the only risk factors associated with development of PPCs in our study were duration of surgery and length of hospital stay.

The most common comorbidities present in our study were HIV and hypertension. These comorbidities have been reported in South Africa (Hanekom, Coetzee and Faure 2006, Pandie et al., 2012). The greatest burden of disease in Africa comes from infectious diseases, with HIV and tuberculosis (TB) dominating the health landscape but now there is an increase in non-communicable diseases, with hypertension and diabetes dominating (Pandie et al., 2012). There is sufficient evidence to support that exercise capacity, diabetes, and HIV infection are independent risk factors for postoperative pulmonary complications (Hulzebos et al., 2003; Rudra and Das 2006). These comorbidities predispose patients to postoperative pulmonary complications as they result in patients having a poor baseline pulmonary function.

Results of our study show that none of the patients received pre-operative physiotherapy and the majority only received post-operative physiotherapy after a complication had developed. Similar findings were obtained in Australia and New Zealand where very few physiotherapists reported involvement in pre-operative physiotherapy despite the significant benefits highlighted in the literature (Reeve 2008). The short period between diagnosis and surgery has often been regarded as an inadequate period of time to sufficiently impact upon exercise capacity in order to improve the outcomes of patients post-surgery (Reeve 2008). Reductions in post-operative pulmonary complications will require development and consensus acceptance of diagnostic criteria and creation of valid standard of measurement of the complications (Romig and Dorman 2011).

Limitations of the study and recommendations

The study design was limiting since a retrospective records review made it difficult to infer causality. The sample size was not large enough hence the need to carry out a similar study, with a bigger sample size in which data is prospectively recorded in a randomized controlled trial especially to determine if HIV status and age affect the outcomes of surgical patients. There are measures that need to be taken so that spirometry tests are done in all patients undergoing abdominal and thoracic surgery to identify the at risk population.

The other limitation was unavailability of severity scores of patients using validated scales like American

Society of Anesthesiologists (ASA), Acute Physiology and Chronic Health Evaluation score (APACHE), or the Sequential Organ Failure Assessment score (SOFA). This limitation was reported in another study by Tadyanemhandu and Manie (2015), and it was recommended that the physicians and anesthetists consider using validated scales to measure the severity of the condition more objectively.

Conclusions

Post-operative pulmonary complications were common and were associated with increased morbidity and mortality and adversely affected clinical outcomes of patients. The presence of the comorbidities which included HIV, hypertension, and diabetes further complicated the management of the patients. The risk factors associated with development of PPCs in our study were duration of surgery and length of hospital stay. Strategies to reduce the rate of the complications have to be implemented by the health practitioners as a team in order to reduce the burden of disease on the patients as well as on hospital management.

Abbreviations

ANOVA: Analysis of variance; CCU: Critical care unit; ICU: Intensive care unit; JREC: Joint research ethics committee; MRCZ: Medical Research Council of Zimbabwe; PPC: Post-operative pulmonary complication

Acknowledgements

Would like to thank all the people who contributed tirelessly to the success of the project, hospital staff from the participating wards and also from the medical records department.

Funding

No funding was received for the study.

Authors' contributions

CT and RM participated in the design of the study. RM was responsible for the collection of the completed questionnaires and data management. CT, VC, and RM participated in the data analysis. FK, CN, SC, and SM contributed to the writing up and editing of the final manuscript. All authors read and approved the final manuscript.

Competing interest

The authors declare that they have no competing interests.

Author details

[1]Department of Rehabilitation, College of Health Sciences, University Of Zimbabwe, PO Box AV 178, Avondale, Harare, Zimbabwe. [2]Department of Community Medicine, College of Health Sciences, University Of Zimbabwe, PO Box AV 178, Avondale, Harare, Zimbabwe. [3]Division of Basic Medical Sciences, Faculty of Medicine, National University of Science and Technology, PO Box AC 939, Ascot, Bulawayo, Zimbabwe. [4]Division of Physiotherapy, Department of Health and Rehabilitation Sciences, Faculty of Health Sciences, University of CapeTown, Anzio Road, Observatory, CapeTown, South Africa.

References

Ärnlöv J. Estimates of global, regional, and national incidence, prevalence, and mortality of HIV, 1980-2015: the global burden of disease study 2015. The Lancet HIV. 2016;3(8):E361–87.

Arozullah AM, Khuri SF, Henderson WG, Daley J. Development and validation of a multifactorial risk index for predicting postoperative pneumonia after major non-cardiac surgery. Ann Intern Med. 2001;135:847–57.

Bhat SA, Shinde V, Chaudhari L. Audit of intensive care unit admissions from the operating room. Indian Journal of Anesth. 2006;50(6):193–200.

Brooks-Brunn J. Postoperative atelectasis and pneumonia. Heart Lung. 1995;24:94–115.

Chalya PL, Gilyoma JM, Dass RM, Mchembe MD, Matasha M, Mabula JB, Mbelenge N, Mahalu W. Trauma admissions to the intensive care unit at a reference hospital in northwestern Tanzania. Scandinavian journal of trauma, resuscitation and. Emerg Med. 2011;19:61.

Denu ZA, Yasin MO, Melekie TB, Berhe A. Postoperative pulmonary complications and associated factors among surgical patients. J Anesth Clin Res. 2015;6:554. doi:10.4172/2155-6148.1000554.

Fisher BW, Majumdar SR, McAlister FA. Predicting pulmonary complications after nonthoracic surgery: a systematic review of blinded studies. Am J Med. 2002;112:219–25.

Frankel H, Sperry J, Kaplan L, Foley A, Rabinovici R. Classification of adverse events occurring in a surgical intensive care unit. Am J Surg. 2007;194:328–32.

Grimes CE, Law RSL, Borgstein ES, Mkandawire NC, Lavy CBD. Systematic review of met and unmet need of surgical disease in rural sub-Saharan Africa. World J Surg. 2012;36:8–23.

Hanekom S, Coetzee AR, Faure M. Outcome evaluation of a south African surgical ICU—a baseline study. South African Journal of Critical Care. 2006;22(1):14–20.

Hulzebos EH, Van Meeteren NL, De Bie RA, Dagnelie PC, Helders PJ. Prediction of postoperative pulmonary complications on the basis of preoperative risk factors in patients who had undergone coronary artery bypass graft surgery. Phys Ther. 2003;83(1):8–16.

Inoue J, Ono R, Makiura D, Kashiwa-Motoyama M, Miura Y, Usami M, Nakamura T, Imanishi T, Kuroda D. Prevention of postoperative pulmonary complications through intensive preoperative respiratory rehabilitation in patients with esophageal cancer. Disease of the Esophagus. 2013;26:68–74.

Jammer I, Wickboldt N, Sander M, Smith A, Schultz MJ, Pelosi P, Leva B, Rhodes A, Hoeft A, Walder B, Chew MS, Pearse RP. Standards for definitions and use of outcome measures for clinical effectiveness research in perioperative medicine: European Perioperative clinical outcome (EPCO) definitions. A statement from the ESA-ESICM joint taskforce on perioperative outcome measures. Eur J Anaesthesiol. 2015;32:88–105.

Jensen L, Yang L. Risk factors for postoperative pulmonary complications in coronary artery bypass graft surgery patients. Eur J Cardiovasc Nurs. 2007;6:241–6.

Kelkar KV. Post-operative pulmonary complications after non-cardiothoracic surgery. Indian J Anaesth. 2015 Sep;59(9):599–605.

Kodra N, Shpata V, Ohri I. Risk factors for postoperative pulmonary complications after abdominal surgery. Open Access Maced J Med Sci. 2016;4(2):259–63.

Lavy C, Tindall A, Steinlechner C, Mkandawire N, Chimangeni S. Surgery in Malawi—a national survey of activity in rural and urban hospitals. Ann R Coll Surg Engl. 2007;89:722–4. doi:10.1308/003588407X209329.

Nthumba PM, Juma PI. HIV infection: implications on surgical practice, HIV-infection - impact, awareness and social implications of living with HIV/AIDS, 2011. Eugenia Barros (Ed.), ISBN: 978-953- 307-343-9.

Odimba BFK. The impact of HIV infection on the surgical disease burden in Africa. East and Central Journal of Surgery. 2010;15(1):3–8.

Okafor UV. An audit of unplanned postoperative intensive care unit admissions in Enugu, Nigeria: causes and outcome. South African Journal of Critical Care. 2009;25:1.

Ozgediz D, Riviello R. The "other" neglected diseases in global public health: surgical conditions in sub-Saharan Africa. PLoS Med. 2008;5(6):e121. doi:10. 1371/journal.pmed.0050121.

Pandie M, van der Plas H, Maartens G, Mendelson M. The role of the infectious diseases unit at Groote Schuur hospital in addressing South Africa's greatest burden of disease. S Afr Med J. 2012;102(6):528–31.
Pearse RM, Moreno RP, Bauer P, Pelosi P, Metnitz P, Spies C, Vallet B, Vincent JL, Hoeft A, Rhodes A, for the European Surgical Outcomes Study (EuSOS) group for the Trials groups of the European Society of Intensive Care Medicine and the European Society of Anaesthesiology. Mortality after surgery in Europe: a 7 day cohort study. Lancet. 2012;380:1059–65.
Qaseem A, Snow V, Fitterman N, Hornbake ER, Lawrence VA, Smetana GW, Weiss K, Owens DK. Risk assessment for and strategies to reduce perioperative pulmonary complications for patients undergoing noncardiothoracic surgery: a guideline from the American College of Physicians. Ann Intern Med. 2006;144:575–80.
Reeve J. Physiotherapy interventions to prevent postoperative pulmonary complications following lung resection. What is the evidence? What is the practice? N Z J Physiother. 2008;36(3):118–30.
Rock P, Rich PB. Postoperative pulmonary complications. Curr Opin Anaesthesiol. 2003;16:123–31.
Romig MC, Dorman T. Opening your eyes to postoperative pulmonary complications. Crit Care Med. 2011;39:9.
Rudra A, Das S. Postoperative pulmonary complications. Indian Journal of Anesthetics. 2006;50(2):89–98.
Sawyer R, Leon A. Common complications in the surgical intensive care unit. Crit Care Med. 2010;38:9.
Semer NB, Sullivan SR, Meara JG. Plastic surgery and global health: how plastic surgery impacts the global burden of surgical disease. J Plast Reconstr Aesthet Surg. 2010;63(8):1244–8.
Sharafkhaneh A, Falk JA, Minai OA, Lipson DA. Overview of the perioperative management of lung volume reduction surgery patients. Proc Am Thorac Soc. 2008;5:438–41.
Smetana GW. Postoperative pulmonary complications: an update on risk assessment and reduction. Cleve Clin J Med. 2009;76(suppl 4):S60–5.
Tadyanemhandu C, Manie S. Profile of patients and physiotherapy patterns in intensive care units in public hospitals in Zimbabwe: a descriptive cross-sectional study. BMC Anesthesiol. 2015;15:136.

18

The rising tide of opioid use and abuse: the role of the anesthesiologist

Elena J. Koepke[1], Erin L. Manning[2], Timothy E. Miller[1], Arun Ganesh[3], David G. A. Williams[1] and Michael W. Manning[1*]

Abstract

Opioid use has risen dramatically in the past three decades. In the USA, opioid overdose has become a leading cause of unintentional death, surpassing motor vehicle accidents. A patient's first exposure to opioids may be during the perioperative period, a time where anesthesiologists have a significant role in pain management. Almost all patients in the USA receive opioids during a surgical encounter. Opioids have many undesirable side effects, including potential for misuse, or opioid use disorder. Anesthesiologists and surgeons employ several methods to decrease unnecessary opioid use, opioid-related adverse events, and side effects in the perioperative period. Multimodal analgesia, enhanced recovery pathways, and regional anesthesia are key tools as we work towards optimal opioid stewardship and the ideal of effective analgesia without undesirable sequelae.

Keywords: Perioperative medicine, Multimodal analgesia, Opioid-free anesthesia, Opioid-reduced anesthesia, Opioid epidemic, Enhanced recovery pathways

Background

Opioids are an effective form of analgesia for acute pain but, with over-prescription, have become detrimental to public health in the USA. In the 1990s, a patient advocacy movement focused on pain control was born, and physician, patient advocacy, and professional societies began to promote aggressive treatment of both acute and chronic pain with opioids. The movement was propagated by many well-intentioned clinicians; however, the pharmaceutical industry had a hand in its creation and distribution. Although not a comprehensive summation of the causes of the opioid epidemic, the following events illustrate that a multitude of parties were complicit in its evolution:

1. In 1996, the American Pain Society declared that pain should be assessed "with the same zeal (as) other vital signs…"
2. In 1999, the VA Hospital System declared pain as "the fifth vital sign."
3. JCAHO, the hospital credentialing agency, followed suit and educated health professionals to perform a consistent assessment and treatment of pain, as well as mandated the documentation of pain scores (Alam 2016).
4. During this time, the Federation of State Medical Boards also released a pain control policy that encouraged the use of opioids in the treatment of chronic pain.

Incidentally, the educational media promoted by JCAHO and the FSMB policy on chronic pain were funded by the pharmaceutical industry, or written by members who were on the payroll of a prominent pharmaceutical company. As a result, use and prescriptions for opioids began to multiply. The misleading claims and treatment guidelines were not brought to light until the USA was in the midst of an opioid epidemic.

Since 1999, there has been a steady increase in the number of opioids sold and opioid-related deaths (Manchikanti et al. 2012) (Fig. 1). In 2015, more than 40% of the world's supply of thebaine, a main ingredient in hydrocodone and oxycodone, was consumed by the USA. Gram for gram, people in the USA consume more narcotic medication than other nations worldwide. By

* Correspondence: Michael.manning@duke.edu
[1]Division of General, Vascular and Transplant Anesthesiology, Department of Anesthesiology, Duke University, Box 3094, 2301 Erwin Road, Durham, NC 27710, USA
Full list of author information is available at the end of the article

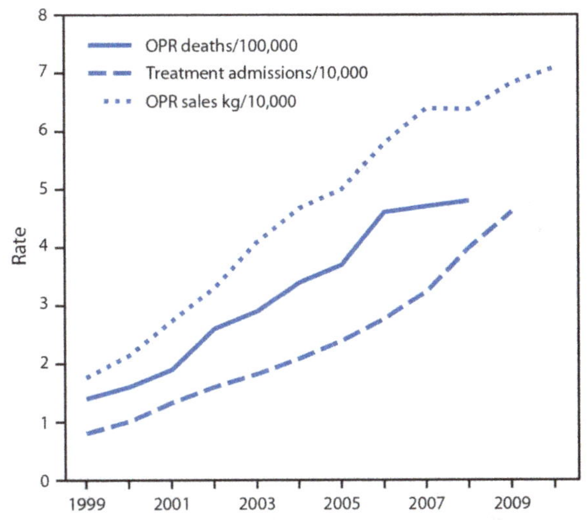

Fig. 1 Rates of opioid pain reliever overdose death, opioid pain relief treatment admissions, and kilograms of opioid pain relievers sold—United States, 1999–2010. Age-adjusted rates per 100,000 population for opioid pain reliever (OPR) deaths, crude rates per 10,000 population for OPR abuse treatment admissions, and crude rates per 10,000 population for kilograms of OPR sold. From Centers for Disease Control and Prevention (2011)

2017, the number of opioid-related deaths has continued to increase (Hedegaard et al. 2017) and the US government has declared the opioid epidemic as a public health emergency.

In this review, we will briefly describe the opioid burden within the USA, with emphasis on the emerging evidence of a link between acute exposure to opioids and chronic opioid dependence. We will then highlight alternative approaches to the management of intraoperative and acute postoperative surgical pain which emphasize multimodal analgesics and thereby decrease the need for opioid use in the acute hospital setting.

Perioperative use of opioids

In a recent survey of adult surgical patients, 75% had pain they rated as moderate/extreme during the immediate post-surgical period (Gan et al. 2014). Approximately 99% of all surgical patients in the USA receive opioids perioperatively at some point during their care (Kessler et al. 2013). Some argue, however, that opioids are used more frequently than needed due to increasing use of quality metrics that use pain control as a measure of quality of care (Zgierska et al. 2012). Despite the fact that opioids have significant side effects, they have historically been the primary treatment for post-surgical pain as they are very effective with a quick onset of action and no analgesic ceiling.

Opioid use, however, begets opioid use. Patients who received opioids for their primary pain therapy in the acute perioperative period are commonly to require increased doses to maintain the same analgesic effects (Chia et al. 1999). This is usually attributed to the development of "acute tolerance" to the analgesic effects of opioids, although this loss of analgesic efficacy may also be the result of opioid-induced hyperalgesia. Opioid-induced hyperalgesia has been defined as a state of nociceptive sensitization caused by exposure to opioids (Chu et al. 2008). Hyperalgesia and tolerance are very different pharmacologic phenomena that can lead to similar net increases in opioid dosing over time. This has been referred to as the *opioid paradox*: the more opioids used intraoperatively, the more opioids required postoperatively. The paradox has been measured in surgical patients up to 2 days postoperatively (Joly et al. 2005). Both acute opioid tolerance and opioid-induced hyperalgesia are the postulated mechanisms behind this phenomenon.

Postoperative use of opioids and chronic opioid use

Using opioids to treat acute post-surgical pain was not originally believed to increase the risk of long-term opioid dependence or addiction in patients. An infamous letter published in a 1980's *New England Journal of Medicine* quotes: "We conclude that despite widespread use of narcotic drugs in hospitals, the development of addiction is rare in medical patients with no history of addiction" (Porter and Jick 1980). However, recent literature suggests that some opioid-naïve patients became chronic users of opioids after surgery, chronic being defined as opioid use lasting > 90 days postoperatively. In a retrospective study of over 36,000 opioid-naïve patients undergoing elective surgery in the USA between 2013 and 2014, the incidence of chronic opioid use after surgery was ~ 6%. This did not differ between major and minor surgical procedures (Brummett et al. 2017).

Another study of opioid-naive patients undergoing short-stay surgery also found significant rates of chronic opioid dependence 1 year after surgery (Lee et al. 2017). Focusing on curative-intent cancer surgery in the USA from 2010 to 2014, Lee et al. found approximately 10% of patients were still using opioids 1 year after surgery.

The perioperative use of benzodiazepines, selective serotonin reuptake inhibitors (SSRIs), diabetes, younger age, lower income, higher intraoperative use, and the duration of acute postoperative opioid use have all been identified as factors which carry increased risk of prolonged postoperative opioid use (Clarke et al. 2014). A study by Shah et al. analyzed a one million patient sample of a large health insurance claim database which represented the US-insured population from 2005 to 2015. They found that postoperative prescribing patterns can effect the incidence of chronic opioid use disorder. Starting on the third postoperative day, every day of opioid therapy increases the risk of a patient becoming a chronic consumer of opioids—with the most dramatic increases after the fifth and 31st day of therapy. Cumulative prescription dose of ≥700 morphine milligram equivalents, initial prescription for a 10- or 30-day supply, or a second prescription or refill were also associated with an increased incidence of chronic opioid use disorder at 1 year postoperative. Moreover, the incidence of long-term usage is approximately 15% in patients whose first episode of consumption is for > 8 days, and this rises as high as 30% for patients whose initial acute opioid use lasts 31 days or more (Shah et al. 2017). This study may underestimate the true incidence of long-term usage as it focused on the American commercially insured population and did not include patients who paid for their prescriptions out of pocket or obtained opioids illicitly. Additionally, this study included all types of patients and was not limited to the perioperative population.

Given that a significant proportion of opioid-naïve patients entering surgery may ultimately become chronic opioid users, minimizing opioids during the perioperative period should be an important goal of anesthesiologists. Identifying the patients that are high risk for opioid misuse or opioid use disorder in perioperative clinics enables the perioperative team to construct a plan to minimize the length of time the patient is exposed to opioids inside and outside of the hospital.

Acute side effects of perioperative opioids

Beyond increasing the risk of developing opioid use disorder, perioperative opioid consumption may produce undesirable side effects such as nausea/vomiting, constipation/ileus, pruritus, altered mental status, urinary retention, respiratory complications, and increased length of stay (Oderda et al. 2007). While many of these side effects are frustrating to patients in the immediate postoperative period, the most dangerous effects are those that affect the respiratory system.

Opioid-induced respiratory depression (ORD) is a significant cause of brain damage and death in the postoperative period. Cashman and Dolin reported their meta-analysis of almost 20,000 patients who underwent thoracic, abdominal, major gynecological, or major orthopedic surgery using a single postoperative analgesic technique with observation for adverse events for at least 24 h postoperatively (Cashman and Dolin 2004). The authors reported incidence of ORD varying from 0.1 to 37% based on their analysis, depending on the route of administration of the opioid, the type of opioid, the definition and method of monitoring ORD, and the prospective versus retrospective nature of the study. Lee et al. analyzed the Anesthesia Closed Claims Project Database and found that over 88% of ORD occurred within 24 h of the surgical procedure, and 13% of these occurred after the patients had been discharged from the PACU to the ward (Lee et al. 2015). The most common outcome for these ORD was death (55%) followed by recoverable injury (23%) and brain damage (22%).

Postoperative prescribing: public health considerations

A small selection of studies has explored the quantity of opioids prescribed for various surgeries and the amount actually taken by patients following hospital discharge. Surgeons at Dartmouth found that 67% of prescribed opioids after common general surgeries were not taken by the patient (Hill et al. 2017). The quantity of pills prescribed was inconsistent and ranged from 0 to 120 pills.

Unused medications, including opioids, can subsequently be used for nonmedical purposes by the patient, his or her family, or others who may have access to improperly stored medications. In a survey of heroin users, approximately 75% reported that they initially started with a prescription opioid, often from another patient's prescription (Jones 2013). In a study examining patients undergoing either cesarean section or thoracic surgery, investigators found that patients took fewer than five doses after discharge, and almost 80% of patients left their leftover pills in an unsecured location in their homes (Bartels et al. 2016; Rodgers et al. 2012). Almost none of the patients receiving opioids were given information on how to properly dispose these unused pills (Brummett et al. 2017).

Further research is needed to determine the appropriate amount of post-discharge opioids for each individual patient and procedure. We recommend that anesthesiologists assist their surgeon colleagues to establish institution-wide guidelines for postoperative opioid prescription. As anesthesiologists, we can provide verbal and written education on proper disposal techniques of opioids at perioperative clinic visits in an effort to decrease the distribution of leftover pills (Bicket et al. 2017). The perioperative anesthesia clinic visits are also an appropriate time to educate patients about the benefits of multimodal analgesia. A conversation should be held about our duty to ensure patient safety, and subsequently, we may avoid high doses of opioids with multimodal analgesia.

In addition, all physicians or providers who write for opioid prescriptions outside of the initial surgery encounter should be educated on the expected course length of an opioid prescription after a given surgery or injury. This will prevent primary care physicians from unnecessarily refilling prescriptions outside the normal time window and will also give them an idea as to when a patient is not healing properly or may be having a complication from surgery.

Despite the notoriety of the epidemic, it is still commonplace to use large amounts of opioids in the perioperative setting. Both anesthesiologists and surgeons are well-positioned to partner together to decrease the total amount of opioid used and prescribed in the preoperative, intraoperative, and postoperative settings. However, a multidisciplinary and multifaceted approach is needed to address the problem of the prescription opioid epidemic successfully. An important goal should be to start from the beginning and to ensure as many opioid-naïve patients remain opioid-naïve while having adequate pain control throughout their recovery.

Contribution of multimodal analgesia

Since the 1990s, a significant amount of research has gone into multimodal analgesia, as a methodology of pain control which utilizes non-opioid medications which target different pain receptors to better manage and control pain. The synergistic effect of the multiple medications also reduces the amount of opioid needed to control pain postoperatively, as opposed to using an opioid mono-therapy. Medications such as acetaminophen, gabapentin/pregabalin, ketamine, magnesium, dexamethasone, non-steroidal anti-inflammatory drugs (NSAIDs), duloxetine, and lidocaine are among those that have been studied as components of the multimodal approach (Fig. 2).

Acetaminophen has shown in systemic reviews (Macario and Royal 2011; Smith 2011) and clinical trials to reduce postoperative opioid use by as much as 30% at 4 h postoperatively (Aryaie et al. 2018; Memis et al. 2010; Saurabh et al. 2015; Sinatra et al. 2005). Although most trials concentrate on IV acetaminophen, a 2015 systematic review concluded that there is little evidence for using IV acetaminophen over oral acetaminophen in patients that are able to take medications by mouth perioperatively—which is useful when considering overall medication costs (Jibril et al. 2015).

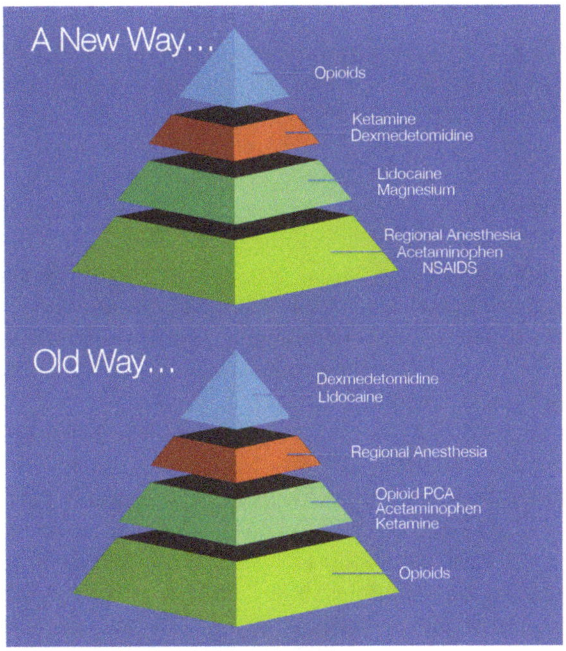

Fig. 2 New paradigm in analgesia management. The old way of management of pain has relied on opioids as the foundation of pain control, with non-opioid adjuncts added if necessary due to patient condition. In the new way, management of pain begins with non-opioid-based techniques that are evidence based and demonstrated to decrease opioid use

There is conflicting evidence on whether or not the reduced opioid doses reduce opioid-related side effects or opioid-related adverse events in studies with concurrent opioid use (McNicol et al. 2011; Memis et al. 2010). A recent study using a nationwide database reported that in spine surgery patients, IV acetaminophen did not reduce inpatient use of opioids or opioid-related adverse events (Mörwald et al. 2018). The effectiveness of acetaminophen may be related to procedure and patient specifics. Additional trials are needed to make a definite conclusion about the ability of acetaminophen to reduce opioid-related adverse events.

Gabapentin and pregabalin are also commonly used in multimodal analgesia and have shown to reduce opioid consumption in the perioperative period. Randomized, placebo-controlled, and double-blind studies have shown that 1200 mg of perioperative gabapentin reduces postoperative morphine equivalents in various types of major procedures (Wick et al. 2017). A meta-analysis in 2007 showed that preoperative gabapentin doses ranging from 300 to 1200 mg decreased opioid use by 30 mg of morphine in the first 24 h post-procedure (Tiippana et al. 2007). Pregabalin has been shown in a meta-analysis to have similar effects on postoperative opioid reduction as well as reducing opioid-related side effects postoperatively (Engelman and Cateloy 2011; Mörwald et al. 2018).

NSAIDs are a very potent pain reliever and are often overlooked as an immediate perioperative medication due to concerns of side effects. When used in scheduled doses and in the correct patient population, they can be a powerful adjunct to any pain regimen. In their 2017 review on multimodal anesthesia, Wick et al. highlighted the findings that 600 mg of ibuprofen is efficacious as 15 mg of oxycodone hydrochloride (Wick et al. 2017). A long-held belief has been that NSAIDs, particularly ketorolac, increase the risk of surgical bleeding. However, Gobble et al. reported findings that ketorolac was not shown to increase incisional or GI bleeding in patients under 75 years old (Gobble et al. 2014). Recent meta-analyses in pediatric neurosurgery patients (Richardson et al. 2016) and plastic surgery patients (Stephens et al. 2015) both found no increased risk of postoperative bleeding.

A 2005 meta-analysis reported that NSAIDs in conjunction with opioid treatment significantly decreased pain scores at 24 h (Elia et al. 2005). It also reported that it decreased morphine consumption at 24 h by 50% with the COX-2 inhibitor rofecoxib and by 40% with other NSAIDs (Elia et al. 2005). The addition of NSAIDs or COX-2 inhibitor to an opioid pain regimen also decreased the incidence of nausea, vomiting, and sedation in both small and large surgeries. Although morphine consumption was significantly reduced, there was no reduction in opioid-adverse events (Elia et al. 2005). However, these trials reviewed within the meta-analysis were focused on efficacy of pain control. More focused studies are needed to show how a multimodal perioperative pain regimen can reduce opioid-related adverse events.

Perioperative administration of the alpha-2-agonists, clonidine and dexmedetomidine, has been shown to reduce postoperative opioid consumption by 4–15 mg of morphine equivalents, respectively, as well as reduced the pain intensity and nausea in patients (Blaudszun et al. 2012).

N-Methyl-D-aspartate (NMDA) antagonists are also commonly used medications in a multimodal pain regimen. Ketamine, a NMDA receptor antagonist, has long been known to decrease acute post-surgical pain and analgesic consumption. It is a very effective in helping to decrease tolerance to postoperative opiate use as well as being an effective analgesic ± opiates, non-steroidal anti-inflammatory medications, and acetaminophen (Katz 1993; McQuay 1992). Loftus et al. found that ketamine reduced opioid consumption in the postoperative period 0 to 48 h (Loftus et al. 2010). Moreover, these investigators found that opioid-dependent patients treated with ketamine had reduced pain up to 6 weeks after surgery compared to controls (Loftus et al. 2010).

More recently, Nielsen and colleagues reported that ketamine administered intraoperatively during spinal fusion surgery significantly decreased opioid use during the first 24 h postoperatively (Nielsen et al. 2017). In addition, these chronic pain patients with chronic opioid use receiving intraoperative ketamine had significantly less sedation and significantly improved pain scores at 6 months (Nielsen et al. 2017). This highlights ketamine's long reaching effects at improving pain while achieving reduced use of opioids.

A 2015 meta-analysis by King et al. concluded that the low-affinity noncompetitive NMDA receptor antagonist dextromethorphan, a common ingredient in cough syrup, significantly decreased postoperative opioid consumption 24–48 h after surgery (King et al. 2016). This review of 14 trials and 848 patients found that preoperative dextromethorphan reduced morphine consumption by 10.5 mg postoperatively. It also decreased pain scores up to 24 h postoperatively.

Dexamethasone, long-used for inflammation and nausea/vomiting prophylaxis, is now gaining popularity as an adjunct in perioperative pain management. In 2011, De Oliveira et al. published a study that showed that doses of 0.11–0.2 mg/kg of dexamethasone were optimal for postoperative pain reduction and decreasing opioid consumption postoperatively (De Oliveira Jr. et al. 2011). This study was particularly important because, before this, less than 0.1 mg/kg dexamethasone was commonly given perioperatively for nausea/vomiting prophylaxis purposes. Additional studies continue to show the postoperative pain benefits of dexamethasone. A 2017 meta-analysis by Meng et al. found that dexamethasone significantly reduced opioid consumption for the entire 48 h after total joint arthroplasty as well as resulted in reduced pain scores (Meng and Li 2017).

In 2013, a systemic review concluded that magnesium significantly decreased early (3 h) postoperative and late (24 h) postoperative pain (De Oliveira et al. 2013). It also significantly reduced nausea and vomiting. Patients that received magnesium infusions intraoperatively and postoperatively had a greater reduction of pain score and greater reduction of morphine use than both control group and intraoperative magnesium use without accompanying postoperative administration (Bolcal et al. 2005; De Oliveira et al. 2013). Morphine use decreased on average more than 10 mg in the immediate postoperative period, although the total magnesium dose did not affect total postoperative opioid consumption. This may be due to the fact that magnesium was given intraoperatively and did not continue into the postoperative period. Despite the large decrease in postoperative opioid, magnesium did not decrease systemic adverse effects of morphine such as nausea or vomiting.

IV lidocaine infusions have been shown to reduce opioid consumption decrease postoperative pain, reduce hospital length of stay, and have earlier return of bowel function in open abdominal procedures (Vigneault et al. 2011). In some surgeries, this begs the question whether or not epidural infusions of local anesthetic are necessary. A study by Terwaki et al. reported that IV lidocaine infusion in major abdominal surgery was inferior to epidural analgesia with respect to opioid consumption. However, lidocaine was associated with improvements in several important aspects of recovery (Terkawi et al. 2016).

Duloxetine has been shown to significantly decrease morphine requirements after total abdominal hysterectomy, total knee arthroscopy, and spine surgery (Bedin et al. 2017). Studies differed on whether or not duloxetine reduced pain scores 48 h after surgery, but one could argue that opioid consumption is an objective measure of pain control as opposed to the subjective nature of pain scores. An animal-model trial in 2016 showed that it significantly reduced incisional pain in rats as well as allodynia and hyperalgesia (Wang et al. 2016). A review by Helander in 2017 on multimodal analgesia concluded that additional randomized controlled trials on duloxetine's effect on postoperative reduction of opioids should be completed (Helander et al. 2017b).

Regional anesthesia

The use of regional anesthesia is essentially a universally utilized component of any perioperative multimodal analgesia or enhanced recovery after surgery (ERAS) pathway (Grant et al. 2017). Both neuraxial and peripheral nerve blocks can be used concurrently with an opioid-free anesthetic. A patient may be able to remain opioid free from the first few hours after surgery and possibly for days depending on the type of block and surgery performed.

Epidural catheters play an important role in opioid reduction in ERAS pathways, as well as enhancing early recovery (Grant et al. 2017). One of the benefits cited for epidural use in open abdominal surgery ERAS pathways relates to the role epidural catheters play in reducing opioid-related adverse events (Grant et al. 2017). Specifically, adequate pain control through opioid-sparing analgesic techniques aids in the reduction of postoperative nausea and vomiting, ileus, somnolence, hyperalgesia, and postoperative delirium (Kim et al. 2016).

More recently, some of the focus on regional anesthesia/analgesia for a variety of abdominal surgical procedures (both as part of ERAS pathways and independently) has shifted to truncal fascial plane blocks, including transversus abdominal plane (TAP), rectus sheath, and quadratus lumborum blocks (Bashandy and Elkholy 2014; Garg et al. 2017; Helander et al. 2017a; Hutchins et al. 2015; Kadam 2013; Kim et al. 2016). While many of these fascial plane blocks have been performed as single injection with ropivacaine and bupivacaine, a desire to prolong the time to rescue with opioid analgesia (or to completely avoid opioids altogether) has led to use of both continuous indwelling regional catheters and liposomal bupivacaine (Hutchins et al. 2015; Mitra and Sinatra 2004; Stokes et al. 2017). Recent studies of transversus abdominis plane (TAP) blocks with liposomal bupivacaine for robotic-assisted hysterectomy and colorectal surgery showed lower pain scores, decreased postoperative opioid requirements in the first 72 and 36 h respectively (Hutchins et al. 2015; Stokes et al. 2017).

Additionally, regional anesthetic techniques are quite useful for opioid-tolerant patients who often have poorly controlled postoperative pain. In fact, it has been suggested that regional anesthesia/analgesia procedures be offered to opioid-tolerant patients whenever feasible (Mitra and Sinatra 2004). With the variety of regional techniques available and the flexibility of these techniques regarding different surgical procedures, regional anesthesia/analgesia uniquely positions the anesthesiologist to have a significant impact in the reduction of opioids in the perioperative period.

Enhanced recovery pathways

Enhanced recovery pathways (ERPs) are multidisciplinary pathways aimed at reducing the stress of surgery, and thereby accelerating functional recovery. A key principle of ERPs is that anesthesia, surgery, and nursing team work together to decrease perioperative opioid use by implementing a multifaceted analgesia technique through all phases of perioperative care.

The goal is to deliver optimal analgesia. Optimal analgesia can be defined as "a technique that optimizes patient comfort and facilitates recovery of physical function, while minimizing the adverse effects of analgesics" (McEvoy et al. 2017).

To facilitate this goal, preoperative patient education is key. As pain is a complex and subjective biopsychosocial experience, optimal analgesia cannot be achieved without management of patient expectations and education regarding realistic goals of pain treatment. It is critical for the patients to understand that "pain-free" is not the primary goal of optimal analgesia.

The exact components of an enhanced recovery pathway will vary from institution to institution based on local factors, as well as the surgical and patient population. Importantly, there are many ways to achieve optimal analgesia that are efficacious. Each pathway should include a well-structured and planned multimodal approach from the preoperative period into the post-discharge recovery phase. It is also recommended that each pathway should have a "plan B" to allow for individual patient variation and a rescue analgesia pathway to troubleshoot breakthrough pain while continuing enhanced recovery principles and minimizing the negative effects of intravenous opioids.

High compliance with a variety of standardized non-opioid ERP bundles is strongly associated with a significant decrease in primary inpatient opioid consumption and improved outcomes in a variety of surgical procedures. Although multimodal analgesia routinely continues after hospital discharge, at present, most current care pathways in the USA do not include any guidelines on discharge opioid prescribing. With recent data showing that ERP implementation has not reduced the amount of opioid prescribed at discharge, this appears to be a missed opportunity and should be addressed as ERPs evolve (Brandal et al. 2017).

Opioid-free anesthesia: present and future

Prior to the widespread adoption of opioids into anesthesia practice in the late 1960s, anesthesia (hypnosis, amnesia, and immobility) was obtained through the use of inhaled anesthetics and/or high-dose Pentothal. Unfortunately, this brought with it the complication of hemodynamic instability and suppression of hemodynamics requiring additional support.

With the introduction of opioids, came the concept of "balanced anesthesia" which was widely embraced for its lack of effect on the cardiovascular system. Opioids provide hemodynamic stability through suppressing the sympathetic system which is why they are preferred at induction. In addition, opioids are among the strongest analgesics, and analgesia then came to be an essential part of balanced anesthesia (Mulier 2017; Mulier 2016).

The introduction of opioids was important because hypnotics at the time were strong cardiovascular depressants. Many patients had undiagnosed or untreated cardiovascular coronary diseases, as understanding was limited at that time. So, by giving high doses of opioids allowed the anesthesiologists to reduce the doses of hypnotics and muscle relaxants (Bovill et al. 1984; Sebel and Bovil 1982). Today, hypnotics and neuromuscular blocking agents are much more stable and can be titrated to achieve a sufficient depth of hypnosis and muscle relaxation with minimal risk. And almost all patients today have been diagnosed and treated for their cardiovascular problems prior to presenting for elective surgery.

Now, there are drugs which can act to stabilize the sympathetic nervous system, including alpha-2 agonists such as clonidine and dexmedetomidine, local anesthetics given intravenously (lidocaine) (De Oliveira et al. 2012), and magnesium (De Oliveira et al. 2013). Drugs such as gamma-aminobutyric acid modulators such as gabapentin can decrease opioid requirements (Tiippana et al. 2007). Given alone, almost all of them will reduce the intraoperative opioid use when given in a sufficiently high dose, which may result in prolonged sedation. If, however, these are given together in a multimodal approach, it may be possible to avoid all intraoperative opioids and avoid excessive sedation. The advantage of such a multimodal approach is that postoperative opioids given as analgesics are then also dramatically reduced. It is worth noting that although primary care and pain physicians commonly combine many of these medications safely, we do not yet have literature on the safety of each of the different combinations among various age groups or procedures.

From an anesthetic perspective, one can perform an opioid-free anesthetic (OFA) while still providing satisfactory pain control. Jan Mulier and colleagues at Algemeen Ziekenhuis Sint-Jan Brugge-Oostende, Bruges, Belgium, have found that opioids can be completely eliminated from the anesthetics of patients undergoing bariatric surgery with improved outcomes especially in the area of obstructive sleep apnea (Mulier 2016). Mulier et al. performed a retrospective cohort of 5000 patients within their institution; a dramatic reduction in postoperative opioid use in the first 24 h (mean and standard deviation [SD] of morphine equivalents 21 mg and SD 0.99 versus 6 mg and SD 0.48) was reported, with fewer complications and a shorter length of stay (LOS). In this cohort, patients with obstructive sleep apnea (OSA) were not found to have more complications compared with non-OSA patients after OFA.

Similar reports have demonstrated that multimodal adjuncts can be utilized with similar outcomes to those of opioid use (Bakan et al. 2015; Steyaert and Lavand'homme 2018). We are left to wonder, why is not this approach adopted by the anesthesia community at large? OFA is something one has to learn. OFA is also a paradigm shift in thinking for many practitioners. At our own institution, our first OFA pathway was met with a healthy degree of skepticism; however, it is now become established for many minor-moderate pain procedures (Table 1) and has significantly reduced, if not altogether eliminated the requirement for opioids to control pain. Importantly, while opioids are not routinely given intraoperatively in any of our ERPs, they are always available postoperatively if needed. Our goal is not to leave patients in pain, but for many patients to complete their surgical journey with satisfactory pain relief without the need for opioids.

In summary, the available evidence suggests that avoiding opioids during anesthesia is feasible without hemodynamic instability. Further studies are needed that look at long-term outcomes such as total postoperative opioid use, duration of this use, and return to function, as well as the incidence of chronic pain. In the current setting of the opioid crisis, we should lead the charge to change our clinical practice to minimize or eliminate the use of perioperative opioids which can potentially have more far reaching effects than simply length of stay or reduced nausea. The new approach in anesthesia can provide hypnosis with amnesia and muscle relaxation at the moment the anesthesiologist or surgeon requires it, while also maintaining sufficient tissue perfusion and sympathetic stability to protect organs.

Conclusion

Anesthesiologists are leading experts in pain medicine, and through evidence-based implementations such as ERAS and multimodal anesthesia, the specialty is helping to address the opioid crisis by reducing the amount of opioid used in the perioperative period while still maintaining adequate acute pain control. The time has come to change the foundations of our practice from that of an opioid-based one to that of a multimodal practice (Fig. 2), wherein analgesia is managed with non-opioid-based agents first, then layering on additional layers of analgesics saving opioids as the capstone in analgesic management.

Perioperative physicians and anesthesiologists should continue to pursue evidence-based research to assist

Table 1 Opioid-reducing enhanced recovery pathway. This is the protocol used at the authors' institution for multimodal, opioid-reducing analgesia

Drug	Duration of surgery		Notes
	Short (1–2 h)	Long (> 2 h)	
Preoperative (day prior)			
Tylenol	975 mg TID	975 mg TID	
Ibuprofen	800 mg TID	800 mg TID	
Holding room			
Gabapentin	600 mg	600 mg	
Celebrex	450 mg	450 mg	
Tylenol	975 mg	975 mg	
Glycopyrolate	0.2–0.3 mg	0.2–0.3 mg	
Intraoperative			
Induction			
Ketamine	Bolus	Bolus and infusion	Bolus 0.25 mg/kg Infusion 4 μg/kg/min
Lidocaine	Bolus	Infusion	Bolus 1 mg/kg Infusion 1 mg/kg/h
Dexmetatomidine		Bolus and infusion	Bolus 1 μg/kg Infusion 0.1 μg/kg/h
Magnesium	Bolus	Bolus and infusion	Bolus 2 g Infusion 1 g/h
Analgesics (provider discretion)			
Toradol	Bolus	Bolus	15–30 mg
Hydromorphone	Bolus	Bolus	0.2–0.4 mg
Morphine	Bolus	Bolus	0.06–0.1 mg/kg
PACU			
Analgesics			
Fentanyl	25 μg/dose	25 μg/dose	
Hydromorphone	0.2–0.4 mg/dose	0.2–0.4 mg/dose	
Morphine	4 mg/dose	4 mg/dose	
Antiemetics			
Zofran	4 mg	4 mg	
Dexamethasone	4–8 mg	4–8 mg	
Haldol	1–2 mg	1–2 mg	
Benadryl	6.25 mg	6.25 mg	

with the opioid epidemic from a broad, perioperative population health approach. We share the responsibility with the rest of the medical community to not only decrease the financial burden on society and on hospitals but to assist in solving the epidemic, which has now become the number one accidental cause of death in the USA.

Abbreviations
ERAS: Enhanced recovery after surgery; ERP: Enhanced recovery pathway; IV: Intravenous; LOS: Length of stay; NMDA: *N*-Methyl-D-aspartate; NSAIDs: Non-steroidal anti-inflammatory drugs; OFA: Opioid-free anesthetic; ORD: Opioid-induced respiratory depression; SD: Standard deviation; SSRI: Selective serotonin reuptake inhibitor; TAP: Transversus abdominis plane

Authors' contributions
All authors contributed to the development of the manuscript, agree to its contents, and approved its final version.

Competing interests
The authors declare that they have no competing interests.

Author details
[1]Division of General, Vascular and Transplant Anesthesiology, Department of Anesthesiology, Duke University, Box 3094, 2301 Erwin Road, Durham, NC 27710, USA. [2]Division of Regional Anesthesiology, Department of Anesthesiology, Duke University, Durham, USA. [3]Division of Pain, Department of Anesthesiology, Duke University, Durham, USA.

References

Alam A, Juurlink DN. The prescription opioid epidemic: an overview for anesthesiologists. Can J Anesth. 2016;63(1):61–8. https://doi.org/10.1007/s12630-015-0520-y.

Aryaie AH, Lalezari S, Sergent WK, Puckett Y, Juergens C, Ratermann C, et al. Decreased opioid consumption and enhance recovery with the addition of IV acetaminophen in colorectal patients: a prospective, multi-institutional, randomized, double-blinded, placebo-controlled study (DOCIVA study). Surg Endosc. 2018.

Bakan M, Umutoglu T, Topuz U, Uysal H, Bayram M, Kadioglu H, et al. Opioid-free total intravenous anesthesia with propofol, dexmedetomidine and lidocaine infusions for laparoscopic cholecystectomy: a prospective, randomized, double-blinded study. Braz J Anesthesiol. 2015;65(3):191–9.

Bartels K, Mayes LM, Dingmann C, Bullard KJ, Hopfer CJ, Binswanger IA. Opioid use and storage patterns by patients after hospital discharge following surgery. PLoS ONE. 2016;11(1):e0147972.

Bashandy GMN, Elkholy AHH. Reducing postoperative opioid consumption by adding an ultrasound-guided rectus sheath block to multimodal analgesia for abdominal cancer surgery with midline incision. Anesth Pain Med Kowsar. 2014;4(3):e18263.

Bedin A, Caldart Bedin RA, Vieira JE, Ashmawi HA. Duloxetine as an analgesic reduces opioid consumption after spine surgery. Clin J Pain. 2017;33(10):865–9.

Bicket MC, Long JJ, Pronovost PJ, Alexander GC, Wu CL. Prescription opioid analgesics commonly unused after surgery a systematic review. JAMA Surg. 2017;152(11):1066–71. American Medical Association.

Blaudszun G, Lysakowski C, Elia N, Tramer MR. Effect of perioperative systemic α2 agonists on postoperative morphine consumption and pain intensity: systematic review and meta-analysis of randomized controlled trials. Anesthesiology. 2012;116(6):1312–22.

Bolcal C, Iyem H, Sargin M, Mataraci I, Yildirim V, Doganci S, et al. Comparison of magnesium sulfate with opioid and NSAIDs on postoperative pain management after coronary artery bypass surgery. J Cardiothorac Vasc Anesth. 2005;19(6):714–8.

Bovill JG, Sebel PS, Stanley TH. Opioid analgesics in anesthesia—with special reference to their use in cardiovascular anesthesia. Anesthesiology. 1984; 61(6):731–55.

Brandal D, Keller MS, Lee C, Grogan T, Fujimoto Y, Gricourt Y, et al. Impact of enhanced recovery after surgery and opioid-free anesthesia on opioid prescriptions at discharge from the hospital: a historical-prospective study. Anesth Analg. 2017;125(5):1784–92.

Brummett CM, Waljee JF, Goesling J, Moser S, Lin P, Englesbe MJ, et al. New persistent opioid use after minor and major surgical procedures in US adults. JAMA Surg. 2017;152(6):e170504. American Medical Association.

Cashman JN, Dolin SJ. Respiratory and haemodynamic effects of acute postoperative pain management: evidence from published data. Br J Anaesth. 2004;93(2):212–23.

Centers for Disease Control and Prevention. Vital signs: overdoses of prescription opioid pain relievers—United States, 1999–2008. MMWR. Morb. Mortal Wkly. Rep. 60, 1487–1492 (2011) (160).

Chia Y-Y, Liu K, Wang J-J, Kuo M-C, Ho S-T. Intraoperative high dose fentanyl induces postoperative fentanyl tolerance. Can J Anesth. 1999;46(9):872–7.

Chu LF, Angst MS, Clark D. Opioid-induced hyperalgesia in humans: molecular mechanisms and clinical considerations. Clin J Pain. 2008;24(6):479–96.

Clarke H, Soneji N, Ko DT, Yun L, Wijeysundera DN. Rates and risk factors for prolonged opioid use after major surgery: population based cohort study. BMJ. 2014;348(feb11 3):g1251.

de Oliveira GS, Castro-Alves LJ, Khan JH, McCarthy RJ. Perioperative systemic magnesium to minimize postoperative pain: a meta-analysis of randomized controlled trials. Anesthesiology. 2013;119(1):178–90. Available from: http://eutils.ncbi.nlm.nih.gov/entrez/eutils/elink.fcgi?dbfrom=pubmed&id=23669270&retmode=ref&cmd=prlinks.

De Oliveira GS, Fitzgerald P, Streicher LF, Marcus R-J, McCarthy RJ. Systemic lidocaine to improve postoperative quality of recovery after ambulatory laparoscopic surgery. Anesth Analg. 2012;115(2):262–7.

De Oliveira GS Jr, Almeida MD, Benzon HT, McCarthy RJ. Perioperative single dose systemic dexamethasone for postoperative pain. Anesthesiology. 2011; 115(3):575–88.

Elia N, Lysakowski C, Tram r MR. Does multimodal analgesia with acetaminophen, nonsteroidal antiinflammatory drugs, or selective cyclooxygenase-2 inhibitors and patient-controlled analgesia morphine offer advantages over morphine alone? Anesthesiology. 2005;103(6):1296–304.

Engelman E, Cateloy F. Efficacy and safety of perioperative pregabalin for post-operative pain: a meta-analysis of randomized-controlled trials. Acta Anaesthesiologica Scandinavica. 2011;55(8):927–43. Blackwell Publishing Ltd.

Gan TJ, Habib AS, Miller TE, White W, Apfelbaum JL. Incidence, patient satisfaction, and perceptions of post-surgical pain: results from a US national survey. Curr Med Res Opin. 2014;30(1):149–60.

Garg C, Khanna S, Mehta Y. Quadratus lumborum block for post-operative pain relief in patient with Prune belly syndrome. Indian J Anaesth. 2017;61(10): 840–2. Medknow Publications.

Gobble RM, Hoang HLT, Kachniarz B, Orgill DP. Ketorolac does not increase perioperative bleeding: a meta-analysis of randomized controlled trials. Plast Reconstr Surg. 2014;133(3):741–55. Available from: http://journals.lww.com/plasreconsurg/Abstract/2014/03000/Ketorolac_Does_Not_Increase_Perioperative.55.aspx.

Grant MC, Sommer PM, He C, Li S, Page AJ, Stone AB, et al. Preserved analgesia with reduction in opioids through the use of an acute pain protocol in enhanced recovery after surgery for open hepatectomy. Reg Anesth Pain Med. 2017;42(4):451–7.

Hedegaard H, Warner M, Miniño AM. Drug overdose deaths in the United States, 1999-2016. NCHS Data Brief. 2017;294:1–8.

Helander EM, Menard BL, Harmon CM, Homra BK, Allain AV, Bordelon GJ, et al. Multimodal analgesia, current concepts, and acute pain considerations. Curr Pain Headache Rep. 2017a;21(1):267. 8 ed.

Helander EM, Webb MP, Bias M, Whang EE, Kaye AD, Urman RD. A comparison of multimodal analgesic approaches in institutional enhanced recovery after surgery protocols for colorectal surgery: pharmacological agents. J Laparoendosc Adv Surg Tech A. 2017b;27(9):903–8. Mary Ann Liebert, Inc. 140 Huguenot Street, 3rd Floor New Rochelle, NY 10801 USA.

Hill MV, McMahon ML, Stucke RS, Barth RJ Jr. Wide variation and excessive dosage of opioid prescriptions for common general surgical procedures. Ann Surg. 2017;265(4):709–14.

Hutchins J, Delaney D, Vogel RI, Ghebre RG, Downs LS, Carson L, et al. Ultrasound guided subcostal transversus abdominis plane (TAP) infiltration with liposomal bupivacaine for patients undergoing robotic assisted hysterectomy: a prospective randomized controlled study. Gynecol Oncol. 2015;138(3):609–13.

Jibril F, Sharaby S, Mohamed A, Wilby KJ. Intravenous versus oral acetaminophen for pain: systematic review of current evidence to support clinical decision-making. Can J Hosp Pharm. 2015;68(3):238–47.

Joly V, Richebe P, Guignard B, Fletcher D, Maurette P, Sessler DI, Chauvin M. Remifentanil-induced postoperative hyperalgesia and its prevention with small-dose ketamine. Anesthesiol. 2005;103(1):147–55.

Jones CM. Heroin use and heroin use risk behaviors among nonmedical users of prescription opioid pain relievers—United States, 2002–2004 and 2008–2010. Drug Alcohol Depend. 2013;132(1–2):95–100.

Kadam VR. Ultrasound-guided quadratus lumborum block as a postoperative analgesic technique for laparotomy. J Anaesthesiol Clin Pharmacol. 2013;29(4):550–2.

Katz J. George Washington Crile, anoci-association, and pre-emptive analgesia. Pain. 1993;53(3):243–5.

Kessler ER, Shah M, Gruschkus SK, Raju A. Cost and quality implications of opioid-based postsurgical pain control using administrative claims data from a large health system: opioid-related adverse events and their impact on clinical and economic outcomes. Pharmacotherapy. 2013;33(4):383–91.

Kim N, Matzon JL, Abboudi J, Jones C, Kirkpatrick W, Leinberry CF, et al. A prospective evaluation of opioid utilization after upper-extremity surgical procedures. J Bone Joint Surg. 2016;98(20):e89.

King MR, Ladha KS, Gelineau AM, Anderson TA. Perioperative dextromethorphan as an adjunct for postoperative pain: a meta-analysis of randomized controlled trials. Anesthesiology. 2016;124(3):696–705.

Lee JS-J, Hu HM, Edelman AL, Brummett CM, Englesbe MJ, Waljee JF, et al. New persistent opioid use among patients with cancer after curative-intent surgery. J Clin Oncol. 2017;35(36):4042–9.

Lee LA, Caplan RA, Stephens LS, Posner KL, Terman GW, Voepel-Lewis T, et al. Postoperative opioid-induced respiratory depression. Anesthesiology. 2015; 122(3):659–65.

Loftus RW, Yeager MP, Clark JA, Brown JR, Abdu WA, Sengupta DK, et al. Intraoperative ketamine reduces perioperative opiate consumption in opiate-dependent patients with chronic back pain undergoing back surgery. Anesthesiology. 2010;113:639–46.

Macario A, Royal MA. A literature review of randomized clinical trials of intravenous acetaminophen (paracetamol) for acute postoperative pain. Pain Pract. 2011;11(3):290–6.

Manchikanti L, Helm SI, Fellows B, Janata JW, Pampati V, Grider JS, et al. Opioid

epidemic in the United States. Pain Physician. 2012;15(3):ES9–ES38.
McEvoy MD, Scott MJ, Gordon DB, Grant SA, Thacker JKM, Wu CL, et al. American Society for Enhanced Recovery (ASER) and Perioperative Quality Initiative (POQI) joint consensus statement on optimal analgesia within an enhanced recovery pathway for colorectal surgery: part 1-from the preoperative period to PACU. Perioper Med (Lond). 2017;6:8.
McNicol ED, Tzortzopoulou A, Cepeda MS, Francia MBD, Farhat T, Schumann R. Single-dose intravenous paracetamol or propacetamol for prevention or treatment of postoperative pain: a systematic review and meta-analysis. Br J Anaesth. 2011;106(6):764–75. Available from: https://academic.oup.com/bja/article-lookup/doi/10.1093/bja/aer107.
McQuay HJ. Preemptive analgesia. Br J Anaesth. 1992;69(1):1–3.
Memis D, Inal MT, Kavalci G, Sezer A, Sut N. Intravenous paracetamol reduced the use of opioids, extubation time, and opioid-related adverse effects after major surgery in intensive care unit. J Crit Care. 2010;25(3):458–62.
Meng J, Li L. The efficiency and safety of dexamethasone for pain control in total joint arthroplasty: a meta-analysis of randomized controlled trials. Medicine. 2017;96(24):e7126.
Mitra S, Sinatra RS. Perioperative management of acute pain in the opioid-dependent patient. Anesthesiology. 2004;101(1):212–27.
Mörwald EE, Poeran J, Zubizarreta N, Cozowicz C, Mazumdar M, Memtsoudis SG. Intravenous acetaminophen does not reduce inpatient opioid prescription or opioid-related adverse events among patients undergoing. Spine Surgery, Anesth Analg. 2018. https://doi.org/10.1213/ANE.0000000000003344.
Mulier J. Opioid free general anesthesia: a paradigm shift? Revista Española de Anestesiología y Reanimación (English Edition). 2017;64(8):427–30.
Mulier JP. Perioperative opioids aggravate obstructive breathing in sleep apnea syndrome: mechanisms and alternative anesthesia strategies. Curr Opin Anaesthesiol. 2016;29(1):129–33.
Nielsen RV, Fomsgaard JS, Siegel H, Martusevicius R, Nikolajsen L, Dahl JB, et al. Intraoperative ketamine reduces immediate postoperative opioid consumption after spinal fusion surgery in chronic pain patients with opioid dependency: a randomized, blinded trial. Pain. 2017;158(3):463–70.
Oderda GM, Said Q, Evans RS, Stoddard GJ, Lloyd J, Jackson K, et al. Opioid-related adverse drug events in surgical hospitalizations: impact on costs and length of stay. Ann Pharmacother. 2007;41(3):400–6. 5 ed.
Porter J, Jick H. Addiction rare in patients treated with narcotics. N Engl J Med. 1980;302(2):123.
Richardson MD, Palmeri NO, Williams SA, Torok MR, O'Neill BR, Handler MH, et al. Routine perioperative ketorolac administration is not associated with hemorrhage in pediatric neurosurgery patients. J Neurosurg Pediatr. 2016;17(1):107–15.
Rodgers J, Cunningham K, Fitzgerald K, Finnerty E. Opioid consumption following outpatient upper extremity surgery. J Hand Surg Am. 2012;37A(4):645–50.
Saurabh S, Smith JK, Pedersen M, Jose P, Nau P, Samuel I. Scheduled intravenous acetaminophen reduces postoperative narcotic analgesic demand and requirement after laparoscopic Roux-en-Y gastric bypass. Surg Obes Relat Dis. 2015;11(2):424–30.
Sebel PS, Bovil JG. Cardiovascular effects of sufentanil anesthesia. Anesth Analg. 1982;61(2):115.
Shah A, Hayes CJ, Martin BC. Characteristics of initial prescription episodes and likelihood of long-term opioid use—United States, 2006-2015. MMWR Morb Mortal Wkly Rep. 2017;66(10):265–9.
Sinatra RS, Jahr JS, Reynolds LW, Viscusi ER, Groudine SB, Payen-Champenois C. Efficacy and safety of single and repeated administration of 1 gram intravenous acetaminophen injection (paracetamol) for pain management after major orthopedic surgery. Anesthesiology. 2005;102(4):822–31.
Smith HS. Perioperative intravenous acetaminophen and NSAIDs. Pain Med. 2011; 12(6):961–81.
Stephens DM, Richards BG, Schleicher WF, Zins JE, Langstein HN. Is ketorolac safe to use in plastic surgery? A critical review. Aesthet Surg J. 2015;35(4):462–6.
Steyaert A, Lavand'homme P. Prevention and treatment of chronic postsurgical pain: a narrative review. Drugs. 2018;76(3):167–16. Springer International Publishing.
Stokes AL, Adhikary SD, Quintili A, Puleo FJ, Choi CS, Hollenbeak CS, et al. Liposomal bupivacaine use in transversus abdominis plane blocks reduces pain and postoperative intravenous opioid requirement after colorectal surgery. Dis Colon Rectum. 2017;60(2):170–7.
Terkawi AS, Tsang S, Kazemi A, Morton S, Luo R, Sanders DT, et al. A clinical comparison of intravenous and epidural local anesthetic for major abdominal surgery. Reg Anesth Pain Med. 2016;41(1):28–36.
Tiippana EM, Hamunen K, Kontinen VK, Kalso E. Do surgical patients benefit from perioperative gabapentin/pregabalin? A systematic review of efficacy and safety. Anesth Analg. 2007;104(6):1545–56.
Vigneault L, Turgeon AF, Côté D, Lauzier F, Zarychanski R, Moore L, et al. Perioperative intravenous lidocaine infusion for postoperative pain control: a meta-analysis of randomized controlled trials. Can J Anaesth. 2011;58(1):22–37.
Wang C-F, Russell G, Wang S-Y, Strichartz GR, Wang GK. R-duloxetine and N-methyl duloxetine as novel analgesics against experimental postincisional pain. Anesth Analg. 2016;122(3):719–29.
Wick EC, Association AM, Grant MC, Wu CL. Postoperative multimodal analgesia pain management with nonopioid analgesics and techniques. JAMA Surg. 2017;152(7):691.
Zgierska A, Miller M, Rabago D. Patient satisfaction, prescription drug abuse, and potential unintended consequences. JAMA. 2012;307(13):1377–8.

Preoperative fluid retention increases blood loss during major open abdominal surgery

Robert G. Hahn[1*], Hans Bahlmann[2,3] and Lena Nilsson[2,3]

Abstract

Background: Quantification of renal fluid conservation is possible by urine analysis, and the results can indicate dehydration. The present report sought to determine whether this fluid retention correlates with fluid requirements during major abdominal surgeries that have estimated operating times ≥ 2 h.

Methods: Urine colour, specific weight, osmolality and creatinine concentration were used to calculate a composite "fluid retention index" (FRI) in 97 patients prior to major abdominal surgery. Goal-directed fluid volume optimization, with hydroxyethyl starch supplemented with a background administration of crystalloid fluid, was used.

Results: The median preoperative FRI was 3.0. Fluid retention, considered as present when FRI ≥ 3.5, was found in 37% of the patients. Fluid retention was followed by a significantly larger blood loss (+ 125%; 450 vs. 200 ml), higher haemorrhage rate (+ 41%; 123 vs. 87 ml/h) and greater need for both colloid (+ 43%; 1.43 vs. 1.00 l) and crystalloid (+ 18%; 1.28 vs. 1.08 l) fluids. Despite the larger blood loss, the total fluid balance was more positive after surgery in the dehydrated patients (+ 26%; 1.91 vs. 1.51 l; $P < 0.02$).

Conclusions: Preoperative fluid retention, as detected in a urine sample, was associated with a greater blood loss and a more positive fluid balance during major abdominal surgery.

Keywords: Surgery, Abdominal, Dehydration, Urine specimen collection, Blood loss

Background

Fluid therapy is an inherent component in the management of major abdominal surgery. How the kidneys are currently set to excrete or conserve fluid is of importance to the body's handling of infusion fluids (Hahn et al. 2016), and marked variability is common, both in everyday life (Hahn and Waldréus 2013) and before surgery (Hahn et al. 2014).

A measure of the kidney's state of fluid retention can be obtained by calculating an index based on four analyses of metabolic waste products in the urine (Hahn and Waldréus 2013). A high urinary content of waste products is associated with a longer half-life of crystalloid fluid (Hahn et al. 2014), greater need for fluid optimization (Li et al. 2014), greater rise in the urinary concentration of neutrophil gelatinase-associated lipocalin (NGAL) (Hahn 2015) and more complications after hip fracture surgery (Ylinenvaara et al. 2014), as well as a higher 30-day mortality in acute geriatric care (Johnson et al. 2015). However, little is known about how preoperative fluid retention affects intraoperative fluid balance and the need for infusion fluids.

The aim of the present study was to explore the relationship between preoperative dehydration and fluid requirements during major abdominal surgery. The data was derived from a recently performed clinical trial. The hypothesis was that fluid retention, which might reflect dehydration, would necessitate the infusion of greater amounts of fluid during the surgery.

Methods

Adult patients, ASA I–III, were screened for inclusion if they were scheduled for elective open abdominal surgery (upper or lower gastrointestinal (GI) surgery, urology or gynaecology) with an expected duration of at least 2 h and age ≥ 18 years. Exclusion criteria were American Society of Anesthesiologists class IV, laparoscopic surgery,

* Correspondence: r.hahn@telia.com; robert.hahn@sll.se
[1]Research Unit, Södertälje Hospital, SE-152 86 Södertälje, Sweden
Full list of author information is available at the end of the article

cardiac arrhythmias, aortic or mitral insufficiency resulting in haemodynamic impairment, severe renal and hepatic failure, or pulmonary disease that prevented a ventilation volume of 7 ml/kg ideal body weight or the use of PEEP. The study was conducted every time that a suitable patient and the research team were available.

Procedure

From 195 patients screened for eligibility, 150 were randomized between the use of oesophageal Doppler and pulse oximetry (Pleth Variability Index) techniques to guide the goal-directed fluid therapy, which influence on postoperative outcome was a primary aim of the study. Randomization was performed by using opaque envelopes prepared from a computerized procedure. There were 4 drop-outs. From the remaining 146 patients, a preoperative urine sample had been obtained from 112. The results from the first half of this trial have been published elsewhere and show that the amount of fluid infused in the two groups was quite similar throughout the study (Bahlmann et al. 2016).

The patients were allowed to ingest clear fluids up to 2 h before the anaesthesia. Thirty of them had been instructed to be in the complete fasting state since midnight and underwent a preoperative experiment in which they received 5 ml/kg of Ringer's acetate by intravenous infusion (Hahn et al. 2014). All patients were operated under general anaesthesia and ventilated using volume control with tidal volumes of 7 ml/kg ideal body weight. The gynaecological operations were usually hysterectomy with salpingo-oophorectomy. The most common upper GI surgeries were resection of the stomach, duodenum and pancreas. The most common lower GI operations were colonic resection and rectum amputation. Urology operations were nephrectomies and cystectomies. The maintenance crystalloid infusion consisted of 2 ml/kg/h of buffered dextrose 2.5% with 75 mmol/l of sodium. Details on the types of operations performed and the anaesthetic management are provided as supplements on the journal's website (Additional file 1).

Fluid volume optimization was guided by either oesophageal Doppler or Pleth Variability Index and consisted of intravenous bolus infusions of 3 ml/kg (up to 250 ml) of tetrastarch, either Venofundin (B Braun Medical AB, Danderyd, Sweden) or Volulyte (Fresenius Kabi AB, Uppsala, Sweden), over 3–5 min, using a 50-cm^3 syringe. Volume optimization in the Doppler group (CardioQ, Deltex Medical, Chichester, UK) was guided by stroke volume changes in accordance with published protocols (Challand et al. 2012). For the alternative method, a fluid bolus was given when the Pleth Variability Index exceeded 9%. Details of these measurements have been presented elsewhere (Bahlmann et al. 2016).

Measurements

Two urine samples were taken from all patients in the morning, just before surgery. Urine colour was assessed by holding a 10-ml tube of urine next to a colour scale, which is available at www.hydrationcheck.com (Armstrong et al. 1998). One urine tube was used to measure the concentration of metabolic waste products, which can be used to quantify the degree of dehydration-induced renal water conservation (Hahn and Waldréus 2013; Hahn et al. 2014; Li et al. 2014; Hahn 2015).

The urinary albumin and albumin/creatinine ratio were measured on a DCA Vantage Analyser (Siemens Healthcare Diagnostics, Mölndal, Sweden). The urine-specific gravity was determined using Multistix®10 SG reagent strips and a Clinitek Status®+ Analyser (Siemens Healthcare Diagnostics).

The second tube was sent to the certified clinical chemistry laboratory at Linköping University Hospital for analysis of osmolality.

As a quality measure, blood was obtained for measurement of the high-sensitivity troponin T (hsTnT) and the N-terminal fragment of B-type natriuretic peptide (NT-proBNP), before surgery and on the first and second mornings after surgery. The haemoglobin (Hb) concentration was measured invasively just before the induction of anaesthesia, at the end of the surgery, and on the first morning after the surgery. The Hb concentration was monitored by pulse oximetry during the surgery (Radical 7, Masimo Corp., Irvine, CA).

Fluid retention index (FRI)

The use of a composite index for fluid retention that is based on several markers of renal water conservation has the benefit of reducing confounding influences, such as diet, disease and medication, which typically change only one of the markers. The urine colour is due to end products arising from the fairly stable breakdown of erythrocytes, and it darkens with progressive dehydration. The specific gravity of the urine also increases with dehydration, as do the creatinine concentration and the osmolality.

The ranges of colour, osmolality and creatinine concentrations have been published for subjects aged 17–69 years, and each range paralleled the specific gravity scale (Hahn and Waldréus 2013). These ranges were assigned a score, where a higher value indicated more severe dehydration (Table 1). The mean of the four scores was termed the *fluid retention index* (*FRI*). This term is more appropriate than the previously used "dehydration index" because fluid retention may occasionally be due to other causes than dehydration, in particular in hospital patients.

Exclusion of FRI scores

The composition of the FRI index was then checked for outliers, which were determined by calculating the

Table 1 Scheme for calculating the fluid retention index (FRI), which is the mean of the dehydration scores for 4 urinary indexes of fluid retention

Fluid retention score	1	2	3	4	5	6
Specific gravity	≤ 1.005	1.010	1.015	1.020	1.025	1.030
Osmolality (mOsmol/kg)	< 250	250–450	450–600	600–800	800–1000	> 1000
Creatinine(mmol/l)	< 4	4–7	7–12	12–17	17–25	> 25
Colour (shade)	1	2	3	4	5	6

From Hahn and Waldréus 2013

standard deviation (SD) for the mean of the four scores. An outlier typically raised the SD to > 1.0. The individual scores were then reviewed and any single outlier was omitted, followed by recalculation of the index. The new value was accepted if SD ≤ 1.0, whereas the index was discarded as being inconclusive if the SD was still > 1.0 (Hahn and Waldréus 2013; Hahn et al. 2014).

Fluid balance

Blood loss during surgery was calculated from the sum of the volume in suction tubes and an estimation of the blood absorbed on swabs and dressings.

The *fluid balance* was obtained as the sum of the infused crystalloid and colloid fluid volumes, including blood products, minus the blood loss and excreted urine. Hence,

Fluid balance = (crystalloid + colloid + blood products) − (blood loss + urine).

The *fluid balance in blood volume equivalents* was calculated by dividing the crystalloid and the urine volumes by 3 before entering the figures into this equation.

Statistics

Continuous and categorical demographic, perioperative and biochemical data were compared using analysis of variance (ANOVA), the Mann-Whitney *U* test or the chi^2 test, as appropriate. Correlations between parameters were evaluated by simple and multiple linear regression analysis. P values < 0.05 were considered significant.

Results

Fluid retention index

Preoperative urine samples for analysis of FRI were obtained from 112 patients. The results were incomplete in 6 and inconclusive in 9 cases (see the "Exclusion of FRI scores" in the "Methods" section), which left 97 patients for the final analysis.

The median (IQR) of the FRI was 3.0 (2.2–3.8) for those 97 patients.

FRI varied depending on the type of scheduled surgery: gynaecological 2.3 (1.5–3.5), upper GI surgery 3.3 (2.5–3.8), lower GI surgery 3.0 (1.8–4.1) and urological surgery 3.4 (2.5–4.0) (ANOVA on log-transformed data; $P < 0.008$). There was no indication that dehydrated patients were less well before the surgery.

Fluid retention groups

A cut-off for fluid retention of 3.5 was implemented in accordance with previous work with this cohort (Hahn et al. 2014).

FRI ≥ 3.5 was associated with greater blood loss (+ 125%), blood loss per operating hour (+ 41%), need for colloid fluid (+ 43%), positive fluid balance (+ 27%) and greater positive fluid balance when expressed in blood volume equivalents (+ 29%; Table 2).

Even when controlling for the type of surgery, FRI ≥ 3.5 was still significantly associated with greater blood loss ($P < 0.03$), blood loss/operating time ($P < 0.03$), total fluid balance ($P < 0.03$) and the fluid balance in blood units ($P < 0.02$) (two-way ANOVA based on logarithm-transformed data). The real data for all patients is shown in Table 2 and for the sub-groups in Table 3.

Nine patients (15%) of the patients with FRI < 3.5 were treated with diuretics on a daily basis (treatment withdrawn on the day of the operation) while 6 received such treatment in the other group (17%). Other chronic medications are listed in Additional file 1.

Four out of the 14 patients undergoing pancreatectomy including Whipple's procedure had preoperative serum bilirubin levels above the reference value. Two of them had FRI < 3.5 and two had ≥ 3.5.

Fluid balance

The fluid balance during surgery correlated with FRI (linear regression $r = 0.35$, $P < 0.001$), which was due to the gynaecological and urological surgeries ($r = 0.58$, $P < 0.001$), while this relationship was not statistically significant for the GI operations alone ($P = 0.10$; Fig. 1a).

The fluid balance expressed in blood volume equivalents also correlated with FRI ($r = 0.36$, $P < 0.001$). Again, the linear relationship was mostly due to the gynaecological and urological surgeries ($r = 0.54$, $P < 0.001$), while this relationship was not statistically significant for the GI surgeries alone ($P = 0.10$; Fig. 1b).

Table 2 Data on the surgical operations depending on a high or low fluid retention index (FRI) prior to anaesthesia induction

Parameter	FRI < 3.5 (n = 61)	FRI ≥ 3.5 (n = 36)	Statistics
Preoperatively			
Age (years)	65 (57–72)	67 (50–73)	$P = 0.59$
Body weight (kg)	75 (68–89)	75 (60–85)	$P = 0.42$
ASA class I/II/III (%)[a]	28/59/13	38/52/8	$P = 0.48$
B-Hb concentration (g/l)	126 (118–134)	127 (120–135)	$P = 0.61$
U-albumin/creatinine (mg/mmol)	1.87 (1.15–5.04)	1.02 (0.65–1.83)	$P < 0.002$
Preoperative fluid experiment (n, %)[a]	19 (31%)	11 (31%)	$P = 0.30$
During surgery			
Operating time (h)	2.3 (1.4–4.1)	3.3 (2.2–4.2)	$P = 0.07$
Blood loss (ml)	200 (75–413)	450 (150–738)	$P < 0.01$
Blood loss/operating time (ml/h)	87 (41–154)	123 (74–225)	$P < 0.03$
Erythrocyte transfusion (N patient)	4	5	
Erythrocytes transfused (ml)	863 (552–1408)	1389 (313–1670)	$P = 0.62$
B-Hb concentration (g/l)	106 (93–112)	104 (95–115)	$P = 0.76$
Urine (ml)	245 (171–500)	350 (149–500)	$P = 0.95$
Urine/operating time (ml/h)	92 (62–174)	96 (48–143)	$P = 0.34$
Crystalloid fluid (ml)	1081 (688–1430)	1279 (954–1950)	$P = 0.05$
Colloid fluid (ml)	1000 (700–1400)	1430 (953–1956)	$P < 0.04$
Infused fluid volume (ml)	2140 (1567–2816)	2594 (2248–3461)	$P < 0.02$
Fluid balance (ml)	+ 1506 (1210–2041)	+ 1913 (1439–2403)	$P < 0.02$
Fluid balance, blood equivalents (ml)	+ 954 (729–1401)	+ 1235 (979–1494)	$P < 0.03$
Postoperatively			
Δ S-troponin T, day 0 vs. 1–2 (%)[b, c]	+ 20 (0–66)	0 (− 6 to + 8)	$P < 0.02$
Δ S-NT-proBNP, day 0 vs. 1–2 (%)[b, c]	+ 161 (31–357)	+ 150 (41–462)	$P = 0.43$
B-Hb concentration (g/l)	113 (102–122)	114 (104–124)	$P = 0.74$
Length of hospital stay (days)	7 (5–11)	9 (6–14)	$P = 0.15$

Mann-Whitney's test was used for statistics
[a] contingency table analysis
[b]Repeated-measures ANOVA based on log-transformed data
[c]The means of the values on days 1 and 2 were compared with the preoperative value

Blood loss

The log-transformed blood loss correlated with FRI ($r = 0.23$, $P < 0.03$), which was due to the gynaecological and urological surgeries ($r = 0.44$, $P < 0.005$), while this relationship was not statistically significant for the GI surgeries alone ($P = 0.13$; Fig. 2a).

The blood loss per hour operating time also correlated with FRI for gynaecological and urological surgeries ($r = 0.38$, $P < 0.02$; Fig 2b), while this relationship was not statistically significant for the GI surgeries ($P = 0.13$; Fig. 2c).

Troponin T

Blood for analysis of troponin T and NT-proBNP was obtained from 36 patients. The serum concentration of troponin T before surgery was 8 (5–11) ng/l and the NT-proBNP was 145 (57–250) ng/l.

No increase in troponin T occurred in patients with a high FRI, but the NT-proBNP doubled regardless of whether the FRI had a low or high value. Moreover, there were no differences in B-Hb concentration between the groups (Table 2).

ASA class and fluid monitoring

In a multiple regression model, only the FRI value, but not the ASA class or the mode of monitoring fluid responsiveness (oesophageal Doppler and pulse oximetry), served as a statistically significant predictor of the total fluid balance.

Similarly, only the FRI value was a significant predictor of the surgical blood loss.

Discussion

The result confirms that fluid retention, expressed as a high FRI, is associated with a greater need for fluid

Table 3 Data on the surgical operations depending on high or low fluid retention index (FRI) prior to anaesthesia induction

Parameter	FRI < 3.5 (*n* = 61)	FRI ≥ 3.5 (*n* = 36)	Statistics
Blood loss (ml)			
Gynaecology (*n* = 27)	175 (100–300)	200 (113–513)	*P* < 0.03
Upper GI surgery (*n* = 27)	225 (50–575)	250 (63–725)	
Lower GI surgery (*n* = 31)	150 (81–375)	525 (150–1000)	
Urology (*n* = 12)	1000 (100–1800)	850 (500–1300)	
Blood loss/operating time (ml/h)			
Gynaecology	120 (44–148)	106 (79–163)	*P* < 0.03
Upper GI surgery	55 (29–145)	129 (72–282)	
Lower GI surgery	57 (32–120)	84 (42–217)	
Urology	164 (71–248)	204 (171–229)	
Total fluid balance (ml)			
Gynaecology	1361 (1032–1740)	1674 (1395–2210)	*P* < 0.03
Upper GI surgery	1569 (1362–2095)	1778 (1372–2887)	
Lower GI surgery	1506 (1014–2047)	1913 (1537–2194)	
Urology	1559 (560–1814)	2122 (1489–2938)	
Fluid balance in blood units (ml)			
Gynaecology	915 (791–1113)	1186 (818–1577)	*P* < 0.02
Upper GI surgery	1105 (858–1467)	1223 (902–1455)	
Lower GI surgery	954 (690–1456)	1266 (1172–1447)	
Urology	845 (413–1214)	1289 (1063–1542)	

Two-way analysis of variance was performed on ln-transformed data using the type of surgery and FRI ≥ 3.5 as predictors. The levels of significance for FRI ≥ 3.5 are shown

during surgery to maintain the patients in a fluid optimized state using either oesophageal Doppler or the Pleth Variability Index. The most plausible explanation to this finding is that fluid retention indicated preoperative dehydration, which had to be overcome by infusing larger volumes of fluid.

In contrast, the relationship between blood loss and FRI was a surprising post hoc finding. The explanation is unclear, but infusion of a small volume of Ringer's acetate in these preoperative patients showed that the plasma dilution was greater and the half-life of the fluid twice as long in those with FRI ≥ 3.5 (Hahn et al. 2014).

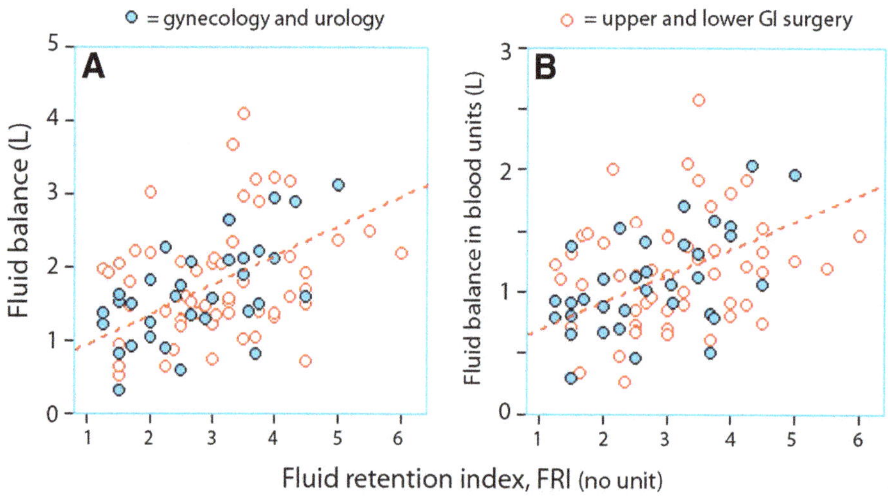

Fig. 1 Fluid retention index (FRI) versus fluid balance parameters (**a**, **b**). The regression lines refer to the gynaecological and urological operations only (*r* = 0.58 and 0.54, respectively)

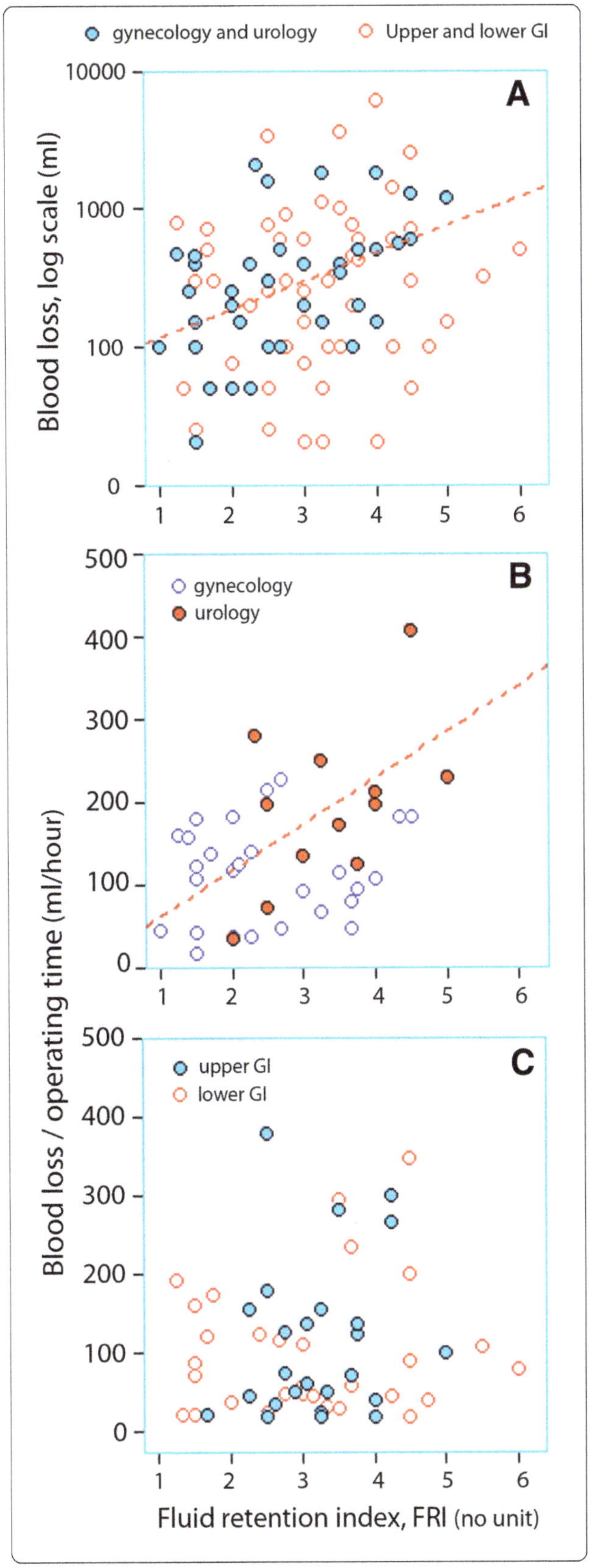

Fig. 2 Fluid retention index (FRI) versus the surgical blood loss in all patients (**a**; note the log scale) and the rate of the haemorrhage in gynaecological and urological patients (**b**; *r* = 0.38) and GI surgeries (**c**; no significant linear relationship)

In elderly urological patients, concentrated urine tripled the plasma volume expansion following infusion of Ringer's acetate and isotonic saline, when compared to patients without concentrated urine (Hahn et al. 2016). A greater haemodilution occurring in patients with concentrated urine might then have impaired coagulation, thereby promoting a greater blood loss. If so, a rapid correction of preoperative dehydration would be at risk of increasing the surgical blood loss.

Another possibility is that the larger volumes of colloid required to maintain an optimized plasma volume caused the greater haemodilution, thereby increasing the blood loss. Hence, the actual cause and effect between infused fluid volume and blood loss remains unclear.

How the kidneys were set to excrete or retain fluid was of relevance to the results and particularly for the gynaecological or urological surgeries. The blood loss, the need for intravenous fluid and the positive fluid balance all increased with greater preoperative fluid retention (Table 2). However, the volume optimization guided by measures of fluid responsiveness required a more positive fluid balance in patients with fluid retention, despite the fact that the blood loss also was greater.

The baseline infusion (2 ml/kg/h) and the GDT optimization as given in this trial resulted in a positive fluid balance of between 1.5 and 2 l. When expressed in blood units, the positive balance averaged 1.1 l, despite a blood loss that was only one third as large. Hence, the recommended "zero balance" (Brandstrup et al. 2012) was not possible to achieve in these patients if an optimized plasma volume according to GDT was to be maintained.

The positive fluid balance was about 1 l when the urine was not concentrated, while twice as large a volume was needed when the urine was concentrated to a degree consistent with dehydration (Fig. 1a). Likewise, the figures for the fluid balance, when expressed in blood volume equivalents, were + 750 ml and + 1.5 l (Fig. 1b). Other data suggest that one could expect a fourfold increase in blood loss rate when FRI increases from 1 to 4 for gynaecological and urological surgery (Fig. 2b).

Several mechanisms may explain why a positive fluid balance was required to maintain the central blood flow. Vasodilatation caused by the anaesthesia, as well as transudation into injured tissue, remains the best acknowledged reasons. Fluid retention oedema becomes more pronounced when crystalloid fluid is infused sometime after hydroxyethyl starch (Hahn et al. 2013, Hahn 2017);

this probably reflects the oncotic properties of leaking starch molecules that bind the crystalloid fluid in extravascular areas. In contrast, evaporation is only ≈ 30 ml/h in an open abdominal surgery (Lamke et al. 1977), and this could therefore explain only 100 ml of the positive balance.

Despite the administration of larger volumes of fluid, the rise in NT-proBNP was not greater in patients with concentrated urine (Table 2). The average patient had at least a doubled plasma concentration of NT-proBNP after the surgery; the upper 25% showed a quadrupled concentration after the surgery. This precursor of BNP is released in response to stretching of the myocytes of the ventricles. The rise shows that cardiac strain was not uncommon during these surgeries, which is surprising given that flow-guided monitoring of the fluid administration should prevent marked fluid overload. In contrast, the small postoperative rise in troponin T seen in many patients was also absent in those with concentrated urine (Table 2).

Limitations of this study were the inclusion of different types of operations, which restricted the possibility of performing statistics. Major surgery is a very complex medical situation, and the mechanisms that govern various parameters, such as urinary excretion, require simpler situations to be readily understood. Among the benefits of the present study is that it was conducted in a standardized way and consistently relied on modern approaches to guide the fluid therapy, although there may be concerns that the oesophageal Doppler and pulse oximetry may not indicate fluid responsiveness correctly.

The algorithm used to calculate FRI is based on assessment of urine colour, specific gravity, osmolality and creatinine, which represent metabolic waste products that appear in higher concentrations when the kidneys conserve fluid. The adopted exclusion process ensured that the finally reported FRI values were robust measures of fluid retention. For example, isolated darkening of the urine due to a catheter-induced haematuria or a high serum bilirubin concentration was not allowed to affect the result.

Conclusions

Preoperative fluid retention, as given by a urine sample indicating dehydration, was associated with greater fluid requirements during major open abdominal surgery. Fluid retention was also followed by greater blood loss and a need for a more positive fluid balance. These effects were most apparent in gynaecological and urological operations. These results suggest that more fluid should routinely be prescribed to those patients who have concentrated urine before an operation. However, more studies are first needed to determine if more fluid given for this reason result in any benefit for the outcome of the patients.

Acknowledgements
Research nurses Susanne Lind and Gunilla Gagnö assisted with the collection of the data.

Funding
The work was supported by the Department of Anaesthesiology and Intensive Care, Linköping University Hospital, by the County Council of Östergötland and by the Mats Kleberg Foundation.

Authors' contributions
HB and LN performed the data collection, and RH performed the calculations and wrote the manuscript. All authors read and approved the final version of the manuscript.

Competing interests
The authors have no competing interests to declare.

Author details
[1]Research Unit, Södertälje Hospital, SE-152 86 Södertälje, Sweden. [2]Department of Anaesthesiology and Intensive Care, Linköping University, Linköping, Sweden. [3]Department of Medical and Health Sciences, Linköping University, Linköping, Sweden.

References

Armstrong LE, Soto JA, Hacker FT, Casa DJ, Kavouras SA, Maresh CM. Urinary indices during dehydration, exercise and rehydration. Sport Nutr & Exerc Metab. 1998;8:345–55.
Bahlmann H, Hahn RG, Nilsson L. Agreement between Pleth Variability Index and oesophageal Doppler to predict fluid responsiveness. Acta Anaesthesiol Scand. 2016;60:183–592.
Brandstrup B, Svendsen PE, Rasmussen M, Belhage B, Rodt SÅ, Hansen B, et al. Which goal for fluid therapy during colorectal surgery is followed by the best outcome: near-maximal stroke volume or zero fluid balance? Br J Anaesth. 2012;109:191–9.
Challand C, Struthers R, Sneyd JR, Erasmus PD, Mellor N, Hosie KB, et al. Randomized controlled trial of intraoperative goal-directed fluid therapy in aerobically fit and unfit patients having major colorectal surgery. Br J Anaesth. 2012;108:53–562.
Hahn RG. Renal injury during hip fracture surgery: an exploratory study. Anaesthesiol Intensive Ther. 2015;47:284–90.
Hahn RG. Renal water conservation determines the increase in body weight after moderate-sized surgery; a randomized controlled trial. Saudi J Anaesth. 2017; 11:144–51.
Hahn RG, Waldréus N. An aggregate urine analysis tool to detect acute dehydration. Int J Sport Nutr Exerc Metab. 2013;23:303–11.
Hahn RG, Bergek C, Gebäck T, Zdolsek J. Interactions between the volume effects of hydroxyethyl starch 130/0.4 and Ringer's acetate. Crit Care. 2013;17:R104.
Hahn RG, Bahlmann H, Nilsson L. Dehydration and fluid volume kinetics before major open abdominal surgery. Acta Anaesthesiol Scand. 2014;58:1258–66.

Hahn RG, Nyberg Isacson M, Fagerström T, Rosvall J, Nyman CR. Isotonic saline in elderly men; an open-labelled controlled infusion study of electrolyte balance, urine flow and kidney function. Anaesthesia. 2016;71:155–62.

Johnson P, Waldreus N, Hahn RG, Stenström H, Sjöstrand F. Fluid retention index predicts the 30-day mortality in geriatric care. Scand J Clin Lab Invest. 2015; 75:444–51.

Lamke LO, Nilsson GE, Reithner HL. Water loss by evaporation from the abdominal cavity during surgery. Acta Chir Scand. 1977;143:279–84.

Li Y, He R, Ying X, Hahn RG. Dehydration, hemodynamics and fluid volume optimization after induction of general anesthesia. Clinics. 2014;69:809–16.

Ylinenvaara SI, Elisson O, Berg K, Zdolsek JH, Krook H, Hahn RG. Preoperative urine-specific weight and the incidence of complications after hip fracture surgery. A prospective, observational study. Eur J Anaesthesiol. 2014;31:85–90.

Pre- to postoperative coagulation profile of 307 patients undergoing oesophageal resection with epidural blockade over a 10-year period in a single hospital: implications for the risk of spinal haematoma

Owain Thomas[1,2*], Emanuel Lybeck[3], Per Flisberg[1,4] and Ulf Schött[1,5]

Abstract

Background: Epidural anaesthesia and analgesia are indicated for oesophageal surgery. A rare but serious complication is spinal haematoma, which can occur on insertion, manipulation or withdrawal of catheters. Evidence and guidelines are vague regarding which tests are appropriate and how to interpret their results. We aimed to describe how routine coagulation test results change during oesophagectomy's perioperative course.

Methods: Following ethical approval, we retrospectively identified patients who had undergone oesophagectomy between 2002 and 2012. Blood test results and details of operations, haemorrhage and complications were recorded and analysed with Excel and R. A literature search was conducted using the PubMed terms 'epidural' AND 'coagulation' AND English language. Relevant articles published in 2000 and after were included.

Results: Three hundred and seven patients received a thoracic epidural infusion with bupivacaine and morphine while 51 received an intravenous morphine infusion. Tests taken preoperatively and before the planned withdrawal of the epidural catheter demonstrated increases in all three measures: aPTT (activated partial thromboplastin time), PT-INR (prothrombin international normalised ratio) and platelet count (Plc). Postoperative thrombocytopenia was almost non-existent while aPTT or PT-INR was elevated above the reference range in 129/307 patients: aPTT was elevated in 116/307 while PT-INR was elevated in 32/307. This is too small a sample to allow meaningful estimation of risk of spinal haematoma: it may be as high as 2.3%. The literature search returned 275 articles, of which 57 were relevant. Twenty-one concerned the natural history of postoperative coagulation; 16, the incidence of and risk factors for spinal haematoma; and 5, evaluation of specific blood tests. Postoperative coagulation is characterised by thrombocytosis and transient moderately abnormal routine coagulation test results. Viscoelastic tests are not validated in the stable postoperative setting.
(Continued on next page)

* Correspondence: odt@cantab.net
[1]Department of Anaesthesiology and Intensive Care Medicine, Institute of Clinical Sciences, Lund, Medical Faculty, University of Lund, 221 00 Lund, Sweden
[2]Department of Paediatric Anaesthesia and Intensive Care, SUS Lund University Hospital, 22185 Lund, Sweden
Full list of author information is available at the end of the article

(Continued from previous page)

Conclusions: Screening for coagulopathy before removal of epidural catheters is of unclear benefit since elevated aPTT and PT-INR are usual and may not indicate hypocoagulation. A thorough clinical assessment is important. We nevertheless recommend caution when being presented with elevated routine tests of coagulation before withdrawing an epidural catheter: viscoelastic haemostatic tests may have a role in testing before withdrawal of epidural catheters but they are so far not validated. Future research should include advanced coagulation analysis as soon as a patient is unfortunate enough to have a spinal haematoma.

Keywords: Epidural anaesthesia, Routine coagulation testing, Spinal haematoma

Background

Epidural anaesthesia and analgesia may reduce the risk of morbidity and mortality in patients undergoing oesophageal surgery, which can be a major insult for patients who are often already frail (Merritt et al. 2011; Watson and Allen 1994). An uncommon but serious complication of epidural catheterization is spinal haematoma, which most often occurs at the time of catheterization or withdrawal of catheters (Moen et al. 2004). For this reason, guidelines generally recommend withdrawal of catheters when routine tests of coagulation, prothrombin time international normalised ratio (PT-INR), activated partial thromboplastin time (aPTT) and platelet count (Plc), are within their normal ranges (Breivik et al. 2010; Horlocker et al. 2010; Gogarten et al. 2010).

The problem with these recommendations is that it is unclear what to do when results indicate mild hypocoagulation: should treatments such as vitamin K, plasma transfusion or prothrombin complex concentrate be given to normalise a PT-INR of 1.5? Should thrombosis prophylaxis be withheld or the catheter be left in place because of a slightly prolonged aPTT, potentially exposing the patient to the risk of venous thrombosis or catheter infection? And should a platelet transfusion and its side-effects be given to correct a Plc of 99×10^6/ml before withdrawal of an epidural catheter in a patient otherwise recovering well?

Most published articles concerning coagulation and postoperative epidural analgesia after major surgery concern hepatic resection where liver function may be affected. In this study, we present pre- and postoperative coagulation status from patients who underwent oesophageal resection over a period of 10 years. Our hypotheses were that postoperative coagulation tests would indicate hypocoagulation, and that postoperative serum creatinine would be correlated to elevated aPTT suggesting an accumulation of thrombosis prophylaxis.

We also present a review of the literature aiming to establish whether our results agreed with previous research, whether there is evidence that current coagulation tests can be used to estimate the risk of spinal haematoma and why coagulation parameters may be elevated in the postoperative period.

Methods

We included patients who had between 2002 and 2012 received epidural or intravenous analgesia after oesophageal surgery at our tertiary hospital, which is a regional centre for treatment of oesophageal cancer. Patients were identified using filed prescription sheets from epidural or intravenous infusion pumps. The data shown in Table 1 was recorded for each patient, which included routine coagulation status before surgery, and before withdrawal of epidural catheters.

Patients were attributed an identification number and masked data was entered in to a spreadsheet using Microsoft Excel before export to R for statistical analysis (R version 3.3.1, www.r-project.org). Original data is available in Additional file 1 but we have removed patients' ages and the date of operation to preserve anonymity. The significance of differences between pre- and postoperative test results were tested using the paired Student's *t* test.

Figure 1 summarises the literature search. A PubMed search was carried out using the terms "epidural" AND "coagulation" AND English language. Articles concerning coagulation in the context of perioperative epidural analgesia published in 2000 or later were retrieved. Articles were sorted into the topics shown in Fig. 1.

Results

Three hundred and seven patients, 69 women and 238 men, who received a thoracic epidural catheter immediately before induction of general anaesthesia for oesophageal surgery were included. Additional file 1 displays patient and quality data: the median length of time between insertion and withdrawal of catheters was 8.5 days (range 1–38). The mean level of placement was T8 (range T4–T12). The median intraoperative haemorrhage was 500 ml (range 50–3800 ml). Forty-one of the patients who had received an epidural catheter were postoperatively given a patient-controlled intravenous morphine infusion, for reasons which are shown in Table 2. This represents 13% of the patients enrolled. All patients were treated with thrombosis prophylaxis (enoxaparin 40 mg daily other than four patients who received 80 mg). No serious complication of epidural catheterization was recorded.

Table 1 Summary of data collected for each patient

Patient details	Preoperative data	Data prior to withdrawal of epidural catheter
Age	Time of epidural catheterization	Time of withdrawal of epidural catheter
Sex	Time of blood testing	Time of blood testing
Epidural or intravenous analgesia	Activated partial thromboplastin time (aPTT)	Time and dosage of the last dose of low molecular weight heparin (LMWH) before withdrawal of epidural catheter
Reason for intravenous analgesia if applicable	Prothrombin time international normalised ratio (PT-INR)	Activated partial thromboplastin time (aPTT)
Level of epidural catheterization	Platelet count (Plc)	Prothrombin time international normalised ratio (PT-INR)
	Blood haemoglobin level (Hb)	Platelet count (Plc)
	Serum albumin (Alb)	Blood haemoglobin level (Hb)
	Serum creatinine (Crea)	

An additional 51 patients who underwent oesophageal resection were identified, who did not receive an epidural catheter. Six proved difficult to catheterize such that the attempt to insert an epidural catheter was given up. Nine of the 51 did not receive an epidural because of abnormal preoperative routine coagulation test results while one had known von Willebrand's Disease, one scleroderma and one renal failure. Ten had relative anatomical contraindications.

Figure 2 shows the dynamics of routine coagulation test results between insertion and withdrawal of catheters. Mean PT-INR increased significantly from 1.0 ± 0.11 to 1.1 ± 0.14: mean aPTT increased significantly from 32 ± 4.0 to 38 ± 6.7 s and mean Plc increased significantly from 269 ± 83 × 10^6 to 339 ± 196 × 10^6. 32/307 patients' PT-INR was elevated above the reference range at the time of catheter withdrawal; for aPTT, this figure was 129/307; and there was only one patient whose Plc was below the reference range at this time. There was no relationship between the amount of intraoperative haemorrhage and any of the postoperative coagulation parameters.

Applying Hanley's simple formula to the 129 patients whose aPTT or PT-INR was elevated above the reference range, the upper 95% confidence interval for the true risk of spinal haematoma in these patients is estimated to be 3/129 = 2.3% (Hanley and Lippman-Hand 1983).

Results for preoperative serum albumin, and serum creatinine and blood haemoglobin preoperatively and at the time of withdrawal, are shown in Additional file 1. Mean serum creatinine decreased significantly from 78 ± 38 to 67 ± 31 μmol/l. There was no correlation between postoperative aPTT and serum creatinine.

Figure 3 shows which coagulation parameters indicate hypocoagulation in the 237 patients for whom data was complete. Half of the patients had an aPTT above the upper limit of the reference range while only 10% had a PT-INR above the reference range. Thrombocytopenia was almost non-existent at the time of withdrawal of epidural catheters.

Results of the literature search

Summaries of the relevant articles described in this section are available in Additional file 2.

Articles concerning the evaluation of tests in the specific context of epidural analgesia

Five articles were found. All are relatively small (between 10 and 52 subjects). The authors of this study are responsible for two of these articles (Thomas et al. 2013; Thomas et al. 2015). Four of the five articles compare whole-blood assays of coagulation to routine test results. Two of the articles find that viscoelastic tests (ROTEM®, TEG® and free-oscillation rheometry) can likely be used to monitor the effect of LMWHs on initiation of coagulation, although they cannot be considered to be validated (Thomas et al. 2015; Klein et al. 2000). Two of the articles compare PT-INR to ROTEM® or TEG® and conclude that although PT-INR is prolonged in the

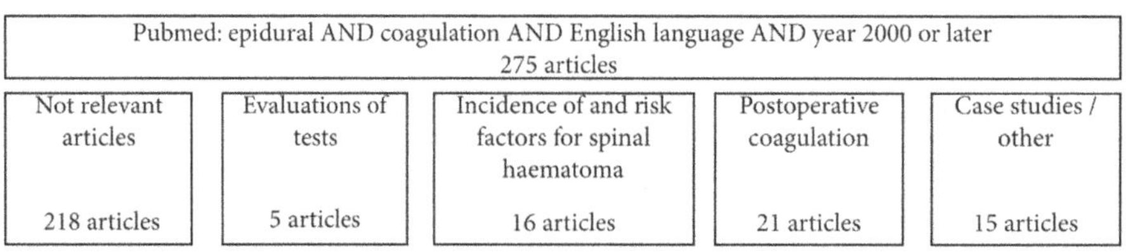

Fig. 1 Search strategy for the literature review presented in this article

Table 2 Reasons for replacing epidural analgesia with intravenous analgesia with an intravenous patient-controlled morphine infusion

Inadequate analgesia provided by epidural catheter	23
Unclear from patient notes	7
Accidental withdrawal of the catheter	7
Elective transition from epidural to IV-PCA	6
Leakage around the catheter	2
Suspected infection around the catheter	2
'Sudden chest pain', epidural catheter presumably withdrawn before antiplatelet drugs	1

postoperative period after major gastrointestinal and orthopaedic surgery with or without warfarin as thrombosis prophylaxis, the viscoelastic tests indicate normo- or hypercoagulation (Thomas et al. 2013; Hepner et al. 2002). Finally, one study compared a patient-near method of measuring PT with routine laboratory results and found good concordance between the methods such that patient-near PT-INR measurement in the operating theatre or intensive care unit is realistic (Nishiyama et al. 2011).

Articles concerning the incidence of and risk factors for spinal haemorrhage

Sixteen articles were found. Many are prospective or retrospective studies in which routine care is given. No or few spinal haematomas are found in the population being studied, and 95% confidence limits for the true risk of haematoma are calculated. For example, among over 11,000 patients who were included, Gulur et al. identified 351 patients with abnormal routine coagulation test results when their epidural catheters were removed: two developed spinal haematomas such that the 95% confidence interval for the actual risk of spinal haematoma can be calculated to be between 1:87 and 1:2597. This statistic is complicated by the two patients developing spinal haematoma having also had spinal drains, one of which was placed because of spinal ischaemia, and that it was 'technically difficult', and therefore presumably traumatic, to place the catheter (Gulur et al. 2015; Ho et al. 2000). Other studies reporting series of 'non-events' are shown in Additional file 2: Davis et al. (2012), Franchi et al. (2011), Pumberger et al. (2013), Volk et al. (2012) and Pace et al. (2014). The results of articles lie within the interval identified from insurance claims in Sweden by Moen in 2004: the risk of spinal haematoma after epidural analgesia for orthopaedics in elderly women may be as high as 1:3600 whereas the risk in obstetrics is nearer 1:200,000. Franchi concludes that the frequency of abnormal PT-INR and aPTT in pregnant women presenting for elective neuraxial blockade is so low that these tests should not be taken (Franchi et al. 2011). Pace reaches a similar conclusion for aPTT after various operations, concluding that extremely few patients without risk factors for coagulopathy have a prolonged aPTT (Pace et al. 2014).

There are two articles which use laboratory studies to provide relevant knowledge: Kassis et al. (2000) measured aPTT and anti-FXa and anti-FIIa activity before subcutaneous heparin was given, then repeated measurements 2 and 4 h later to conclude that epidural catheters can safely be withdrawn 2 h after a subcutaneous injection of unfractionated heparin. Leonard conducted an in vitro experiment concluding that the systemic antiplatelet effect of levobupivacaine given epidurally ought not to affect coagulation, but that it may affect coagulation locally, for example in a blood patch (Leonard et al. 2000).

Two articles identify risk factors for spinal haematoma by using large retrospective studies to find and analyse relatively small numbers of patients who have had spinal haematomas. Risk factors for spinal haematoma at the time of epidural withdrawal, other than abnormal laboratory test results, include liver failure or undergoing hepatic resection, major intraoperative haemorrhage or transfusion of blood products (Pace et al. 2014), taking drugs that may affect haemostasis, such as aspirin, NSAIDs, tricyclic antidepressants or antiplatelet drugs, having abnormal anatomy, in particular spinal stenosis (Pumberger et al. 2013) but also female sex, impaired renal function and type of surgery (Volk et al. 2012).

The last category of study that sheds light on the risk and incidence of spinal haematoma is the studies which investigate epidural catheterization in categories of patient in which there is a relative contraindication for neuraxial blockade: Pastor et al. (2003) and his colleague Canto et al. (2002) describe epidural catheterization 60 min before full heparinization for extracorporteal circulation in heart surgery: over 1000 patient cases are reported without complication, giving an upper 95% confidence interval for risk of epidural haematoma of around 1:300, see Additional file 2. Similarly, Singh reports a case series of patients with FXI deficiency who received uncomplicated epidural analgesia. The most controversial study found in this review is by Liu et al. (2011), who withdrew epidural catheters from patients who had just started warfarin thrombosis prophylaxis despite the PT-INR values of up to 7. The rationale for doing this was that Benzon et al. (2010) reasons that the most important factor antagonised by warfarin is FVII and that this antagonization lags behind the PT-INR becoming prolonged. The clinical appropriateness of this reasoning is strongly questioned by Horlocker et al. (2010). Although Liu included 4365 patients, the small number of patients with PT-INR over 2 means that the upper 95% confidence limit for the actual risk of spinal haematoma can be as high as 1:250 if epidural catheters

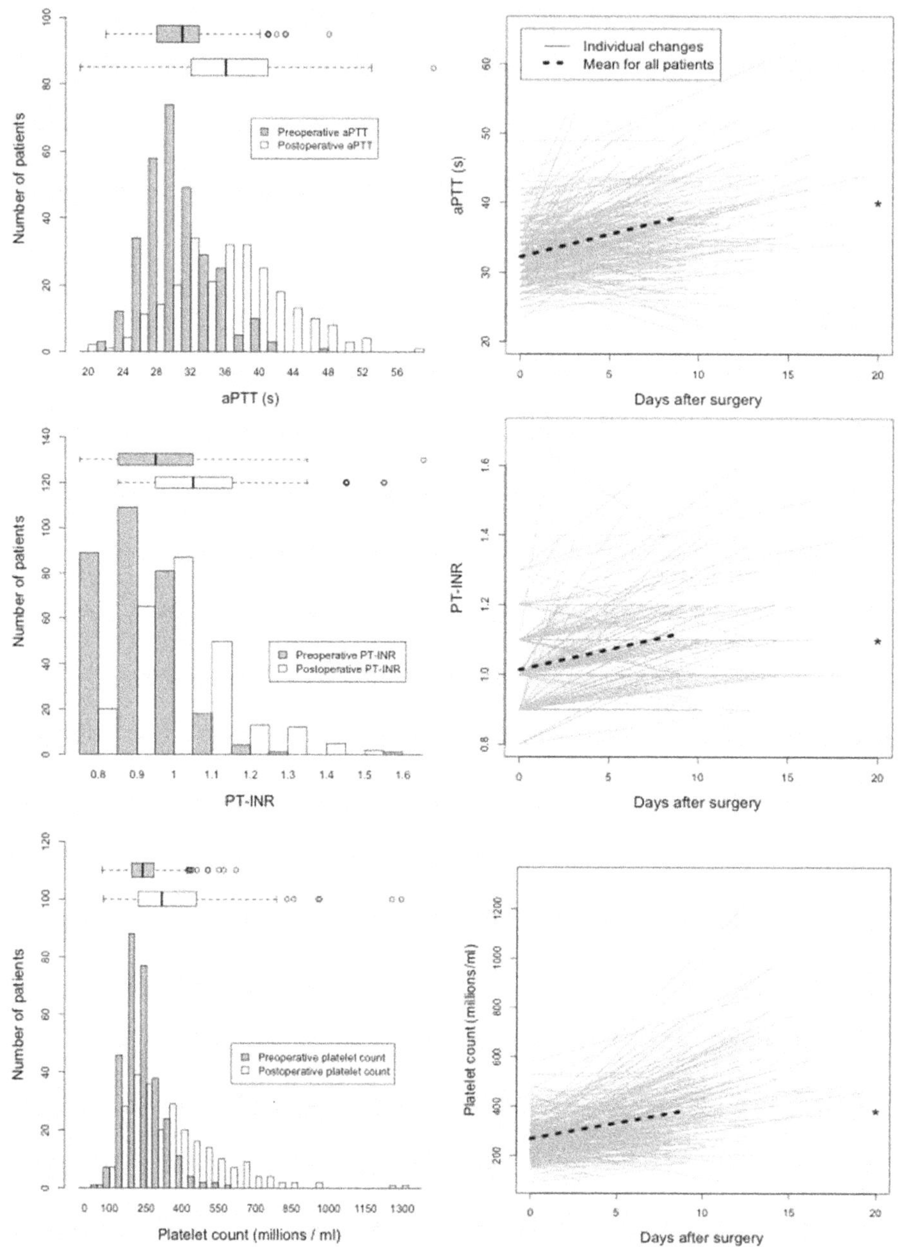

Fig. 2 Dynamics of routine coagulation status between insertion and withdrawal of epidural catheters. Each solid grey line represents a patient. The beginning of the line at time = 0 represents results taken preoperatively, while each line ends at the time at which the patients' epidural catheter was taken. Note that only two data points are shown for each patient. The dotted black lines show mean pre- to postoperative changes for the whole patient group and stars indicate a significant pre- to postoperative difference using the paired Student's *t* test ($P < 0.05$). aPTT, activated partial prothrombin time. PT-INR, prothrombin time international normalised ratio

are withdrawn when PT-INR is > 2 and 1:33 when the PT-INR is > 3 (Carvalho et al. 2011).

Articles concerning the clinical pathophysiology of postoperative coagulation in the context of epidural analgesia

Nineteen articles were found. Fourteen studied postoperative coagulation in patients who had undergone hepatectomy. One of these also included other categories of patients. Almost all the studies recorded PT or PT-INR, aPTT and Plc daily for the first week after surgery. Almost without exception they found a transient dip in Plc during the first two to three postoperative days, accompanied by a slightly shorter prolongation of the PT and sometimes aPTT.

Tsui et al. (2004) investigated the proportion of patients with coagulopathy necessitating delaying withdrawal of an epidural catheter. The risk was highest after

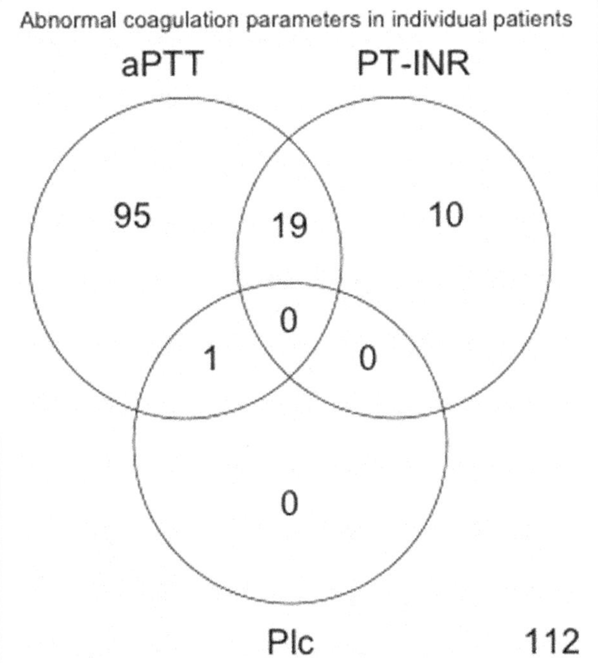

Fig. 3 Venn diagram showing the frequency of routine coagulation tests outside their reference range at the time of withdrawing epidural catheters, indicating hypocoagulation. Only including the 237 patients for whom complete data are available: activated partial thromboplastin time (aPTT), prothrombin time international normalised ratio (PT-INR) and platelet count (Plc)

hepatic resection, lower in major abdominal surgery and lowest in orthopaedics. This is consistent with the other studies in this review. Risk factors for derangements in tests of coagulation were the size of liver resection, duration of surgery, preoperative liver failure, amount of intraoperative haemorrhage, requirement for blood product transfusion and low body mass index (Borromeo et al. 2000; Choi et al. 2007; Elterman and Xiong 2015; Jolly et al. 2011; Karna et al. 2015; Matot et al. 2002; Ramspoth et al. 2014; Schumann et al. 2004; Siniscalchi et al. 2004; Stamenkovic et al. 2011; Yuan et al. 2012).

Bergman and Young (2007) reply to Weinberg et al. (2006) that 'prothrombin is not the whole story' in postoperative coagulation after hepatic resection and point out that these patients are prone to thrombosis despite an elevated PT-INR and aPTT. This may be due to deficiencies in antithrombin or protein C, which are not detected by the PT assay. Mohammed et al. (2013) describe a prospective study of patients undergoing hepatectomy for liver donation, in which ROTEM® is compared with routine tests of coagulation. The transient hypocoagulability indicated by routine tests was not demonstrated by ROTEM® but ROTEM® did not indicate postoperative hypercoagulability either.

Articles presenting case reports or other relevant research

Nine relevant case studies, four reviews and a report from a postal survey were found, see Additional file 2. Two reports describe complications arising as a result of treating a laboratory test indicative of hypocoagulability, in an attempt to reduce the risk of spinal haematoma: Chaney and Labovsky (2005) describe administering vitamin K to a patient to correct an elevated PT-INR 5 days after cardiac surgery, after which the patient had a thromboembolic stroke. Lim et al. (2006) describe a series of patients who received plasma transfusions to correct elevated PT-INRs: one developed anaphylaxis.

Chung et al. (2011), Fakouri et al. (2009) and Goswami et al. (2011) describe patients who would not be expected to be at a high risk of spinal haematoma, but who developed one anyway. Ladha et al. (2013) present a case of a patient with elevated liver function tests but not coagulopathy before gastrectomy with epidural analgesia. She developed a postoperative deficiency of vitamin K-dependent coagulation factors and required urgent decompression of a spinal haematoma.

Finally, there are two studies describing cases where spinal haematoma was not expected, but was preceded by an abnormal course of events: Ozdemir et al. (2009) describe a patient who developed a late chronic intracranial subdural haematoma after inadvertent dura puncture at epidural catheterization. Walker et al. (2011) describes a spinal haematoma in a patient with normal routine coagulation status but various other risk factors for spinal haematoma: major haemorrhage with massive transfusion, multiple attempts at epidural catheterization including a bloody tap and ROTEM® parameters indicative of coagulopathy.

Discussion

General trends of coagulation

This study concerns coagulation after oesophagectomy, which is not as well researched as coagulation after hepatic resection. Nevertheless, our results (Fig. 2) are in concordance with the studies found in the literature review: postoperative coagulation is characterised by moderate increases in PT-INR and aPTT despite these patients being known to be prone to thrombosis. Postoperative inflammation is characterised by thrombocytosis and hyperfibrinogenaemia, which likely compensate for potential deficiencies in coagulation factors that can affect PT-INR and aPTT. Our own research concerning coagulation after major upper gastrointestinal surgery suggest that increases in PT-INR may be caused by postoperative decreases in factor VII while increases in aPTT may be caused by decreases in factor XII. Deficiency of FXII in otherwise healthy individuals is not associated with coagulopathy (Thomas et al. 2016). Given the questionable relevance of standard coagulation parameters, we would agree with other authors, in that an individual assessment of patients' clinical coagulative states is warranted when routine coagulation parameters are mildly elevated and an epidural catheter needs withdrawing (Gulur et al. 2015).

The increase in aPTT would not appear to be caused by postoperative renal failure causing accumulation of LMWH

Half of our patients' postoperative aPTT was above the upper reference limit, which is a greater proportion of patients than that seen in the literature search. The only measure we have of renal function in this study is serum creatinine, which actually decreased over the perioperative period, so it does not explain the prolonged aPTT. A problem with the aPTT assay is that it is not standardised in the same way as PT-INR, so that different methods and reagents can give varying results from a single blood sample (Thomas et al. 2015).

There was an increase in coagulative complications when LMWH was introduced in the USA in a much higher dosage than the one we use (Horlocker and Wedel 1998). It is, however, of note that we give enoxaparin in a standard dose of 40 mg once daily regardless of weight. The patient category most likely to develop spinal haematoma is elderly women undergoing orthopaedic surgery; these patients are much more likely to be small and have renal failure than young patients without significant comorbidity.

Risk of spinal haematoma

Calculating the risk of an uncommon complication from a set of uncomplicated events is notoriously difficult, as described by Ho et al. (2000) and Hanley and Lippman-Hand (1983). We observed only 130 patients with elevated coagulation results, mainly aPTT, without complication, meaning that we cannot with certainty say that the risk of spinal haematoma was lower than 2.3%; we cannot from the data in this study come to any clinical conclusion regarding whether it is safe to withdraw catheters when the aPTT or PT-INR are mildly elevated.

Is there a place for viscoelastic tests in identifying patients at risk of spinal haematoma on withdrawal of epidural catheters? Two of the studies in the literature review provide cases where ROTEM® or TEG® gave an indication of hypocoagulability when routine tests did not (Simons and Mallett 2007; Walker et al. 2011). On the other hand, ROTEM® is insensitive to anticoagulation with warfarin up to a PT-INR of at least 3.0 (manufacturer's information) even if viscoelastic tests using specially adapted and, as yet, not commercially available reagents can be used to monitor clinical vitamin K antagonism (Sorensen et al. 2003). Platelet count is recommended in the ASRA guidelines because of the risk of heparin-induced thrombocytopenia after a few days' treatment with LMWH (Horlocker et al. 2011).

What is next in this area of research?

The recurring theme of most research in this area since the middle of the 1990s is that the risk of epidural haematoma is small and that routine laboratory tests' role in risk stratification is unclear. Even the rather large study by Liu et al. (2011), in which epidural catheters were withdrawn from patients with test results that would in most institutions would have been prohibitive, has insufficient power to come to any definitive conclusion about how to interpret abnormal standard test results.

We do not think that more small prospective studies are going to provide us with adequate data allowing a definition of a 'magic' values for aPTT or PT-INR which allow withdrawal of epidural catheters without the risk of spinal haematoma. It would be more meaningful to analyse all cases of spinal haematoma such that a definitive identification of risk factors for spinal haematoma could be produced. As already described in the ASRA guidelines, patients at high risk should be clinically monitored much more vigilantly than those at low risk. We propose that patients, who develop spinal haematomas after epidural catheterization or withdrawal of a catheter, should be included in continent-wide studies coordinated by professional bodies, in which blood should be taken and sent for advanced coagulation analysis that is too expensive to be run on patients in prospective studies. It is of great interest to define exactly which, if any, coagulopathy causes spinal haematoma: if non-coagulative factors are more important than blood test results, attention should be paid to these to prevent unnecessary haemorrhagic complications of neuraxial blockade.

Conclusion

This is a difficult subject to research and deserves considerable respect since epidural catheterization is a procedure that may reduce morbidity and mortality after high-risk operations, but which is rarely immediately life-saving. The data presented in this study support previous research which indicates that major operations are followed by thrombocytosis combined with aPTT and PT-INR suggesting mild coagulopathy. The implications for the risk of spinal haematoma when epidural catheters are removed are still unclear, which is why a prospective and at least continental-wide study investigating patients who have actually had spinal haematoma should be conducted.

Additional files

Additional file 1: Graphical representation of epidemiological, quality and other laboratory data. Stars indicate significant differences between pre- and postoperative results as tested using Student's *t* test ($P < 0.05$). aPTT, activated partial prothrombin time. PT-INR, prothrombin time international normalised ratio. Plc, platelet count. EPI, epidural analgesia. IV-PCA, intravenous patient-controlled analgesia with morphine. (TIFF 1498 kb)

Additional file 2: Summaries of the individual articles included in the literature search (Vandermeulen et al. 1994; Sandhu et al. 2000; Greaves 1997; Liu and Mulroy 1998; Horlocker 2003; Moen and Irestedt 2008; Singh et al. 2009; Davies 2007; Shontz et al. 2009; Cwik 2012; Ladha et al. 2013; Okuda and Kitajima 2001; Schulz-Stubner et al. 2005; Tyagi and Bhattacharya 2002; Unic-Stojanovic et al. 2012). (PDF 99 kb)

Additional file 3: Raw data presented as a tabulated text file (.txt). Patients' ages and the dates of operation have been removed to preserve anonymity. (TXT 91 kb)

Abbreviations

Alb: Serum albumin; aPTT: Activated partial thromboplastin time; Crea: Serum creatinine; EPI: Epidural analgesia; Hb: Blood haemoglobin; IV-PCA: Intravenous patient-controlled analgesia; LMWH: Low molecular weight heparin; NSAID: Non-steroidal anti-inflammatory drug; Plc: Platelet count; PT-INR: Prothrombin time international normalised ratio; ROTEM®: Rotational thromboelastometry; TEG®: Thromboelastography

Acknowledgements

For the data collection, we thank Elisabet Eldh, Pain Nurse, SUS Lund University Hospital, Sweden, and Christian Schaub, resident in general medicine, Torsten Born's Specialist Practice for Diabetology, Berlin, Germany.

Funding

Data collection was mainly carried out by Christian Schaub (see Acknowledgements) who was funded by the ERASMUS programme (https://ec.europa.eu/programmes/erasmus-plus/).

Authors' contributions

OT carried out the study design, data collection, statistical analysis and the manuscript. EL contributed to the statistical analysis and the manuscript. PF took part in the study design and manuscript. US had a hand in the study design, statistical analysis and the manuscript. All authors read and approved the final manuscript.

Authors' information

N/A

Competing interests

The authors declare that they have no competing interests.

Author details

[1]Department of Anaesthesiology and Intensive Care Medicine, Institute of Clinical Sciences, Lund, Medical Faculty, University of Lund, 221 00 Lund, Sweden. [2]Department of Paediatric Anaesthesia and Intensive Care, SUS Lund University Hospital, 22185 Lund, Sweden. [3]Oskarshamn Hospital, 572 28 Oskarshamn, Sweden. [4]Department of Anaesthesia and Intensive Care, Helsingborg Hospital, Södra Vallgatan 5, 254 37 Helsingborg, Sweden. [5]Department of Anaesthesia and Intensive Care, SUS Lund University Hospital, 221 85 Lund, Sweden.

References

Benzon HT, Avram MJ, Benzon HA, Kirby-Nolan M, Nader A. Factor VII levels and international normalized ratios in the early phase of warfarin therapy. Anesthesiology. 2010;112(2):298–304.

Bergman I, Young Y. Prothrombin time is not the whole story. Anaesth Intensive Care. 2007;35(1):140–1. author reply 141-142

Borromeo CJ, Stix MS, Lally A, Pomfret EA. Epidural catheter and increased prothrombin time after right lobe hepatectomy for living donor transplantation. Anesth Analg. 2000;91(5):1139–41.

Breivik H, Bang U, Jalonen J, Vigfusson G, Alahuhta S, Lagerkranser M. Nordic guidelines for neuraxial blocks in disturbed haemostasis from the Scandinavian Society of Anaesthesiology and Intensive Care Medicine. Acta Anaesthesiol Scand. 2010;54:16–41.

Canto M, Casas A, Sanchez MJ, Lorenzo A, Bataller L. Thoracic epidurals in heart valve surgery: neurologic risk evaluation. J Cardiothorac Vasc Anesth. 2002;16(6):723–6.

Carvalho B, Mariano ER, Butwick AJ. Epidural catheter removal in patients on warfarin thromboprophylaxis: a more cautious interpretation of results required? Reg Anesth Pain Med. 2011;36(6):632. author reply 632-633

Chaney MA, Labovsky JK. Thoracic epidural anesthesia and cardiac surgery: balancing postoperative risks associated with hematoma formation and thromboembolic phenomenon. J Cardiothorac Vasc Anesth. 2005;19(6): 768–71.

Choi SJ, Gwak MS, Ko JS, Kim GS, Ahn HJ, Yang M, Hahm TS, Lee SM, Kim MH, Joh JW. The changes in coagulation profile and epidural catheter safety for living liver donors: a report on 6 years of our experience. Liver Transpl. 2007;13(1):62–70.

Chung JH, Hwang J, Cha SC, Jung T, Woo SC. Epidural hematoma occurred by massive bleeding intraoperatively in cesarean section after combined spinal epidural anesthesia—a case report. Korean J Anesthesiol. 2011; 61(4):336–40.

Cwik J. Postoperative considerations of neuraxial anesthesia. Anesthesiol Clin. 2012;30(3):433–43.

Davies MJ. Perioperative epidural anaesthesia and analgesia—an appraisal of its role. Anaesth Intensive Care. 2007;35(4):593–600.

Davis JJ, Bankhead BR, Eckman EJ, Wallace A, Strunk J. Three-times-daily subcutaneous unfractionated heparin and neuraxial anesthesia: a retrospective review of 928 cases. Reg Anesth Pain Med. 2012;37(6):623–6.

Elterman KG, Xiong Z. Coagulation profile changes and safety of epidural analgesia after hepatectomy: a retrospective study. J Anesth. 2015;29(3):367–72.

Fakouri B, Srinivas S, Magaji S, Kunsky A, Cacciola F. Spinal epidural hematoma after insertion of a thoracic epidural catheter in the absence of coagulation disorders—a call for raised awareness. Neurol India. 2009;57(4):512–3.

Franchi F, Ibrahim B, Rossi F, Maspero ML, Morabito O, Asti D, Bucciarelli P, Biguzzi E. Coagulation testing before epidural analgesia at delivery: cost analysis. Thromb Res. 2011;128(1):18_20.

Gogarten W, Vandermeulen E, Van Aken H, Kozek S, Llau JV, Samama CM. Regional anaesthesia and antithrombotic agents: recommendations of the European Society of Anaesthesiology. Eur J Anaesthesiol. 2010;27:999–1015.

Goswami D, Das J, Deuri A, Deka AK. Epidural haematoma: rare complication after spinal while intending epidural anaesthesia with long-term follow-up after conservative treatment. Indian J Anaesth. 2011;55(1):71–3.

Greaves JD. Serious spinal cord injury due to haematomyelia caused by spinal anaesthesia in a patient treated with low-dose heparin. Anaesthesia. 1997;52(2):150–4.

Gulur P, Tsui B, Pathak R, Koury KM, Lee H. Retrospective analysis of the incidence of epidural haematoma in patients with epidural catheters and abnormal coagulation parameters. Br J Anaesth. 2015;114(5):808–11.

Hanley JA, Lippman-Hand A. If nothing goes wrong, is everything all right? Interpreting zero numerators. JAMA. 1983;249(13):1743–5.

Hepner DL, Concepcion M, Bhavani-Shankar K. Coagulation status using thromboelastography in patients receiving warfarin prophylaxis and epidural analgesia. J Clin Anesth. 2002;14(6):405–10.

Ho AM, Chung DC, Joynt GM. Neuraxial blockade and hematoma in cardiac surgery: estimating the risk of a rare adverse event that has not (yet) occurred. Chest. 2000;117:551–5.

Horlocker TT. Thromboprophylaxis and neuraxial anesthesia. Orthopedics. 2003;26(2 Suppl):s243–9.

Horlocker TT, Heit JA, Wedel DJ, Enneking FK, Rowlingson JC. Safe epidural catheter removal in the patient receiving warfarin: does anybody really know what (prothrombin) time it is? Anesthesiology. 2010;113(3):759–61. author reply 761

Horlocker TT, Neal JM, Rathmell JP. Practice advisories by the American Society of Regional Anesthesia and Pain Medicine: grading the evidence and making the grade. Reg Anesth Pain Med. 2011;36:1–3.

Horlocker TT, Wedel DJ. Spinal and epidural blockade and perioperative low molecular weight heparin: smooth sailing on the Titanic. Anesth Analg. 1998;86(6):1153–6.

Horlocker TT, Wedel DJ, Rowlingson JC, Enneking FK. Executive summary: regional anesthesia in the patient receiving antithrombotic or thrombolytic therapy: American Society of Regional Anesthesia and Pain Medicine Evidence-Based Guidelines (Third Edition). Reg Anesth Pain Med. 2010;35:102–5.

Jolly A, Vohra V, Bhalotra S. 4 postoperative changes in coagulation parameters in 105 patients undergoing live donor hepatectomies-implications for epidural analgesia. J Clin Exp Hepatol. 2011;1(2):134.

Karna ST, Pandey CK, Sharma S, Singh A, Tandon M, Pandey VK. Postoperative coagulopathy after live related donor hepatectomy: incidence, predictors and implications for safety of thoracic epidural catheter. J Postgrad Med. 2015;61(3):176–80.

Kassis J, Fugere F, Dube S. The safe use of epidural anesthesia after subcutaneous injection of low-dose heparin in general abdominal surgery. Can J Surg. 2000;43(4):289–94.

Klein SM, Slaughter TF, Vail PT, Ginsberg B, El-Moalem HE, Alexander R, D'Ercole F, Greengrass RA, Perumal TT, Welsby I, et al. Thromboelastography as a perioperative measure of anticoagulation resulting from low molecular weight heparin: a comparison with anti-Xa concentrations. Anesth Analg. 2000;91(5):1091–5.

Ladha A, Alam A, Idestrup C, Sawyer J, Choi S. Spinal haematoma after removal of a thoracic epidural catheter in a patient with coagulopathy resulting from unexpected vitamin K deficiency. Anaesthesia. 2013;68(8):856–60.

Leonard SA, Walsh M, Lydon A, O'Hare B, Shorten GD. Evaluation of the effects of levobupivacaine on clotting and fibrinolysis using thromboelastography. Eur J Anaesthesiol. 2000;17(6):373–8.

Lim HJ, Koay CK, Lee LS. Postoperative coagulopathy after liver resection—implications for epidural analgesia. Anaesth Intensive Care. 2006;34(1):118–9.

Liu SS, Buvanendran A, Viscusi ER, Hutton E, Lubenow T, Zhou J, Shaw PM, Moric M, Lenart S. Uncomplicated removal of epidural catheters in 4365 patients with international normalized ratio greater than 1.4 during initiation of warfarin therapy. Reg Anesth Pain Med. 2011;36(3):231–5.

Liu SS, Mulroy MF. Neuraxial anesthesia and analgesia in the presence of standard heparin. Reg Anesth Pain Med. 1998;23(6 Suppl 2):157–63.

Matot I, Scheinin O, Eid A, Jurim O. Epidural anesthesia and analgesia in liver resection. Anesth Analg. 2002;95(5):1179–81. table of contents

Merritt RE, Whyte RI, D'Arcy NT, Hoang CD, Shrager JB. Morbidity and mortality after esophagectomy following neoadjuvant chemoradiation. Ann Thorac Surg. 2011;92:2034–40.

Moen V, Dahlgren N, Irestedt L. Severe neurological complications after central neuraxial blockades in Sweden 1990–1999. Anesthesiology. 2004;101:950–9.

Moen V, Irestedt L. Neurological complications following central neuraxial blockades in obstetrics. Curr Opin Anaesthesiol. 2008;21(3):275–80.

Mohammed M, Fayed N, Hassanen A, Ahmed F, Mourad W, El Sheikh M, Abofetouh F, Yassen K, Khalil M, Marwan I, et al. Rotational thromboelastometry and standard coagulation tests for live liver donors. Clin Transpl. 2013;27(2):E101–8.

Nishiyama J, Matsuda M, Urimoto G, Sakamoto R, Ito K, Suzuki T. Applicability of a compact PT-INR measuring device CoaguChek XS to perioperative management. Tokai J Exp Clin Med. 2011;36(4):134–8.

Okuda Y, Kitajima T. Epidural hematoma in a parturient who developed disseminated intravascular coagulation after epidural anesthesia. Reg Anesth Pain Med. 2001;26(4):383–4.

Ozdemir N, Ari MK, Gelal MF, Bezircioglu H. Intracranial chronic subdural haematoma as a complication of epidural anesthesia. Turk Neurosurg. 2009;19(3):285–7.

Pace M, Koury K, Gulur P. Epidurals in patients receiving thromboprophylaxis with unfractionated heparin three times a day: the value of activated partial thromboplastin time testing. Anesth Analg. 2014;119:1215–8.

Pastor MC, Sanchez MJ, Casas MA, Mateu J, Bataller ML. Thoracic epidural analgesia in coronary artery bypass graft surgery: seven years' experience. J Cardiothorac Vasc Anesth. 2003;17(2):154–9.

Pumberger M, Memtsoudis SG, Stundner O, Herzog R, Boettner F, Gausden E, Hughes AP. An analysis of the safety of epidural and spinal neuraxial anesthesia in more than 100,000 consecutive major lower extremity joint replacements. Reg Anesth Pain Med. 2013;38(6):515–9.

Ramspoth T, Roehl AB, Macko S, Heidenhain C, Junge K, Binnebosel M, Schmeding M, Neumann UP, Rossaint R, Hein M. Risk factors for coagulopathy after liver resection. J Clin Anesth. 2014;26(8):654–62.

Sandhu H, Morley-Forster P, Spadafora S. Epidural hematoma following epidural analgesia in a patient receiving unfractionated heparin for thromboprophylaxis. Reg Anesth Pain Med. 2000;25:72–5.

Schulz-Stubner S, Boezaart A, Hata JS. Regional analgesia in the critically ill. Crit Care Med. 2005;33(6):1400–7.

Schumann R, Zabala L, Angelis M, Bonney I, Tighiouart H, Carr DB. Altered hematologic profiles following donor right hepatectomy and implications for perioperative analgesic management. Liver Transpl. 2004;10(3):363–8.

Shontz R, Karuparthy V, Temple R, Brennan TJ. Prevalence and risk factors predisposing to coagulopathy in patients receiving epidural analgesia for hepatic surgery. Reg Anesth Pain Med. 2009;34(4):308–11.

Simons R, Mallett SV. Use of thromboelastography to demonstrate persistent anticoagulation after stopping enoxaparin. Anaesthesia. 2007;62(11):1175–8.

Singh A, Harnett MJ, Connors JM, Camann WR. Factor XI deficiency and obstetrical anesthesia. Anesth Analg. 2009;108(6):1882–5.

Siniscalchi A, Begliomini B, De Pietri L, Braglia V, Gazzi M, Masetti M, Di Benedetto F, Pinna AD, Miller CM, Pasetto A. Increased prothrombin time and platelet counts in living donor right hepatectomy: implications for epidural anesthesia. Liver Transpl. 2004;10(9):1144–9.

Sorensen B, Johansen P, Christiansen K, Woelke M, Ingerslev J. Whole blood coagulation thrombelastographic profiles employing minimal tissue factor activation. J Thromb Haemost. 2003;1(3):551–8.

Stamenkovic DM, Jankovic ZB, Toogood GJ, Lodge JP, Bellamy MC. Epidural analgesia and liver resection: postoperative coagulation disorders and epidural catheter removal. Minerva Anestesiol. 2011;77(7):671–9.

Thomas O, Larsson A, Tynngard N, Schott U. Thromboelastometry versus free-oscillation rheometry and enoxaparin versus tinzaparin: an in-vitro study comparing two viscoelastic haemostatic tests' dose-responses to two low molecular weight heparins at the time of withdrawing epidural catheters from ten patients after major surgery. BMC Anesthesiol. 2015;15:170.

Thomas O, Lybeck E, Strandberg K, Tynngård N, Schött U. Monitoring low molecular weight heparins at therapeutic levels: dose-responses of, and correlations and differences between aPTT, anti-factor XA and thrombin generation assays. PLoS One. 2015;10:1–16.

Thomas O, Rein H, Strandberg K, Schott U. Coagulative safety of epidural catheters after major upper gastrointestinal surgery: advanced and routine coagulation analysis in 38 patients. Perioper Med (Lond). 2016;5:28.

Thomas OD, Gustafsson A, Schott U. Rotational thromboelastometry and multiple electrode platelet aggregometry in four patients with abnormal routine coagulation studies before removal of epidural catheters after major surgery: a case series and research study. J Med Case Rep. 2013;7:282.

Tsui SL, Yong BH, Ng KF, Yuen TS, Li CC, Chui KY. Delayed epidural catheter removal: the impact of postoperative coagulopathy. Anaesth Intensive Care. 2004;32(5):630–6.

Tyagi A, Bhattacharya A. Central neuraxial blocks and anticoagulation: a review of current trends. Eur J Anaesthesiol. 2002;19(5):317–29.

Unic-Stojanovic D, Babic S, Jovic M. Benefits, risks and complications of perioperative use of epidural anesthesia. Med Arch. 2012;66(5):340–3.

Vandermeulen EP, Van Aken H, Vermylen J. Anticoagulants and spinal-epidural anesthesia. Anesth Analg. 1994;79(6):1165–77.

Volk T, Wolf A, Van Aken H, Burkle H, Wiebalck A, Steinfeldt T. Incidence of spinal haematoma after epidural puncture: analysis from the German network for safety in regional anaesthesia. Eur J Anaesthesiol. 2012;29(4):170–6.

Walker C, Ingram M, Edwards D, Wood P. Use of thromboelastometry in the assessment of coagulation before epidural insertion after massive transfusion. Anaesthesia. 2011;66(1):52–5.

Watson A, Allen PR. Influence of thoracic epidural analgesia on outcome after resection for esophageal cancer. Surgery. 1994;115:429–32.

Weinberg L, Scurrah N, Gunning K, McNicol L. Postoperative changes in prothrombin time following hepatic resection: implications for perioperative analgesia. Anaesth Intensive Care. 2006;34(4):438–43.

Yuan FS, Ng SY, Ho KY, Lee SY, Chung AY, Poopalalingam R. Abnormal coagulation profile after hepatic resection: the effect of chronic hepatic disease and implications for epidural analgesia. J Clin Anesth. 2012;24(5):398–403.

21

The relationship between cardiopulmonary exercise test variables, the systemic inflammatory response, and complications following surgery for colorectal cancer

Stephen T. McSorley*, Campbell S. D. Roxburgh, Paul G. Horgan and Donald C. McMillan

Abstract

Background: Both preoperative cardiopulmonary exercise test (CPET)-derived measures of fitness and postoperative C-reactive protein (CRP) concentrations are associated with complications following surgery for colorectal cancer. The aim of the present pilot study was to examine the relationship between CPET and postoperative CRP concentrations in this patient group.

Methods: Patients who had undergone CPET prior to elective surgery for histologically confirmed colorectal cancer in a single centre between September 2008 and April 2017 were included. Preoperative VO_2 at the anaerobic threshold (AT) and peak exercise were recorded, along with preoperative modified Glasgow Prognostic Score (mGPS) and CRP on each postoperative day.

Results: Thirty-eight patients were included. The majority were male (30, 79%), over 65 years old (30, 79%), with colonic cancer (23, 61%) and node-negative disease (24, 63%). Fourteen patients (37%) had open surgery and 24 (63%) had a laparoscopic resection. A progressive reduction in VO_2 at peak exercise was significantly associated with both increasing American Society of Anesthesiology (ASA) grade (median, ml/kg/min: ASA 1 = 22, ASA 2 = 19, ASA 3 = 15, ASA 4 = 12, $p = 0.014$) and increasing mGPS (median, ml/kg/min: mGPS 0 = 18, mGPS 1 = 16, mGPS 2 = 14, $p = 0.039$) There was no significant association between either VO_2 at the AT or peak exercise and postoperative CRP.

Conclusions: The present pilot study reports a possible association between preoperative CPET-derived measures of exercise tolerance, and the preoperative systemic inflammatory response, but not postoperative CRP in patients undergoing surgery for colorectal cancer.

Keywords: Colorectal cancer, Cardiopulmonary exercise testing, Systemic inflammation

Background

Colorectal cancer is a leading cause of death in the developed world (Cancer Research UK, 2016). Surgery continues to form the mainstay of treatment in the majority of cases; however, there is a significant associated degree of morbidity and mortality (Ghaferi et al., 2011). Long-term survival is primarily dictated by tumour differentiation and stage at presentation; however, it is increasingly recognised that postoperative complications have a significant impact on long-term oncologic outcomes (McSorley et al., 2016a).

Cardiopulmonary exercise testing (CPET/CPX) has been developed as a method of assessing a patient's ability to meet the increased oxygen demand of major surgery (Older et al., 1993). It represents a dynamic, non-invasive assessment of a patient's cardiovascular and pulmonary reserve (Smith et al., 2009). Two key measurements relating to oxygen delivery can be derived via CPET; oxygen consumption at the anaerobic threshold (VO_2 at AT) which represents the point at which anaerobic metabolism is required in addition to aerobic metabolism to meet tissue energy demand, and oxygen consumption at peak exercise

* Correspondence: s.mcsorley@doctors.org.uk
Academic Unit of Surgery, School of Medicine, University of Glasgow, R2.06, Level 2, New Lister Building, Glasgow Royal Infirmary, Alexandra Parade, Glasgow G31 2ER, UK

(VO_2 at peak). Patients with VO_2 at AT < 11 ml/min/kg or VO_2 at peak < 19 ml/min/kg are at significant risk of postoperative cardiovascular death and also of surgical complications following major abdominal surgery (Older et al., 1999). Very similar thresholds have also been found to predict the development of postoperative complications in surgery for oesophagogastric cancer (Moyes et al., 2013), in surgery for rectal cancer and colon cancer (West et al., 2014a; West et al., 2014b).

The magnitude of the postoperative systemic inflammatory response is associated with the development of, and severity of, complications following surgery for colorectal cancer (Platt et al., 2012; McSorley et al., 2015). The acute phase reactant C-reactive protein (CRP) has been shown to be a reliable marker of the magnitude of the postoperative systemic inflammatory response (Watt et al., 2015). Indeed, threshold values have been established in the postoperative period which are associated with the development of postoperative complications and the need for investigation (McDermott et al., 2015). The exact mechanism by which poor VO_2 at AT and VO_2 at peak are linked to the development of postoperative complications is incompletely understood. It may be that poor cardiopulmonary exercise tolerance leads to the development of postoperative complications due to an exaggerated postoperative systemic inflammatory response.

Therefore, the aim of the present pilot study was to investigate the relationship between CPET measurements, the preoperative systemic inflammatory response as measured by the modified Glasgow Prognostic Score (mGPS), the postoperative systemic inflammatory response as evidenced by CRP, and complications following surgery for colorectal cancer.

Methods

Patients

This observational pilot study included patients who had undergone CPET prior to elective surgery for histologically confirmed colorectal cancer in a single centre between September 2008 and April 2017.

All patients received prophylactic antibiotics and venous thromboprophylaxis prior to the induction of anaesthesia as per hospital policy. Further postoperative investigation and intervention was at the discretion of the patient's surgical team.

Methods

Clinicopathological data was collected prospectively in a database and anonymised. Recorded information included patient demographics, American Society of Anesthesiology (ASA) grade, body mass index (BMI), smoking status, tumour site, TNM stage (TNM, AJCC), surgical approach, preoperative and postoperative serum CRP and albumin measurements. Data regarding the nature, severity and management of complications was retrospectively categorised using the Clavien Dindo scale (Dindo et al., 2004). Any uncertainties were addressed by review of electronic and/or physical case notes. The study was approved by the West of Scotland Research Ethics Committee, Glasgow.

Serum concentrations of CRP (mg/l) were measured using an autoanalyser (Architect; Abbot Diagnostics, Maidenhead, UK) with a lower detectable limit of 0.2 mg/l as was serum albumin (normal range 35-50 g/l). The preoperative modified Glasgow Prognostic Score (mGPS) was calculated from preoperative serum CRP and albumin (McMillan, 2013).

Cardiopulmonary exercise testing was performed in a single respiratory function laboratory using a ZAN 600 (nSpire Health, Hertford, UK) and Ergoselect bicycle ergometer (Ergoline, Bitz, Germany). A doctor and resuscitation equipment were present during all tests. Several variables were recorded including electrocardiography, blood pressure, oxygen uptake and carbon dioxide output from analysis of inspiratory and expiratory gases. Patients were exposed to an incremental physical exercise protocol to their maximally tolerated level which was determined by exhaustion, symptomatic breathlessness or pain. The measured variables along with the exercise protocol allowed VO_2 at AT and at peak exercise to be quantified.

Statistical analysis

In addition to being analysed as continuous variables, patients were grouped according to the previously described thresholds of VO_2 at AT (< 11 or > 11 ml/min/kg) and at peak exercise (< 19 or > 19 ml/min/kg). Categorical data were compared using the chi-square test or Fisher's exact test where appropriate. Continuous data are presented as median and range and were compared using the Mann-Whitney *U* test or Kruskal-Wallis test in multiple groups. Postoperative CRP concentrations were displayed graphically by postoperative day as median and 95% confidence interval. Correlation between VO_2 at AT and VO_2 at peak exercise and the peak postoperative CRP concentration was assessed using Spearman's correlation coefficients. Statistical analyses were performed using IBM SPSS version 22 for Windows (Chicago, IL, USA).

Results

Patients

Thirty-eight patients completed CPET prior to elective surgery for colorectal cancer at Glasgow Royal Infirmary between 2008 and 2017 (Table 1). The majority were male (30, 79%), over 65 years old (30, 79%), with colonic cancer (23, 61%) and node-negative disease (24, 63%). Fourteen patients (37%) had open surgery and 24 (63%) had a laparoscopic resection. Prior to surgery, 3 patients

Table 1 Patient characteristics and postoperative C-reactive protein levels grouped by VO_2 at the anaerobic threshold and at peak exercise

Characteristic	Cardiopulmonary exercise test variable					
	VO_2 at AT < 11 ml/kg/min (n)	VO_2 at AT > 11 ml/kg/min (n)	*P*	VO_2 at peak < 19 ml/kg/min (n)	VO_2 at peak > 19 ml/kg/min (n)	*P*
Preoperative						
Age (< 65/65–74/> 74)	5/8/11	3/7/4	0.488	4/9/12	4/6/3	0.130
Sex (male/female)	19/5	11/3	1.000	19/6	11/2	0.689
ASA (1/2/3/4)	0/11/12/1	2/8/4/0	0.041	0/10/14/1	2/9/2/0	0.004
BMI (< 20/20–25/36–30/> 30, kg/m²)	1/4/7/12	1/4/5/4	0.206	1/4/7/13	1/4/5/3	0.106
Smoker (never/ex/current)	11/9/4	6/6/2	0.981	10/12/3	10/12/3	0.912
Site (colon/rectum)	16/8	7/7	0.492	17/8	6/7	0.295
TNM stage (I/II/III/IV)	2/12/9/0	3/7/3/1	0.510	3/13/9/0	2/6/3/1	0.969
Preop mGPS (0/1–2)	14/8	11/2	0.259	13/9	12/1	0.036
Neoadjuvant (yes/no)	1/23	2/12	0.542	0/25	3/10	0.034
Intraoperative						
Approach (open/lap)	6/18	8/6	0.081	4/21	10/3	< 0.001
Stoma (yes/no)	10/13	6/8	1.000	11/13	5/8	0.666
Transfusion (yes/no)	1/20	0.10	1.000	1/20	0/10	1.000
Surgery > 4 h (yes/no)	14/10	6/8	0.503	16/9	4/9	0.087
Postoperative						
Any complication (yes/no)	9/15	6/8	1.000	10/15	5/8	1.000
Clavien Dindo grade 3–5(yes/no)	8/16	2/12	0.268	2/23	1/12	1.000
Length of stay (median, range, days)	8 (3–19)	8 (5–15)	0.790	8 (3–15)	9 (5–19)	0.169
POD 3 CRP > 150 mg/l (yes/no)	11/12	8/4	0.476	12/12	7/4	0.493
POD 4 CRP > 150 mg/l (yes/no)	5/12	5/9	0.709	6/13	4/8	0.919

ASA American Society of Anesthesiology, *BMI* body mass index, *AT* anaerobic threshold, *mGPS* modified Glasgow Prognostic Score, *POD* postoperative day, *CRP* C-reactive protein

with locally advanced or margin threatening rectal cancer underwent neoadjuvant chemoradiotherapy (nCRT); there were no cases of pathological complete response.

Complications

Of the 38 patients, 15 (39%) experienced complications (Table 1). No patients died within 30 days of surgery or during the same admission. Of the patients with complications, 10 (26% of all patients) were infective and 5 (13%) were non-infective. When classified using the Clavien Dindo scale, 12 (32% of all patients) were grade 1 to 2 (i.e. required minor intervention) and 3 (8%) were grade 3 to 4 (i.e. necessitated major intervention).

Associations between CPET variables, co-morbidity and mGPS

There was a significant positive correlation ($r_s = 0.628$, $p < 0.001$) between VO_2 at anaerobic threshold (AT) and VO_2 at peak exercise. An increasing burden of co-morbidity as measured by ASA grade (Fig. 1) was significantly associated with progressively lower median VO_2 at peak exercise (ml/kg/min: ASA 1 = 22, ASA 2 = 19, ASA 3 = 15, ASA 4 = 12, $p = 0.014$), but not VO2 at AT ($p = 0.058$).

When VO_2 at AT was compared as a continuous variable amongst patients grouped by preoperative mGPS 0, 1 and 2 (Fig. 2), there was no significant association ($p = 0.147$). When VO_2 at peak exercise was compared as a continuous variable amongst patients groups by mGPS 0, 1 and 2 (Fig. 2), higher mGPS was significantly associated with progressively lower median VO_2 at peak exercise (ml/kg/min: mGPS 0 = 18, mGPS 1 = 16, mGPS 2 = 14, $p = 0.039$).

There was a non-significant linear trend toward greater preoperative systemic inflammation in patients with higher ASA grade ($p = 0.058$).

VO_2 at anaerobic threshold and the postoperative SIR

Fourteen patients (37%) had VO_2 at AT > 11 ml/min/kg and 24 patients (63%) had VO_2 at AT < 11 ml/min/kg (Table 1). When the two groups were compared, there was a significant association between VO_2 at AT and ASA grade ($p = 0.041$). There was no significant association between VO_2 at AT and other preoperative characteristics including patient age, sex, BMI, smoking status, tumour site, TNM stage, preoperative mGPS or neoadjuvant treatment (Table 1).

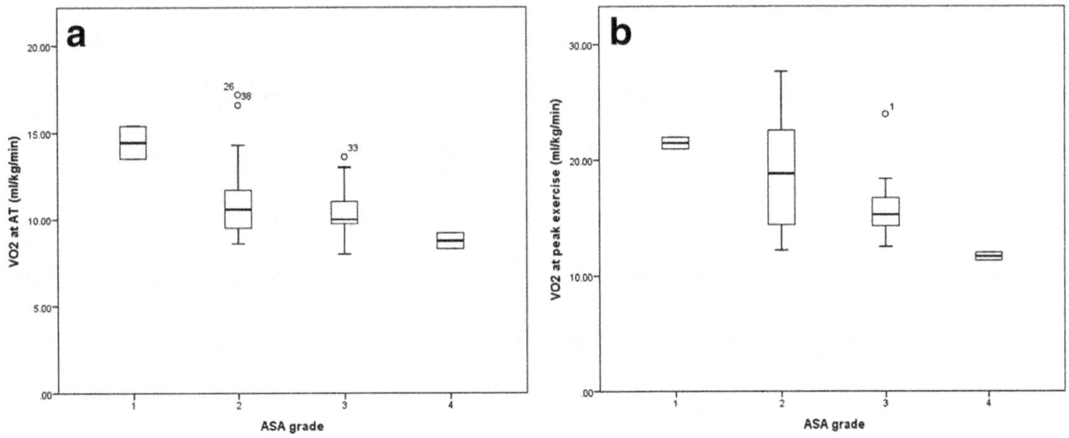

Fig. 1 Boxplots of **a** VO_2 at anaerobic threshold (ml/kg/min) and **b** VO_2 at peak exercise (ml/kg/min) grouped by American Society of Anesthesiology (ASA) grade

There were no significant associations between VO_2 at AT and postoperative complications, established CRP thresholds on postoperative days 3 or 4 (Table 1), or the postoperative CRP trend (Fig. 3). When both VO_2 at AT and peak postoperative CRP (day 4) concentrations were compared as continuous variables, there was no significant correlation ($p = 0.885$).

VO_2 at peak exercise and the postoperative SIR

Thirteen patients (34%) had VO_2 at peak exercise > 19 ml/min/kg and 25 patients (66%) had VO_2 at peak exercise < 19 ml/min/kg (Table 1). When the two groups were compared (Table 1), there was a significant association between VO_2 at peak exercise and ASA ($p = 0.004$). A significantly higher proportion of patients with VO_2 at peak exercise < 19 ml/min/kg had an mGPS of 1–2 (41 vs. 8%, $p = 0.036$). A significantly lower proportion of patients with VO_2 at peak exercise < 19 ml/min/kg underwent nCRT (0 vs. 23%, $p = 0.034$). With regard to intraoperative variables (Table 1), a significantly higher proportion of patients with VO_2 at peak exercise < 19 ml/min/kg underwent laparoscopic surgery (84 vs. 23%, $p < 0.001$).

There was no significant association between VO_2 at peak exercise and postoperative complications, established CRP thresholds on postoperative days 3 or 4 (Table 1), or the postoperative CRP trend (Fig. 3). When VO_2 at peak exercise and peak postoperative CRP (day 3) concentrations were compared as continuous variables, there was no significant correlation ($p = 0.898$).

Discussion

The present pilot study confirms the relationship between CPET-derived measures of exercise tolerance and co-morbidity as measures by ASA grade in patients prior to surgery for colorectal cancer. Moreover, the present

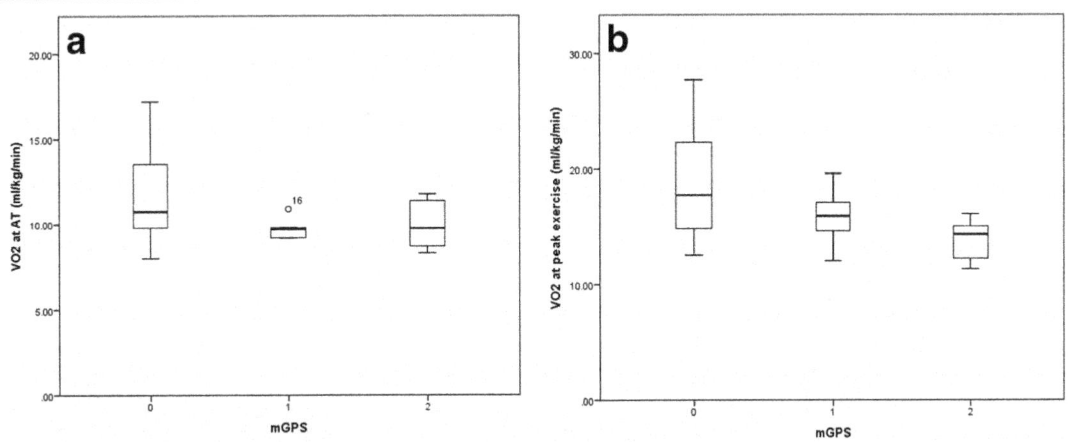

Fig. 2 Boxplots of **a** VO_2 at anaerobic threshold (ml/kg/min) and **b** VO_2 at peak exercise (ml/kg/min) grouped by modified Glasgow Prognostic Score (mGPS)

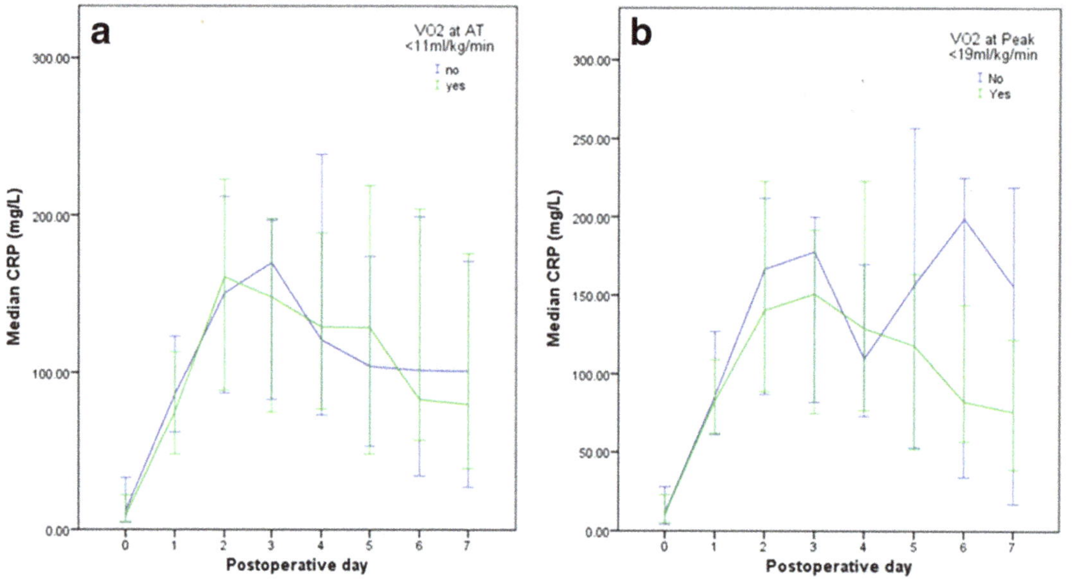

Fig. 3 Median postoperative C-reactive protein (CRP) concentrations (mg/l) in patients grouped by **a** VO_2 at the anaerobic threshold (ml/kg/min) and **b** VO_2 at peak exercise (ml/kg/min)

results show for the first time an inverse relationship between the VO_2 at peak exercise and the preoperative systemic inflammatory response. There was no significant association with the magnitude of the postoperative systemic inflammatory response. However, given the small numbers of patients examined, these relationships warrant further investigation.

The neuroendocrine, metabolic and immune responses to surgical trauma lead to an increase in oxygen requirement from baseline usually supplied by increasing tissue oxygen extraction and cardiac output in the postoperative period, with the aim of increasing oxygen delivery (Shoemaker & Czer, 1979). However, not all patients are able to utilise these mechanisms sufficiently to prevent the accrual of an "oxygen debt", when oxygen delivery is outstripped by tissue oxygen requirement (Waxman et al., 1981). The degree of oxidative stress placed on the patient has been found to be associated with the production of pro-inflammatory cytokines (Rixen & Siegel, 2000). It has been postulated that oxidative stress and resultant tissue hypoxia, especially in the gut, drives a significant proportion of the postoperative systemic inflammatory response (Mainous et al., 1995). Indeed, it is well recognised that tissue hypoxia can lead to activation and augmentation of the innate immune system via hypoxia-inducible factor 1α (HIF-1α) (Peyssonnaux et al., 2005; Nizet & Johnson, 2009). CPET thus uses graded exercise to quantify a given patients' anaerobic threshold and other measures including VO_2 at peak exercise and METs. These CPET variables are associated with postoperative outcomes following abdominal and colorectal surgery (Older et al., 1999; West et al., 2014a; West et al., 2014b).

It was of interest that a significant association was found between VO_2 at peak exercise and the preoperative mGPS at the univariate level. It remains unclear whether this relationship is explained by the association between preoperative systemic inflammation and co-morbid state or other effects. Indeed, the preoperative systemic inflammatory response has previously been shown to be directly associated with preoperative co-morbidity in patients undergoing surgery for colorectal cancer (Richards et al., 2010), and it may be this which links mGPS to reduced peak exercise tolerance. This finding was not confirmed by the results of the present study. However, the trend to association between mGPS and ASA was likely non-significant due to patient numbers. Alternatively, systemic inflammation has a key causal role in the development of the cancer cachexia syndrome, with loss of skeletal muscle quantity and quality, and resultant loss of physical function in patients with cancer (McSorley et al., 2017a). It may be that systemic inflammation exerts its influence on exercise tolerance through this mechanism.

Although previous studies in colorectal surgery have reported an association between patients with VO_2 at AT < 11 ml/min/kg and VO_2 at peak exercise < 19 ml/min/kg and the development of postoperative complications (West et al., 2014a; West et al., 2014b), this was not confirmed in the present study. This is most likely due to the small number of patients in the present study. The magnitude of the postoperative systemic inflammatory response, as evidenced by CRP, is increasingly understood to be associated with the development of postoperative complications following surgery for colorectal cancer (Watt et al., 2017a). These postoperative complications, whether categorised by their type or severity, are associated with poorer long-term oncologic outcomes following surgery for colorectal cancer (McSorley et al., 2016a). Furthermore, studies in surgery for oesophageal, gastric and colorectal cancer suggest that the magnitude of the postoperative systemic inflammatory response is itself a prognostic factor (Matsuda et al., 2015; Saito et al., 2015; McSorley et al., 2016b). Such findings have prompted the investigation of patient and operative factors which influence the postoperative systemic inflammatory response, along with potential methods which might be used to attenuate it, with the aim of reducing postoperative complication rates (Watt et al., 2017b; McSorley et al., 2016c; McSorley et al., 2017b). Indeed, it might be hoped that ongoing studies examining prehabilitation as an intervention to reduce postoperative complication rates may also find an impact on the postoperative systemic inflammatory response.

The main limitation of the present study is the small number of included patients. Preoperative CPET is not routinely used as an evaluation of fitness for colorectal surgery in our unit at present. These small numbers lead to limited ability to make confident statements about the association between CPET, postoperative CRP and complications, and prevented subgroup analysis. Furthermore, the multiple comparisons used in analysis, in the context of the small number of patients, also reduce the confidence in the observed associations or lack thereof.

Conclusions

In conclusion, the present pilot study reports a possible association between preoperative CPET-derived measures of exercise tolerance, and the preoperative systemic inflammatory response in patients undergoing surgery for colorectal cancer. The mGPS may be a surrogate for overall "fitness" in these patients; however, systemic inflammation may well be a causal factor in poor exercise tolerance in this group of patients. No association was found between CPET-derived measures and the magnitude of the postoperative systemic inflammatory response; however, small numbers and the presence of important confounders mean that further work in a larger cohort of patients is warranted.

Abbreviations

AJCC: American Joint Committee on Cancer; ASA: American Society of Anesthesiology; AT: Anaerobic threshold; BMI: Body mass index; CPET/CPX/CPEX: Cardiopulmonary exercise testing; CRP: C-reactive protein; HIF: Hypoxia inducible factor; MET: Metabolic equivalent; mGPS: Modified Glasgow Prognostic Score; nCRT: Neoadjuvant chemoradiotherapy; TNM: Tumour nodes metastasis staging; VO_2: Volume of oxygen consumed

Authors' contributions

STM, CSDR, PGH and DCM are responsible for the study conception and design. STM, CSDR are responsible for the acquisition of data. STM and DCM are responsible for the analysis and interpretation of data. STM, PGH and DCM contributed to the drafting of the manuscript. STM, CSDR, PGH and DCM contributed to the critical revision of the manuscript. All authors read and approved the final manuscript.

Competing interests

The authors declare that they have no competing interests.

References

Cancer Research UK. Bowel cancer statistics. http://www.cancerresearchuk.org/health-professional/cancer-statistics/statistics-by-cancer-type/bowel-cancer. Accessed Aug 2016.

Dindo D, Demartines N, Clavien P. Classification of surgical complications: a new proposal with evaluation in a cohort of 6336 patients and results of a survey. Ann Surg. 2004;240:205–13.

Ghaferi LG, Birkmeyer JD, Dimick JB. Hospital volume and failure to rescue with high-risk surgery. Med Care. 2011;49:1076–81.

Mainous MR, Ertel W, Chaudry IH, et al. The gut: a cytokine-generating organ in systemic inflammation. Shock. 1995;4:193–9.

Matsuda S, Takeuchi H, Kawakubo H, et al. Correlation between intense postoperative inflammatory response and survival of esophageal cancer patients who underwent transthoracic esophagectomy. Ann Surg Oncol. 2015;22(13):4453–60.

McDermott FD, Heeney A, Kelly ME, et al. Systematic review of preoperative, intraoperative and postoperative risk factors for colorectal anastomotic leaks. Br J Surg. 2015;102:462–79.

McMillan DC. The systemic inflammation-based Glasgow Prognostic Score: a decade of experience in patients with cancer. Cancer Treat Rev. 2013;39(5):534–40.

McSorley ST, Black DH, Horgan PG, et al. The relationship between tumour stage, systemic inflammation, body composition and survival in patients with colorectal cancer. Clin Nutr. 2017a. https://doi.org/10.1016/j.clnu.2017.05.017. [Epub ahead of print]

McSorley ST, Horgan PG, McMillan DC. The impact of the type and severity of postoperative complications on long-term outcomes following surgery for colorectal cancer: a systematic review and meta-analysis. Cit Rev Oncol Hematol. 2016a;97:168–77.

McSorley ST, Horgan PG, McMillan DC. The impact of preoperative corticosteroids on the systemic inflammatory response and postoperative complications following surgery for gastrointestinal cancer: a systematic review and meta-analysis. 2016c;101:139–150.

McSorley ST, Ramanathan ML, Horgan PG, et al. Postoperative C-reactive protein measurement predicts the severity of complications following surgery for colorectal cancer. Int J Color Dis. 2015;30(7):913–7.

McSorley ST, Roxburgh CSD, Horgan PG, et al. The impact of preoperative dexamethasone on the magnitude of the postoperative systemic inflammatory response and complications following surgery for colorectal cancer. Ann Surg Oncol. 2017b;24(8):2104–12.

McSorley ST, Watt DG, Horgan PG, et al. Postoperative systemic inflammatory response, complication severity, and survival following surgery for colorectal cancer. Ann Surg Oncol. 2016b;23(9):2832–40.

Moyes LH, McCaffer CJ, Carter RC, et al. Cardiopulmonary exercise testing as a predictor of complications in oesophagogastric cancer surgery. Ann R Coll Surg Engl. 2013;95:125–30.

Nizet V, Johnson RS. Interdependence of hypoxic and innate immune responses. Nat Rev Immunol. 2009;9:609–17.

Older P, Hall A, Hader R. Cardiopulmonary exercise testing as a screening test for perioperative management of major surgery in the elderly. Chest. 1999;116:355–62.

Older P, Smith R, Courtney P, et al. Preoperative evaluation of cardiac failure and ischaemia in elderly patients by cardiopulmonary exercise testing. Chest. 1993;104(3):701–4.

Peyssonnaux C, Datta V, Cramer T. HIF-1 alpha expression regulates the bactericidal activity of phagocytes. J Clin Invest. 2005;115:1806–15.

Platt JJ, Ramanathan ML, Crosbie RA, et al. C-reactive protein as a predictor of postoperative infective complications after curative resection in patients with colorectal cancer. Ann Surg Oncol. 2012;19:4168–77.

Richards CH, Leitch EF, Horgan PG, et al. The relationship between patient physiology, the systemic inflammatory response and survival in patients undergoing curative resection of colorectal cancer. Br J Cancer. 2010;103(9):1356–61.
Rixen D, Siegel JH. Metabolic correlates of oxygen debt predict posttrauma early acute respiratory distress syndrome and the related cytokine response. J Trauma. 2000;49:392–402.
Saito T, Kurokawa Y, Miyazaki Y, et al. Which is a more reliable indicator of survival after gastric cancer surgery: postoperative complication occurrence or C-reactive protein elevation? J Surg Oncol. 2015;112(8):894–9.
Shoemaker WC, Czer LS. Evaluation of the biologic importance of various haemodynamic and oxygen transport variables: which variables should be monitored in postoperative shock? Crit Care Med. 1979;7:424–31.
Smith TB, Stonell C, Purkayastha S, et al. Cardiopulmonary exercise testing as a risk assessment method in non cardiopulmonary surgery: a systematic review. Anaesthesia. 2009;64:883–89365.
Watt DG, Horgan PG, McMillan DC. Routine clinical markers of the magnitude of the systemic inflammatory response after elective operation: a systematic review. Surgery. 2015;157(2):362–80.
Watt DG, McSorley ST, Park JH, et al. A postoperative systemic inflammatory score predicts short- and long-term outcomes in patients undergoing surgery for colorectal cancer. Ann Surg Oncol. 2017a;24(4):1100–9.
Watt DG, Ramanathan ML, McSorley ST, et al. Clinicopathological determinants of an elevated systemic inflammatory response following elective potentially curative resection for colorectal cancer. Ann Surg Oncol. 2017b;24(9):2588–94.
Waxman K, Lazrove S, Shoemaker WC. Physiologic responses to operation in high risk surgical patients. Surg Gynecol Obstet. 1981;152:633–8.
West MA, Lythgoe D, Barben CP, et al. Cardiopulmonary exercise variables are associated with postoperative morbidity after major colonic surgery: a prospective blinded observational study. Br J Anaesthesia. 2014b;112(4):665–71.
West MA, Parry MG, Lythgoe D, et al. Cardiopulmonary exercise testing for the prediction of complications after rectal cancer surgery. Br J Surg. 2014a;101:1166–72.

22

Evaluation of operating room reverse Trendelenburg positioning and its effect on postoperative hypoxemia, aspiration, and length of stay

C. Michael Dunham[1*], Barbara M. Hileman[2], Amy E. Hutchinson[3], Tamara Antonaccio[4], Elisha A. Chance[2], Gregory S. Huang[1], Gregory Szmaj[3], Kristen Calabro[5], Cynthia Bishop[6] and Tyson T. Schrickel[7]

Abstract

Background: In 2014, this group published an investigation of surgical patients from 2012 who had substantial rates of postoperative hypoxemia (POH) and perioperative pulmonary aspiration (POPA). Therefore, we investigated whether intraoperative reverse Trendelenburg positioning (RTP) decreases POH and POPA rates.

Methods: Consecutive ASA I–IV surgical patients who had preoperative pulmonary stability requiring general anesthesia with endotracheal intubation were evaluated. Using pulse oximetry, hypoxemia was documented intraoperatively and during the 48 h following PACU discharge. POPA was the presence of a pulmonary infiltrate with hypoxemia. In early 2015, a multifaceted effort was undertaken to enhance anesthesiologist and operating nurse awareness of RTP to potentially decrease POH and POPA rates. Analyses included (1) combining 2012 and 2015 cohorts to assess risk conditions, (2) comparing post-campaign 2015 (increased RTP) and 2012 cohorts, and (3) comparing 2015 patients with audit-documented RTP during surgery to the other 2015 patients.

Results: Combining the 500 patients in 2012 with the 1000 in 2015 showed that POH had increased mortality (2.3%), compared to no POH (0.2%; $p = 0.0004$). POH had increased postoperative length of stay (LOS) (4.6 days), compared to no POH (2.0 days; $p < 0.0001$). POPA had increased mortality (7.7%) and LOS (8.8 days), compared to no POPA (0.4%; $p = 0.0004$; 2.3 days; $p < 0.0001$). Open aortic, cranial, laparotomy, and neck procedures had greater POH (41.3%) and LOS (4.0 days), compared to other procedures (16.3%; $p < 0.0001$; 2.2 days; $p < 0.0001$). Glycopyrrolate on induction had lower POH (17.4%) and LOS (1.9 days), compared to no glycopyrrolate (21.6%; $p = 0.0849$; 2.7 days; $p < 0.0001$). POH was lower (18.1%) in 2015, than in 2012 (25.6%; $p = 0.0007$). POPA was lower with RTP in 2015 (0.6%), than in 2012 (4.8%; $p = 0.0088$). For the 2015 patients, LOS was lower with audit-documented RTP (2.2 days), compared to other patients (2.7 days; $p = 0.0246$).

Conclusions: These findings are only hypothesis-generating. A randomized clinical trial is needed to confirm whether RTP has an inverse association with POH and POPA, and if RTP and glycopyrrolate are associated with improved outcomes.

Keywords: Aspiration, respiratory, Hypoxemia, Period, perioperative, Operating rooms, Supine position, Reverse Trendelenburg

* Correspondence: dunham.michael@sbcglobal.net
[1]Trauma, Critical Care, and General Surgery Services, St. Elizabeth Youngstown Hospital, 1044 Belmont Ave., Youngstown, OH 44501, USA
Full list of author information is available at the end of the article

Background

In 2014, our group published an investigation of patients who underwent extra-thoracic procedures under general anesthesia and had preoperative pulmonary stability (Dunham et al. 2014). We provided evidence to suggest that the substantial rates of perioperative hypoxemia and perioperative pulmonary aspiration (POPA) may have been related to horizontal recumbency.

It has been established that POPA can lead to death (Cotton and Smith 1984; Morgan 1984; Tiret et al. 1986; Kozlow et al. 2003) and may cause clinically significant morbidities (Cotton and Smith 1984; Kozlow et al. 2003; Kluger and Short 1999). Of importance, there are findings from operating room (OR), intensive care unit, and animal investigations demonstrating that aspiration can occur despite the presence of a cuffed endotracheal tube (Ewig and Torres 2002; Torres et al. 1992; Reali-Forster et al. 1996; Petring et al. 1986; Seegobin and van Hasselt 1986; Kalinowski and Kirsch 2004). Further, clinical evidence demonstrates that horizontal positioning in mechanically ventilated patients is a risk for pulmonary aspiration with lung inflammation (Kalinowski and Kirsch 2004; Smith and Ng 2003) and ventilator-associated pneumonia (Ewig and Torres 2002; Torres et al. 1992; Ferrer and Artigas 2002; Keenan et al. 2002; Koeman et al. 2001; Fernandez-Crehuet et al. 1997; Drakulovic et al. 1999; Kollef 1993). Accordingly, the Institute for Healthcare Improvement recommends elevating the head of the bed during intensive care unit mechanical ventilation to prevent pulmonary aspiration and ventilator-associated pneumonia (Institute for Healthcare Improvement 2012).

Of relevance, previous literature indicates that patients undergoing general endotracheal anesthesia for a surgical procedure are primarily placed in a supine, lithotomy, lateral, or prone position (Blitt et al. 1970; McEwen 1996; Adedeji et al. 2010), where horizontal recumbency is typically enforced (McEwen 1996; Adedeji et al. 2010; Smith 1990). Horizontal recumbency for typical operative body positions is promulgated within the operative nursing literature and teaching circles as common practice (McEwen 1996; Adedeji et al. 2010; Smith 1990). Specifically, horizontal positioning is disseminated by the use of specific narrative description statements (McEwen 1996; Adedeji et al. 2010) and inclusion of illustrations and photographs (McEwen 1996; Smith 1990; Mulier et al. 2010) that portray horizontal recumbency. Four review publications about POPA were evaluated for comments regarding body positioning. The most current review only included a single comment regarding body positioning (Abdulla 2013) and another did not mention body positioning (Engelhardt and Webster 1999). Ng et al. indicated that the Trendelenburg position is a risk for POPA, and lithotomy positioning may be a risk for POPA (Ng and Smith 2001). The greatest attention to body position as a risk for POPA was in a review by Kalinowski et al. in 2004 (Kalinowski and Kirsch 2004). The authors stated that aspiration is common in patients with impaired consciousness in the supine position, and with successful tracheal intubation, pulmonary aspiration seems less frequent if the patient's head is elevated 45° (Kalinowski and Kirsch 2004). When considering reported evidence for the risks for POPA, horizontal recumbency, as a common practice, is counterintuitive.

In a previous work, we reported that the perioperative hypoxemia rate was substantial in all operative procedure categories (Dunham et al. 2014). Although the primary body position during the operative procedure was supine or lithotomy, the standard anesthesia practice was to maintain horizontal recumbency in all patients, except for a few in the sitting position. The previous study findings and literature documentation were consistent with the notion that perioperative hypoxemia, in part, may be a manifestation of occult-pulmonary or micro-pulmonary aspiration during horizontal recumbency.

In response to the earlier study findings and considerations from relevant literature, the primary purpose of the current study was to investigate whether reverse Trendelenburg positioning (RTP) during general anesthesia may have an inverse association with postoperative hypoxemia (POH) and POPA. Specifically, the study institution implemented an endeavor in 2015 to increase RTP awareness as a practice that may be beneficial. The authors compared 500 consecutive surgical patients from the previous investigation in 2012 (with decreased RTP awareness) to a cohort of 1000 consecutive surgical patients in 2015 (with improved RTP awareness). It was hypothesized that RTP would be associated with lower POH and POPA rates.

Methods

The analyses included two cohorts: patients who met the inclusion criteria in 2012 and patients who met the same inclusion criteria in 2015 following OR nursing and anesthesiology staff RTP awareness training. The primary goal was to compare patients in 2012 (with decreased RTP awareness) to patients in 2015 (with improved RTP awareness). The secondary goal was to combine the patient cohorts in 2012 and 2015 and describe clinical associations with mortality, POH, POPA, and length of stay (LOS).

The present study was approved by the Mercy Health Youngstown Institutional Review Board for human investigations (15–023 approved July 16, 2015). The need for written informed consent was waived, because of the study's retrospective nature. Patients' records and information were anonymized and de-identified before analysis.

Inclusion criteria

Inclusion criteria were patients aged 18 years or older, those who had preoperative pulmonary stability, and patients who underwent an operative procedure that required endotracheal intubation and a general anesthetic. Preoperative pulmonary stability criteria included a respiratory rate of 12–24 breaths per minute, and either an oxygen saturation measure by pulse oximetry (SpO_2) ≥ 94% with room air or nasal cannula oxygen with a flow rate of 1 to 2 L/min or partial pressure of oxygen/inspired oxygen (PaO_2/FiO_2) ≥ 300, if greater supplemental oxygen was received. Patients were identified through the surgery case log, and data were collected from the electronic medical record (EMR).

Exclusion criteria

Exclusion criteria were tracheal intubation before emergency department arrival, endotracheal intubation > 24 h before surgery, thoracotomy procedure, any cardiac procedure, Glasgow Coma Scale score < 13, an American Society of Anesthesiologists (ASA) classification V or VI, and patients with more than one surgery requiring tracheal intubation during the same hospitalization.

Preoperative and intraoperative variables

Preoperative variables were age, ASA classification, emergency versus elective procedures, preexisting lung disease (PELD), and weight. PELD was considered present when a patient required any of the following respiratory therapies on a daily basis: home bi-level positive airway pressure, supplemental oxygen, an inhalational bronchodilator, or systemic bronchodilator or steroid. This information was ascertained by reviewing the anesthesia preoperative assessment note and the history and physical examination documented in each patient's EMR. Intraoperative variables were OR duration (OR minutes), operative procedure categories, glycopyrrolate administration during anesthesia induction, and amount of fluid input. These data were gathered from the anesthesia intraoperative record, which had been hand written and scanned into the electronic medical record.

Hypoxemia classification

As perioperative pulse oximetry monitoring is routine at our institution, we used intraoperative hypoxemia (IOH) and/or POH as a potential indicator of POPA. A co-investigator examined each patient's anesthesia operative record and documented the presence of intraoperative SpO_2 < 98%. A co-investigator also screened the EMR for evidence of POH. A positive POH screen was defined as two or more episodes of SpO_2 < 94%, on room air or nasal cannula supplemental oxygen at 1–2 L/min, or SpO_2 < 98% with greater supplemental oxygen within a 24-h period, during the 48 h following surgery. SpO_2 < 94% during the first 2 h following OR extubation was not counted as a POH event, as hypoventilation may be related to post-anesthesia recovery. The first author, a retired board-certified surgical intensivist, reviewed each patient's data whenever a patient had IOH and/or a positive POH screen. FiO_2 was typically 60–100%. Whenever the intraoperative SpO_2 was clearly < 98% and the intraoperative FiO_2 was subsequently increased, the patient was classified as having an episode of IOH. When the postoperative SpO_2 had decreased by ≥ 5% compared to the preoperative value, the patient was categorized as having an episode of POH.

There was no automated SpO_2 data inflow into the electronic medical record (neither in the OR nor outside the OR). Within the OR, any decrement in SpO_2 prompted an investigation that the pulse oximetry probe had proper patient contact. Outside the OR, SpO_2 probe contact was confirmed by the nurse or respiratory therapist and directly entered into the electronic medical record by the nurse or respiratory therapist.

POPA classification

POPA was defined as the presence of an IOH or POH event and an acute pulmonary infiltrate on thoracic radiographic imaging (chest radiograph or computed tomography scan) within the 48-h period following surgery. The first author examined each chest radiographic image available in the EMR in patients categorized with IOH or POH, for a pulmonary infiltrate. When the first author's findings of an infiltrate were corroborated by the radiologist's report, the patient was classified as POPA-positive.

Selection of the RTP target

In early 2015, a literature search for RTP intervention studies identified 18 publications. Of these studies, seven (39%) used an RTP target of 10°, whereas the other studies had five other RTP target levels (5–30°), with a frequency of ≤ 17% each. Following this literature review, the first author and directors of OR nursing and anesthesiology assembled in the OR. The first author was positioned on the OR table, and RTP was adjusted to a level where the chief of anesthesiology believed that the risk for pulmonary aspiration would likely be mitigated. The OR table angle was 8.3°, as measured using a digital protractor (model 320.48295; Craftsman® Digital Torpedo Level, Hoffman Estates, IL). On the basis of this experience and the literature review, we selected a 10° tilt as the RTP target.

Enhancing staff RTP awareness

In early 2015, the director of surgical and perioperative services, the manager and assistant manager of the OR nursing staff, and the chief of anesthesiology endorsed the view that RTP may mitigate POH and POPA. Their support was based on an appraisal of our publication findings from 2014, a review of the relevant literature, and the recommendation by the Institute for Healthcare Improvement.

In early April 2015, formal educational presentations regarding OR RTP were provided to the OR nursing staff, attending anesthesiologists and certified registered nurse anesthetists, general surgical attendings and residents, and orthopedic surgical attendings and residents. The presentations included (1) a literature review demonstrating that aspiration occurs despite the use of cuffed endotracheal tubes, (2) a literature review showing that horizontal positioning is associated with pulmonary aspiration in mechanically ventilated patients, (3) the Institute for Healthcare Improvement recommendation, (4) a review of our study published in 2014 regarding perioperative hypoxemia and aspiration, and (5) pictorials illustrating 10° RTP using a commercial OR table protractor. Additionally, discussions regarding RTP pros and cons took place between the first author and chief of neurosurgery, chief of gynecological surgery, and a senior urologist.

OR RTP was implemented on April 6, 2015. The reinforcement of RTP awareness included daily OR nursing staff rounds, the implementation of OR nursing staff RTP audits, bi-monthly anesthesia staff meetings, and the availability of table protractors (750 Pitch and Slope Locator; Johnson Level & Tool Mfg. Co., Inc., Mequon, WI) for each OR. The principal recommendation for the OR nursing staff was that RTP should be used when clinically reasonable and technically feasible. The primary recommendations made during discussions with the anesthesia staff were that RTP should be used when clinically reasonable and technically feasible, during tracheal intubation, tracheal extubation, and the operative procedure. The OR nursing staff RTP audits were noncompulsory, performed daily, and they indicated the patient's position during the operative procedure: (a) persistent RTP, (b) intermittent RTP, or (c) no RTP. The OR nurse completed the audit form at the end of the surgical procedure. A designated general surgical resident, an orthopedic attending surgeon, and a certified registered nurse anesthetist agreed to foster RTP awareness among their peers. Signs were placed outside of each OR as a reminder that RTP may reduce POH.

RTP surveys

In early 2016 before the study results were released, the OR nursing and anesthesiology staff were given a survey regarding RTP in the OR. The purpose of the survey was to determine the degree to which the staff embraced the notion of RTP. Two statements were included in the OR nursing staff survey: "an intraoperative reverse Trendelenburg position may decrease the risk for postoperative hypoxemia" and "I am inclined to use a reverse Trendelenburg position during the operative procedure when clinically and technically feasible." Four statements were included in the anesthesiology staff survey: "an intraoperative reverse Trendelenburg position may decrease the risk for postoperative hypoxemia"; "I am inclined to use a reverse Trendelenburg position during tracheal intubation when clinically and technically feasible"; "I am inclined to use a reverse Trendelenburg position during the operative procedure when clinically and technically feasible"; and "I am inclined to use a reverse Trendelenburg position during tracheal extubation when clinically and technically feasible." Each statement was followed by Likert scale response options: strongly agree, agree, uncertain, disagree, and strongly disagree.

Cohort analysis organization

Patients from 2012 to 2015 were combined to determine conditions that were associated with mortality, POH, POPA, and the postoperative LOS. Comparisons between 2012 and 2015 represented periods where RTP awareness was negligible or improved, respectively. Relative to the 2012 cohort, the 2015 cohort was also consecutively obtained, with the same inclusion and exclusion criteria. Some inter-group analyses were performed, based on the 2015 OR nursing staff RTP audits that classified patients who had RTP during the operative procedure.

Statistical analysis

Data were entered into a Microsoft Excel® 2010 spreadsheet (Microsoft Corp., Redmond, WA) and imported into SAS System for Windows, release 9.2 (SAS Institute Inc., Cary, NC), for statistical analyses. For the continuous variable cohort data, mean and standard deviation was used. Pearson correlation analysis was performed to assess associations between two continuous variables. The Wilcoxon rank-sum test was used to compare continuous data between two groups. Analysis of variance was applied to compare continuous data involving more than two groups. The Fischer's exact test was used to assess the relationship between two dichotomous variables. Multivariate logistic regression analysis was performed to assess the relationship between a dependent variable that was dichotomous and potential independent variables. Multivariate linear regression analysis was performed to evaluate independent variable relationships with a dependent, continuous variable. The level of significance was considered $p < 0.05$.

Results

Patients

Among patients aged 18 years or older who had an operative procedure that required endotracheal intubation and a general anesthetic, Glasgow Coma Scale score ≥ 13, and ASA classification I–IV and who did not require tracheal intubation before emergency department arrival, endotracheal intubation > 24 h before surgery, thoracotomy procedure, any cardiac procedure, or more than one surgery requiring tracheal intubation during the same hospitalization, the rates of preoperative pulmonary instability were 6.0% (32/532) for the 2012 patient cohort and 9.1% (100/1100) for the 2015 cohort ($p = 0.0332$). From May 14, 2012, through July 13, 2012, 500 consecutive surgical patients were included in the original published study. The most recent consecutive cohort included 1000 patients who had undergone an operative intervention from May 13, 2015, through September 20, 2015.

OR personnel surveys

The OR nursing staff survey was conducted in early June 2016, and it included 41 participants. The anesthesiology staff survey was performed in June 2016, and it included 44 anesthesiologists, certified registered nurse anesthetist staff, and student certified registered nurse anesthetist personnel. Responses to the survey statements indicate that the majority strongly agreed or agreed with the notion that RTP may be useful (Table 1).

Noncompulsory RTP audits

The OR nursing staff submitted 387 RTP audit forms throughout the period during which the 1000 patients in 2015 underwent an operation. The RTP audit process had been operational for several weeks before the study phase. See LOS associations (within 2015 comparison) for results.

Mortality associations (combined 2012 and 2015)

From the combined 2012 and 2015 patient cohorts, the mortality rate was 0.6% (9/1500). Hypothesis-generating associations regarding mortality are depicted in Table 2. Compared to non-dying patients, dying patients had increased POH and POPA, older age, higher ASA classification, and a higher rate of emergency operations.

Table 1 Operating room personnel surveys

	Strongly agree or agree	Uncertain	Disagree or strongly disagree
Nursing staff (*n* = 41)			
RTP may decrease POH	34 (82.9%)		7 (17.1%)
Inclined to use RTP	33 (80.5%)		8 (19.5%)
Anesthesiology staff (*n* = 44)			
RTP may decrease POH	41 (93.2%)	1 (2.3%)	2 (4.5%)
Use RTP during tracheal intubation	41 (93.2%)	1 (2.3%)	2 (4.5%)
Use RTP during the operative procedure	39 (88.6%)	1 (2.3%)	4 (9.1%)
Use RTP during tracheal extubation	39 (88.6%)		5 (11.4%)

RTP reverse Trendelenburg, *POH* postoperative hypoxemia

Table 2 Mortality associations

	Lived	Died	*p* value
Patients	1491 (99.4%)	9 (0.6%)	
Adverse outcomes			
Postoperative hypoxemia	302 (20.3%)	7 (77.8%)	0.0004
Perioperative aspiration	48 (3.2%)	4 (44.4%)	< 0.0001
Postoperative length of stay (days)	2.5 ± 3.4	5.1 ± 5.7	0.2099
Preoperative risk			
Age	56 ± 17	75 ± 14	0.0016
ASA classification	2.8 ± 0.6	3.2 ± 0.7	0.0464
Emergency procedures	120 (8.1%)	3 (33.3%)	0.0058
Preexisting lung disease	221 (14.8%)	1 (11.1%)	0.7546
Weight (kg)	86 ± 24	80 ± 22	0.4037
Intraoperative risk			
Operating room minutes	128 ± 74	149 ± 69	0.3972
Glycopyrrolate on induction	366 (24.6%)	1 (11.1%)	0.3499
Fluid input (L)	1.6 ± 1.0	2.2 ± 2.0	0.3964

ASA American Society of Anesthesiologists

POH associations (combined 2012 and 2015)

From the combined 2012 and 2015 patient cohorts, the POH rate was 20.6% (309/1500). Hypothesis-generating associations regarding POH are shown in Table 3. Compared to patients without POH, those with POH had increased mortality and LOS, older age, higher ASA classification, higher rate of emergency operations and PELD, higher weight, longer time in the OR, and they received less glycopyrrolate and more fluids. POH rates, according to the surgical procedure category, are

Table 3 Postoperative hypoxemia (POH) associations

	POH (No)	POH (Yes)	*p* value
Patients	1191 (79.4%)	309 (20.6%)	
Adverse outcomes			
Mortality	2 (0.2%)	7 (2.3%)	0.0004
Postoperative length of stay (days)	2.0 ± 2.6	4.6 ± 4.8	< 0.0001
Preoperative risk			
Age	55 ± 18	63 ± 15	< 0.0001
ASA classification	2.8 ± 0.6	3.1 ± 0.5	< 0.0001
ASA classification 3 or 4	857 (72.0%)	273 (88.4%)	< 0.0001
Emergency procedures	88 (7.4%)	35 (11.3%)	0.0246
Preexisting lung disease	160 (13.4%)	62 (20.1%)	0.0034
Weight (kg)	86 ± 24	89 ± 23	0.0489
Intraoperative risk			
Operating room minutes	122 ± 68	154 ± 90	< 0.0001
Glycopyrrolate on induction	303 (25.4%)	64 (20.7%)	0.0849
Fluid input (L)	1.5 ± 0.9	2.0 ± 1.5	< 0.0001

ASA American Society of Anesthesiologists

depicted in Table 4. Open aortic, cranial, laparotomy, and non-spinal neck procedures had the highest POH rates, and together they define a high-risk POH group. The POH rate was greater for the POH high-risk group (41.3% [107/259]) than for the lower-risk cohort (16.3% [202/1241]; $p < 0.0001$; relative risk 2.5).

POH associations (2012 versus 2015)

A comparison of the 2012 and 2015 patient cohorts is shown in Table 5, and it demonstrates a reduction in 2015 POH. Compared to the 2012 patient cohort, the 2015 patient cohort had a lower POH rate, higher age and ASA classification, and they received less fluid. Results of the multivariate logistic regression analysis of the 1500 patients inferred that POH was likely simultaneously (independently) increased with greater time in the OR ($p < 0.0001$), age ($p < 0.0001$), ASA classification ($p < 0.0001$), and weight ($p = 0.0078$), and decreased for the year 2015 ($p < 0.0001$), and might be decreased with glycopyrrolate administration ($p = 0.0756$). A model equation was created, using the 2012 logistic regression maximum likelihood estimates to predict the POH rate. Using age 54 and ASA classification 2.8 (2012), the POH rate was predicted to be 23.9%, whereas applying age 57 and ASA classification 2.9 (2015), the predicted POH rate was 25.8%. The difference in the POH rate between 2012 and 2015 was 7.5% (25.6% [–] 18.1%). The relative risk reduction in POH with increased RTP sensitivity (2015) was 29.3% (7.5%/25.6%).

POPA associations (combined 2012 and 2015)

From the combined 2012 and 2015 patient cohorts, the POPA rate was 3.5% (52/1500). Hypothesis-generating associations regarding POPA are depicted in Table 6.

Table 4 POH and POPA rates according to the surgical procedural categories

Procedure	Total	POH	POPA	LOS
Open aortic	17	58.8%	29.4%	3.9
Cranial	55	41.8%	5.5%	4.9
Laparotomy	110	40.9%	11.8%	5.2
Neck	77	37.7%	2.6%	1.6
Spine	285	19.3%	3.5%	2.6
Extremity/pelvis	387	19.1%	2.1%	3.3
Laparoscopy	275	16.0%	2.9%	1.5
Miscellaneous	126	15.9%	1.6%	1.7
Face soft tissue	21	9.5%	0%	1.0
Breast	76	5.5%	0%	0.3
Oral	71	4.2%	1.4%	0.4
	1500	Mean = 20.6%	Mean = 3.5%	Mean = 2.5 days

POH postoperative hypoxemia, *POPA* perioperative pulmonary aspiration, *LOS* postoperative length of stay

Table 5 Comparison of postoperative hypoxemia rates for the 2012 and 2015 patient cohorts

	2012	2015	*p* value
Patients	500	1000	
Postoperative hypoxemia	128 (25.6%)	181 (18.1%)	0.0007
Preoperative risk			
Age	54 ± 17	57 ± 17	0.0021
Age ≥ 75 years	62 (12.4%)	186 (18.6%)	0.0023
ASA classification	2.8 ± 0.7	2.9 ± 0.6	0.0323
ASA classification 3 or 4	359 (71.8%)	771 (77.1%)	0.0248
Emergency procedures	36 (7.2%)	87 (8.7%)	0.3182
Preexisting lung disease	69 (13.8%)	153 (15.3%)	0.4406
Weight (kg)	86 ± 24	86 ± 24	0.9357
Intraoperative risk			
Operating room minutes	129 ± 77	128 ± 73	0.8031
Glycopyrrolate on induction	119 (23.8%)	248 (24.8%)	0.6711
Fluid input (L)	1.8 ± 1.2	1.5 ± 1.0	0.0001

ASA American Society of Anesthesiologists

Compared to patients without POPA, those with POPA had an increased mortality and LOS, older age, higher ASA classification, rate of emergencies, and PELD, and longer time in the OR and they received more fluids.

Open aortic, cranial, and laparotomy procedures had the highest POPA rates and together they define a high-risk POPA group (Table 4). The POPA rate was greater for the POPA high-risk group (11.5% [21/182]) than for

Table 6 Perioperative pulmonary aspiration (POPA) associations

	POPA (No)	POPA (Yes)	*p* value
Patients	1448 (96.5%)	52 (3.5%) 95% CI: 2.7–4.5%	
Adverse outcomes			
Mortality	5 (0.4%)	4 (7.7%)	0.0004
Postoperative length of stay (days)	2.3 ± 3.0	8.8 ± 6.7	< 0.0001
Preoperative risk			
Age	60 ± 17	64 ± 18	0.0012
Age ≥ 75 years	230 (15.9%)	18 (34.6%)	0.0004
ASA classification	2.8 ± 0.6	3.1 ± 0.6	0.0004
ASA classification 3 or 4	1084 (74.9%)	46 (88.5%)	0.0254
Emergency procedures	113 (7.8%)	10 (19.2%)	0.0032
Preexisting lung disease	210 (14.5%)	12 (23.1%)	0.0871
Weight (kg)	86 ± 24	82 ± 24	0.1397
Intraoperative risk			
Operating room minutes	126 ± 71	190 ± 114	0.0002
Glycopyrrolate on induction	354 (24.5%)	13 (25.0%)	0.9274
Fluid input (L)	1.6 ± 0.9	2.9 ± 2.4	0.0003

ASA American Society of Anesthesiologists, *CI* confidence interval

the lower-risk cohort (2.4% [31/1318]; $p < 0.0001$; relative risk 4.8).

POPA associations (2012 versus 2015)

The POPA rate was lower for the 2015 patient cohort (2.8% [28/1000]) than for the 2012 patient cohort (4.8% [24/500]; $p = 0.0459$). Of 28 patients with POPA in 2015, 26 had POH and the other 2 had intraoperative hypoxemia. Of 24 patients with POPA in 2012, 20 had POH and the other 4 had intraoperative hypoxemia. Of 283 patients with IOH or POH in 2015, 81 (28.6%) underwent thoracic imaging, whereas of 150 patients with IOH or POH in 2012, 50 (33.3%) underwent thoracic imaging ($p = 0.3098$). Results of multivariate logistic regression analysis suggested that POPA was simultaneously (independently) increased with greater time in the OR ($p < 0.0001$), higher age ($p = 0.0088$), and emergency procedures ($p = 0.0001$), and decreased with the year 2015 ($p = 0.0171$), and possibly increased with higher ASA classification ($p = 0.0623$).

A comparison of the 2015 patient cohort (documented to be in RTP throughout all or a portion of the operative procedure) and 2012 cohort (decreased RTP) is depicted in Table 7. The two groups are reasonably well matched for preoperative and intraoperative risk criteria. However, the operative procedure RTP group had a substantial reduction of POPA. Findings of multivariate logistic regression analysis implied that POPA was likely simultaneously (independently) increased with emergency procedures ($p = 0.0452$) and PELD ($p = 0.0289$) and decreased with documented operative procedure RTP in 2015 ($p = 0.0290$).

Table 7 Perioperative aspiration comparison of 2015 cohort with documented procedure RTP to 2012 cohort

	RTP (↓) (2012)	RTP (Yes) (2015)	*p* value
Total	500 (74.1%)	175 (25.9%)	
Perioperative aspiration	24 (4.8%)	1 (0.6%)	0.0088
Preoperative risk			
Age	54 ± 17	56 ± 17	0.2310
ASA classification	2.8 ± 0.6	2.9 ± 0.6	0.822
Emergency procedures	36 (7.2%)	5 (2.9%)	0.0384
Preexisting lung disease	69 (13.8%)	41 (23.4%)	0.0030
Weight (kg)	86 ± 24	89 ± 23	0.1571
Intraoperative risk			
Operating room minutes	129 ± 77	126 ± 61	0.5225
Glycopyrrolate on induction	119 (23.8%)	48 (27.4%)	0.3384
Fluid input (L)	1.8 ± 1.2	1.6 ± 0.9	0.0184

RTP reverse Trendelenburg, ↓ decreased RTP, *Yes* RTP throughout or a portion of the operative procedure, *ASA* American Society of Anesthesiologists

LOS associations (combined 2012 and 2015)

From the combined 2012 and 2015 patient cohorts, the mean LOS was 2.5 ± 3.4 days (range 0–37 days). Of 1500 patients, 76.6% ($n = 1149$) were discharged by the third postoperative day. Hypothesis-generating associations regarding LOS are depicted in Table 8. The data inferred that an increased LOS was likely related to POH, POPA, time in the OR, age, ASA classification, emergency status, fluid input, and POH high-risk procedures (i.e., open aortic, cranial, laparotomy, and non-spinal neck procedures). The data suggested that a decreased LOS was associated with glycopyrrolate administration upon induction.

LOS associations (2012 versus 2015)

Despite the decreased POH rate for 2015, the LOS for 2015 (2.6 ± 3.4 days) was similar to that in 2012 (2.3 ± 3.3 days; $p = 0.0714$). Results of multivariate linear regression analysis (combined 2012 and 2015 cohorts) implied that LOS was likely to be simultaneously (independently) increased with increasing age ($p < 0.0001$) and ASA classification ($p < 0.0001$), but it was not different according to the year ($p = 0.2737$).

Table 8 Postoperative length of stay (LOS) associations

	LOS (days)	*R* value	*p* value
POH, no	2.0 ± 2.6		
POH, yes	4.6 ± 7.8		< 0.0001
Perioperative aspiration, no	2.3 ± 3.0		
Perioperative aspiration, yes	8.8 ± 6.7		< 0.0001
Time in operating room		(+) 0.25	< 0.0001
< 150 min	2.1 ± 3.1		
≥ 150 min	3.5 ± 3.7		< 0.0001
Age		(+) 0.20	< 0.0001
< 75 years	2.3 ± 3.1		
≥ 75 years	3.6 ± 4.5		< 0.0001
ASA classification		(+) 0.20	< 0.0001
1 or 2	1.6 ± 2.1		
3 or 4	2.8 ± 3.6		< 0.0001
Elective procedures	2.3 ± 3.2		
Emergency procedures	4.6 ± 4.6		< 0.0001
Glycopyrrolate on induction, no	2.7 ± 3.6		
Glycopyrrolate on induction, yes	1.9 ± 2.3		< 0.0001
Fluid input (L)		(+) 0.25	< 0.0001
< 2.0 L	2.1 ± 3.1		
≥ 2.0 L	3.6 ± 3.8		< 0.0001
POH high risk, no	2.2 ± 3.0		
POH high risk, yes	4.0 ± 4.4		< 0.0001

ASA American Society of Anesthesiologists, *POH* postoperative hypoxemia, *high risk*, open aortic, cranial, laparotomy, and non-spinal neck operative procedures

LOS associations (within 2015 comparison)

The 2015 audit patient categorizations were no RTP, 212 (21.2%) patients; RTP throughout the operative procedure, 64 (6.4%); RTP during a portion of the operative procedure, 111 (11.1%); and no audit, 613 (61.3%). The durations of LOS (days) by patient categorization were no RTP, 2.4 ± 2.8; RTP throughout the operative procedure, 1.8 ± 2.6; RTP during a portion of the operative procedure, 2.4 ± 3.0; and no audit, 2.8 ± 3.7 ($p = 0.0533$).

The four subsets were reorganized into two groups: RTP–Yes (RTP throughout or a portion of the operative procedure) and RTP–No (no RTP or no audit) (Table 9). The RTP–Yes group had fewer emergency procedures but a greater weight and more instances of PELD than the RTP–No group. Findings of univariate analysis suggested that compared to the RTP–No group, the RTP–Yes group had a reduction in postoperative LOS. Results of multivariate linear regression analysis inferred that LOS was likely to simultaneously (independently) increase with the ASA classification ($p < 0.0001$) and decrease with glycopyrrolate administration ($p = 0.0002$) and operative procedure RTP ($p = 0.0399$).

Discussion

Evidence for increased RTP during 2015

Before and during the study period, multiple processes were implemented to foster the use of RTP. The director of surgical and perioperative services, manager and assistant manager of the OR nursing staff, and chief of anesthesiology endorsed the notion that RTP may be beneficial for patients undergoing general anesthesia. Multiple in-service activities were conducted for the OR nursing and anesthesiology staff to encourage the use of RTP, when clinically and technically feasible. Additionally, we gave presentations to and had discussions with surgeons of multiple disciplines regarding the potential benefit of RTP. Daily OR nursing staff rounds were performed to reinforce the use of RTP during the operative procedure. OR table protractors were made available for each room to facilitate RTP and prompt the use of RTP. Signs were placed outside of each OR, as a reminder that RTP may reduce POH. Daily audits served to remind the OR nursing staff to use RTP.

According to the survey results taken before the study results were released, substantial evidence exists that the OR nursing and anesthesiology staff embraced the notion that RTP may be important. Numerous discussions between the OR nurse manager and assistant manager with OR nursing staff typically indicated an understanding by the staff that RTP may be of value. These conversations were supported by the OR nursing staff survey. Several dialogs between the chief of anesthesiology and the anesthesia staff usually indicated an understanding that RTP may be of value. These responses are shown in the anesthesiology staff survey results.

The OR nursing staff audits specifically document the use of RTP during 2015. Similarly, the OR nurse manager and assistant manager observed the use of RTP on numerous occasions during their OR rounds and throughout the day. The managers confirmed that RTP was more commonly used in 2015 than in 2012. The chief of anesthesiology found that RTP during the OR procedure was common, and it was typical for tracheal intubation and extubation. She has an unequivocal sense that RTP was more frequently used in 2015 than in 2012. Importantly, the POH rate in 2015 was substantially decreased, despite the higher ASA classification and age. The increased use of RTP offers a plausible explanation for decreased POH and POPA rates in 2015. On the basis of the aforementioned findings, we conclude that RTP is associated with improved perioperative outcomes. The 2015 audit, which showed that patients with documented RTP had a decrease in LOS, supports this argument.

Table 9 Outcomes according to operative procedure reverse Trendelenburg (RTP) status

Audit	RTP (No)	RTP (Yes)	*p* value
	825 (82.5%)	175 (17.5%)	
Postoperative length of stay (days)	2.7 ± 3.5	2.2 ± 2.8	0.0246
Preoperative risk			
Age	57 ± 18	56 ± 17	0.3479
ASA classification	2.8 ± 0.6	2.9 ± 0.6	0.5627
Emergency procedures	82 (9.9%)	5 (3.0%)	0.0025
Preexisting lung disease	112 (13.6%)	41 (23.4%)	0.0010
Weight (kg)	86 ± 24	89 ± 23	0.0746
Intraoperative risk			
Operating room minutes	129 ± 75	126 ± 61	0.5419
Glycopyrrolate on induction	200 (24.2%)	48 (27.4%)	0.3753
Fluid input (L)	1.5 ± 1.0	1.6 ± 0.9	0.5296

No no operative RTP or no audit, *Yes* RTP throughout or a portion of the operative procedure, *ASA* American Society of Anesthesiologists

OR personnel surveys

After the study period, the anesthesia and OR nursing staff were surveyed regarding their perceptions of RTP. The surveys were conducted before data dissemination to mitigate any bias that may have been fostered by having knowledge of the study results. The intent of the survey was to reveal staff attitudes toward RTP during the study period. Of 85 anesthesia and OR nursing staff members participating in the surveys, more than 75% indicated that they perceived RTP as beneficial and that it should be used when feasible. Disagreement or uncertainty responses were sparse; however, dissenting replies suggest that individual perceptions were volitional and not biased by peer pressure. Results of the surveys indicate that the staff members were receptive to implementing RTP, under appropriate circumstances, during the study period.

Noncompulsory RTP audits

During 2015, nearly 40% of the study patients had a noncompulsory RTP audit completed throughout the study period. The audit indicated whether RTP was used during the surgical procedure (all the time, some of the time, or none of the time). However, it did not indicate whether RTP was used during tracheal intubation or extubation. Importantly, the RTP audit process served as a daily reinforcement that RTP may be beneficial and that it should be considered when appropriate.

Mortality associations (combined 2012 and 2015)

Compared to non-dying patients, dying patients had higher rates of POH, POPA, and emergency surgery and greater age and ASA classification. The higher rates of POH and POPA in dying patients suggest the notion that these outcomes, in particular, and pulmonary complications, in general, are likely to be clinically valid conditions and have an association with adverse outcomes. These findings also propose that the abstraction processes used in this study to categorize patients with POH and POPA may be clinically useful. The higher rate of emergency surgery procedures, older age, and higher ASA classification in non-survivors suggest that these preoperative risk conditions have a relationship with mortality.

POH associations (combined 2012 and 2015)

When the 2012 and 2015 patient cohorts were combined, POH was shown to likely be associated with adverse postoperative outcomes, and preoperative and intraoperative risk conditions. The potential association of POH with increased postoperative mortality and longer LOS indicates the need to substantiate the clinical validity of POH as an entity, and it suggests the credibility of our particular medical record abstraction process. The relationship between POH and intraoperative risk conditions suggests that OR events are linked to the development of POH. Additionally, the data imply that glycopyrrolate administration on anesthesia induction and shortening the surgical duration might be associated with improved outcomes. Further, the hypothesis-generating association of POH with preoperative risk factors suggests that host conditions may affect subsequent POH; however, these are typically not modifiable. The POH rates were substantially increased with open aortic, cranial, laparotomy, and non-spinal neck surgical procedures, compared to other procedural categories. This finding infers that these surgical procedures may need to receive more attention, especially when considering future strategies to mitigate POH. Patients with preoperative $SpO_2 < 94\%$ were excluded in order to enhance the likelihood that hypoxemia, if it were to develop, would have been related to intraoperative risk conditions.

POH associations (2012 versus 2015)

Compared to 2012, the POH rate in 2015 appeared to be substantially decreased, despite a higher age and ASA classification for the 2015 patient cohort. The time in the OR, patient weight, emergency procedures, glycopyrrolate administration, and PELD rates were comparable for the 2012 and 2015 patient cohorts. Findings of multivariate logistic regression analysis suggest that POH is simultaneously (independently) reduced for the year 2015, i.e., the period with increased use of RTP, and might be reduced with glycopyrrolate administration on anesthesia induction. Using the POH prediction model developed from the 2012 patient cohort, the POH rate in 2015 was predicted to be higher due to the higher ASA classification and age. However, the POH rate was significantly decreased during 2015, inferring that there is likely to be an inverse association between POH and RTP. The POH relative risk reduction was nearly 30% for the 2015 patient cohort, compared to the 2012 cohort.

POPA associations (combined 2012 and 2015)

When the 2012 and 2015 cohorts were combined, POPA was shown to likely be associated with adverse postoperative outcomes, and preoperative and intraoperative risk conditions. The hypothesis-generating association of POPA with increased postoperative mortality and longer LOS indicates the need to substantiate the clinical validity of POPA as an entity and to confirm the credibility of our specific medical record abstraction process in a prospective study. The relationship between POPA and intraoperative risk conditions suggests that OR events are linked to the development of POPA. Furthermore, the potential association of POPA with preoperative risk factors suggests that host conditions may affect subsequent POPA; however, these are usually not modifiable. The POPA rates were substantially increased with open aortic, cranial, and laparotomy surgical procedures compared to other procedural categories. These surgical procedures may need to receive greater consideration, when contemplating potential strategies to mitigate POPA.

POPA associations (2012 versus 2015)

The POPA rate in 2015 compared to that in 2012 was significantly decreased. This decrease occurred despite a higher age and ASA for the 2015 patient cohort, factors that are likely to be associated with an increased risk for POPA. Results of multivariate logistic regression analysis suggested that POPA was simultaneously (independently) reduced for the year 2015, i.e., the period with increased use of RTP. Using the OR nursing staff audits for 2015, patients with documented RTP anytime during the surgical procedure had a reduction in POPA. This finding was substantiated by results of univariate and multivariate statistical analyses. In summary, these findings imply that RTP is likely to be associated with a reduction in POPA.

LOS associations (combined 2012 and 2015)

The mean LOS was 2.5 days, with 75% of patients having been discharged by the third postoperative day. After combining the 2012 and 2015 cohorts, LOS was shown to likely be associated with adverse postoperative outcomes, and preoperative and intraoperative risk conditions. As previously stated, POH and POPA appear to have been related to an increased LOS. Patients undergoing high-risk POH procedures (i.e., open aortic, cranial, laparotomy, non-spinal neck procedures) compared to other procedures had a substantially longer LOS. LOS was longer with certain host conditions (increased age and ASA classification and emergency procedures). The following intraoperative conditions are likely to be associated with increased LOS: increased OR time, no glycopyrrolate administration, and more intraoperative fluid administration. These data suggest that administering glycopyrrolate on anesthesia induction and decreasing the duration of the surgical procedure might be useful strategies for decreasing LOS.

LOS associations (2012 versus 2015)

Despite the decreased POH rate for 2015, the LOS was similar for 2015 and 2012. A potential reduction in LOS due to the decrease in the lower POH rate for 2015 was likely offset by the higher age and ASA classification for 2015, as these factors appear to be associated with an increase in LOS.

LOS associations (within 2015 comparison)

Using the OR nursing staff audits for 2015, patients with documented RTP during the surgical procedure had a reduced LOS. This finding is supported by the univariate and multivariate statistical analyses. Specifically, the group with documented RTP likely had fewer emergency procedures but a greater weight and higher PELD rate. Results of multivariate linear regression analysis suggested that LOS was simultaneously (independently) decreased with glycopyrrolate administration on anesthesia induction and with documented RTP during the operative procedure. These data infer that glycopyrrolate administration and RTP are likely strategies to reduce LOS in patients undergoing general anesthesia and endotracheal intubation.

Study limitations

The glycopyrrolate associations with POH had p values of 0.05–0.09 suggesting that subsequent studies may or may not demonstrate an inverse association with POH. Certainly, our investigation may not have been sufficiently powered. The primary study limitation is the failure to document RTP use for every surgical case during 2012 and 2015. Ideally, there would be documentation for all 1500 patients regarding the use or non-use of RTP during tracheal intubation, the surgical procedure, and tracheal extubation. This would have enabled us to precisely and objectively determine RTP use in the OR during 2012 and 2015. Additionally, RTP as a mechanism to reduce POH and POPA was not studied in a randomized, controlled manner. Other factors that may have affected outcomes but were not investigated include the intraoperative tidal volume, positive end-expiratory pressure, tracheal cuff pressure levels, intraoperative body position, volume of secretions aspirated before extubation, and amounts of postoperative narcotic patients received.

Conclusions

This study's findings are hypothesis-generating, not hypothesis-confirming. A randomized clinical trial is needed to confirm (1) whether POH and POPA have an association with mortality and postoperative LOS, (2) if RTP has an inverse association with POH, POPA, and LOS, (3) whether glycopyrrolate administration on anesthesia induction is associated with a lower postoperative LOS and a reduction in POH, and (4) if our particular medical record abstraction process is credible. POH rates, POPA rates, and postoperative LOS are likely to be substantially increased with open aortic, cranial, laparotomy, and non-spinal neck surgical procedures compared to other procedural categories. The study results signal the need to confirm whether RTP, glycopyrrolate administration, and a shorter surgery time are beneficial for improving perioperative outcomes in patients undergoing general anesthesia and endotracheal intubation. Heightened attention may need to be paid to surgical procedures with an increased risk for POH, POPA, and prolonged LOS, when considering future strategies to mitigate pulmonary adverse outcomes. We recommend that future investigations have a prospective design and ideally include group randomization.

Abbreviations

ASA: American Society of Anesthesiology; EMR: Electronic medical record; IOH: Intraoperative hypoxemia; LOS: Postoperative length of stay; OR: Operating room; PELD: Preexisting lung disease; POH: Postoperative hypoxemia; POPA: Perioperative pulmonary aspiration; RTP: Reverse Trendelenburg positioning; SpO_2: Oxygen saturation as measured by pulse oximetry

Acknowledgements

The authors wish to thank Marina C. Hanes, BA, ELS for copyediting the manuscript and Stacy B. Coe and Hassan Aboumerhi, MD for participating in data collection.

Funding

No external source of funding was received.

Authors' contributions
CMD, BMH, AEH, TA, EAC, GSH, and CB conceptualized and designed the study. CMD, BMH, AEH, TA, EAC, GS, KC, CB, and TTS were involved in the day-to-day oversight of the study. CMD, BMH, and EAC performed the data collection. CMD performed the data analysis. All authors interpreted the data. CMD, BMH, EAC, and GSH performed the literature search and drafted the manuscript. All authors critically revised the manuscript for important intellectual content. All authors made substantial contributions to the conception and design, acquisition of data, or analysis and interpretation of data. All authors were involved in drafting the manuscript or revising it critically for important intellectual content. All authors read and approved the final manuscript.

Authors' information
CMD has 35 years experience as a trauma surgeon and is a retired board-certified surgical intensivist and general surgeon. BMH and EAC are experienced full-time research assistants for the Trauma and Neurosciences Research Department. AEH is a board-certified anesthesiologist and the chief of anesthesiology. TA is the assistant nurse manager of the operating room nursing staff. GSH is a board-certified general surgeon, a trauma surgeon, and a board-certified surgical intensivist. GS is an experienced and registered nurse anesthetist. KC is a senior general surgical resident. CB is the director of surgical and perioperative services. TTS is the chief of orthopedic trauma surgery.

Competing interests
The authors declare that they have no competing interests.

Author details
[1]Trauma, Critical Care, and General Surgery Services, St. Elizabeth Youngstown Hospital, 1044 Belmont Ave., Youngstown, OH 44501, USA. [2]Trauma and Neurosciences Research Department, St. Elizabeth Youngstown Hospital, 1044 Belmont Ave., Youngstown, OH 44501, USA. [3]Department of Anesthesiology, St. Elizabeth Youngstown Hospital, 1044 Belmont Ave., Youngstown, OH 44501, USA. [4]OR Nursing Staff, St. Elizabeth Youngstown Hospital, 1044 Belmont Ave., Youngstown, OH 44501, USA. [5]Department of Surgery, St. Elizabeth Youngstown Hospital, 1044 Belmont Ave., Youngstown, OH 44501, USA. [6]Surgical and Perioperative Services, St. Elizabeth Youngstown Hospital, 1044 Belmont Ave., Youngstown, OH 44501, USA. [7]Department of Orthopedic Surgery, St. Elizabeth Youngstown Hospital, 1044 Belmont Ave., Youngstown, OH 44501, USA.

References
Abdulla S. Pulmonary aspiration in perioperative medicine. Acta Anaesthesiol Belg. 2013;64:1–13.
Adedeji R, Oragui E, Khan W, Maruthainar N. The importance of correct patient positioning in theatres and implications of mal-positioning. J Perioper Pract. 2010;20:143–7.
Blitt CD, Gutman HL, Cohen DD, Weisman H, Dillon JB. "Silent" regurgitation and aspiration during general anesthesia. Anesth Analg. 1970;49:707–13.
Cotton BR, Smith G. The lower oesophageal sphincter and anaesthesia. Br J Anaesth. 1984;56:37–46.
Drakulovic MB, Torres A, Bauer TT, Nicolas JM, Nogue S, Ferrer M. Supine body position as a risk factor for nosocomial pneumonia in mechanically ventilated patients: a randomised trial. Lancet. 1999;354:1851–8.
Dunham CM, Hileman BM, Hutchinson AE, Chance EA, Huang GS. Perioperative hypoxemia is common with horizontal positioning during general anesthesia and is associated with major adverse outcomes: a retrospective study of consecutive patients. BMC Anesthesiol. 2014;14:43.
Engelhardt T, Webster NR. Pulmonary aspiration of gastric contents in anaesthesia. Br J Anaesth. 1999;83:453–60.
Ewig S, Torres A. Prevention and management of ventilator-associated pneumonia. Curr Opin Crit Care. 2002;8:58–69.
Fernandez-Crehuet R, Diaz-Molina C, de Irala J, Martinez-Concha D, Salcedo-Leal I, Masa-Calles J. Nosocomial infection in an intensive-care unit: identification of risk factors. Infect Control Hosp Epidemiol. 1997;18:825–30.
Ferrer R, Artigas A. Clinical review: non-antibiotic strategies for preventing ventilator-associated pneumonia. Crit Care. 2002;6:45–51.
Institute for Healthcare Improvement: Prevent ventilator-associated pneumonia. Institute for Healthcare Improvement. 2012. www.ihi.org. Accessed 9 Dec 2013.
Kalinowski CP, Kirsch JR. Strategies for prophylaxis and treatment for aspiration. Best Pract Res Clin Anaesthesiol. 2004;18:719–37.
Keenan SP, Heyland DK, Jacka MJ, Cook D, Dodek P. Ventilator-associated pneumonia. Prevention, diagnosis, and therapy. Crit Care Clin. 2002;18:107–25.
Kluger MT, Short TG. Aspiration during anaesthesia: a review of 133 cases from the Australian Anaesthetic Incident Monitoring Study (AIMS). Anaesthesia. 1999;54:19–26.
Koeman M, van der Ven AJ, Ramsay G, Hoepelman IM, Bonten MJ. Ventilator-associated pneumonia: recent issues on pathogenesis, prevention and diagnosis. J Hosp Infect. 2001;49:155–62.
Kollef MH. Ventilator-associated pneumonia. A multivariate analysis. JAMA. 1993;270:1965–70.
Kozlow JH, Berenholtz SM, Garrett E, Dorman T, Pronovost PJ. Epidemiology and impact of aspiration pneumonia in patients undergoing surgery in Maryland, 1999-2000. Crit Care Med. 2003;31:1930–7.
McEwen DR. Intraoperative positioning of surgical patients. AORN J. 1996;63:1059–63. 66-79; quiz 80-6
Morgan M. Control of intragastric pH and volume. Br J Anaesth. 1984;56:47–57.
Mulier JP, Dillemans B, Van Cauwenberge S. Impact of the patient's body position on the intraabdominal workspace during laparoscopic surgery. Surg Endosc. 2010;24:1398–402.
Ng A, Smith G. Gastroesophageal reflux and aspiration of gastric contents in anesthetic practice. Anesth Analg. 2001;93:494–513.
Petring OU, Adelhoj B, Jensen BN, Pedersen NO, Lomholt N. Prevention of silent aspiration due to leaks around cuffs of endotracheal tubes. Anesth Analg. 1986;65:777–80.
Reali-Forster C, Kolobow T, Giacomini M, Hayashi T, Horiba K, Ferrans VJ. New ultrathin-walled endotracheal tube with a novel laryngeal seal design. Long-term evaluation in sheep. Anesthesiology. 1996;84:162–72. discussion 27A
Seegobin RD, van Hasselt GL. Aspiration beyond endotracheal cuffs. Can Anaesth Soc J. 1986;33:273–9.
Smith KA. Positioning principles. An anatomical review. AORN J. 1990;52:1196-202, 204, 206-8.
Smith G, Ng A. Gastric reflux and pulmonary aspiration in anaesthesia. Minerva Anestesiol. 2003;69:402–6.
Tiret L, Desmonts JM, Hatton F, Vourc'h G. Complications associated with anaesthesia–a prospective survey in France. Can Anaesth Soc J. 1986;33:336–44.
Torres A, Serra-Batlles J, Ros E, Piera C. Puig de la Bellacasa J, Cobos A et al. Pulmonary aspiration of gastric contents in patients receiving mechanical ventilation: the effect of body position. Ann Intern Med. 1992;116:540–3.

23

Clinical and economic impact of goal-directed fluid therapy during elective gastrointestinal surgery

Juying Jin, Su Min*, Dan Liu, Ling Liu and Bixiao Lv

Abstract

Background: Several randomized controlled trials suggest that goal-directed fluid therapy (GDFT) may result in improved postoperative outcomes. The aim of this study was to assess the clinical and financial impact of the real-life implementation of intraoperative GDFT in patients undergoing elective gastrointestinal surgery in a Chinese tertiary medical center.

Methods: This Quality Improvement Program (QIP) study comprised three phases of 5, 1, and 5 months, respectively. During the first phase, we retrospectively collected perioperative data from patients who received standard intraoperative fluid management from January to May 2016. Then a 1-month training period allowed the clinical staff to become familiar with the GDFT protocol. After the training phase, GDFT was used from July to November 2016. In the GDFT group, stroke volume (SV) was continuously monitored and optimized towards the plateau of the Frank-Starling curve. The primary outcome measure was postoperative morbidity (the proportion of patients with one or more complications within 30 days after surgery). Secondary outcomes were total hospital cost, postoperative length of hospital stay, and 30-day mortality.

Results: Data from 200 patients before (control group) and 201 patients after the implementation of GDFT (GDFT group) were collected and compared. There was no significant difference in demographics and surgical procedures between the two groups. Postoperative morbidity was significantly lower in the GDFT group than in the control group (30.8% vs. 44.0%, $p = 0.006$). No significant differences were observed for mean total hospital cost (76,793 RMB vs. 74,444 RMB; $p = 0.430$), median postoperative length of hospital stay (10 days vs. 10 days; $p = 0.104$), and 30-day mortality (1% vs. 0.5%; $p = 0.565$).

Conclusion: In patients undergoing gastrointestinal surgery, the implementation of a GDFT protocol was associated with a reduction in postoperative morbidity without increasing costs.

Keywords: Goal-directed fluid therapy, Gastrointestinal surgery, Postoperative complications, Stroke volume

Background

Intraoperative fluid management is part of everyday anesthesiology practice and a key determinant of postoperative outcome. The advantages and limitations of liberal versus restrictive fluid therapy strategies have been debated for years (Brandstrup et al. 2003, Nisanevich et al. 2005, Futier et al. 2010). Insufficient fluid administration may be responsible for tissue hypoperfusion, organ dysfunction, and postoperative complications (Futier et al. 2010, Myles et al. 2018). Hypovolemia is not easy to detect from variables such as heart rate and blood pressure (Bennett-Guerrero et al. 1999, Thom et al. 2010). On the other hand, large volumes of intravenous fluid may cause complications due to tissue edema such as delayed healing and weaning from mechanical ventilation (Holte et al. 2002). As a result, goal-directed fluid therapy (GDFT) has been proposed to tailor fluid administration to the individual needs of patients undergoing major surgery (Bellamy

* Correspondence: ms1068@outlook.com
Department of Anesthesiology, the First Affiliated Hospital, Chongqing Medical University, 1 Youyi Road, Chongqing 400016, China

2006, Corcoran et al. 2012, Doherty and Buggy 2012, Calvo-Vecino et al. 2018).

Several randomized controlled trials (RCTs) and meta-analyses suggest that GDFT is useful to improve postoperative outcome, namely to decrease postoperative morbidity, hospital length of stay and costs (Pearse et al. 2005, Benes et al. 2010, Hamilton et al. 2011, Grocott et al. 2013, Scheeren et al. 2013, Zakhaleva et al. 2013, Calvo-Vecino et al. 2018). However, a limited number of RCTs have been done in China (Zhang et al. 2013, Zheng et al. 2013, Luo et al. 2017), and very few physicians and institutions have implemented this concept in their day-to-day practice. Importantly, the effectiveness of GDFT remains to be confirmed in real-life conditions. Therefore, we designed a Quality Improvement Program (QIP) to implement GDFT in patients undergoing major abdominal surgery and to study the impact on postoperative morbidity and costs.

Methods

Screening and consent

This study (clinicaltrials.gov Identifier: NCT02507557) was approved by the local ethics committee (registration number: 20160301) and was conducted in a tertiary teaching hospital. We studied consecutive adult patients who were to undergo elective gastrectomy, colorectal surgery, or small bowel resection, before (control group) and after (GDFT group) the implementation of GDFT. Patients less than 18 years old, without any comorbidity (American Society of Anesthesiologists physical status I), and pregnant women were excluded from this study. Patients were followed until 30 days after the operation or death. Written informed consent was obtained from all patients in the GDFT group. The local ethics committee waived the requirement for informed consent in the control group due to the retrospective nature of the analysis. All patients' records/information were anonymized and de-identified prior to analysis.

Study design

Our QIP comprised three phases. During the first phase, from January to May 2016, patients received conventional intraoperative fluid management. In this control group, the use of fluids and vasoactive and inotropic drugs were at the discretion of the anesthesiologist. The second phase was conducted in June 2016. The goal of this training phase was to allow all members of our clinical staff to become familiar with the intraoperative GDFT protocol. After 1 month training, fluid management was conducted according to the GDFT protocol, from July to November 2016 (third phase, GDFT group; see Fig. 1).

Anesthesia management

The patients in both groups were fasted for solid foods for 6 h and clear liquids for 2–3 h before surgery. All patients were given 300 mL oral drink (Outfast, Yichang Humanwell Pharmaceutical Co., Hubei, China) 2 to 3 h preoperatively. No preanesthetic medication was used. All patients received prophylactic antibiotics in accordance with established guidelines (Bratzler et al. 2013). Other principles of enhanced recovery after surgery

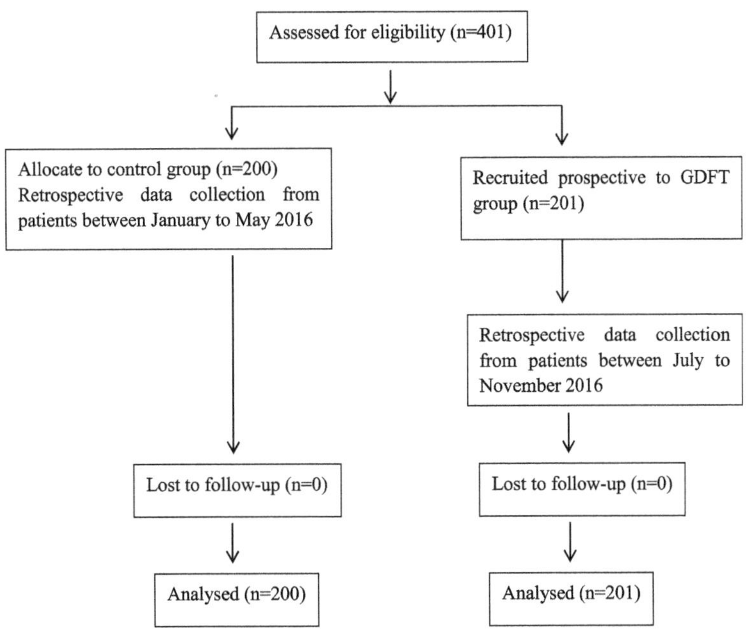

Fig. 1 Flowchart of the patients in this study

(ERAS) protocol were not applied to patients undergoing gastrointestinal surgery within our institution during the execution of this study. In all cases, the anesthetic procedure was decided by the responsible anesthesiologist. General anesthesia was induced by 2–2.5 mg/kg propofol and 0.2–0.4 μg/kg sufentanil followed by 0.6–0.9 mg/kg rocuronium given for neuromuscular blockage. After tracheal intubation, patients' lungs were ventilated (FiO_2 0.5–0.6) with a tidal volume of 8 mL/kg (ideal body weight) and an initial respiratory rate of 12 breaths/min adjusted to achieve an end-tidal CO_2 between 35 and 45 mmHg. Anesthesia was maintained with inhalation of sevoflurane in 40% O_2 in air. Intravenous sufentanil and rocuronium were injected intermittently as needed. Packed red blood cells were administered at the discretion of the anesthesiologist. Our perioperative care protocol suggests using a hemoglobin level of 7 g/dL as a transfusion threshold for healthy patients and 10 g/dL for patients with pulmonary or cardiac disease. Body temperature > 36 °C was maintained during surgery in both groups. Postoperative pain control was achieved with intravenous patient-controlled analgesia devices with tramadol.

GDFT protocol

In the GDFT group, an arterial line was inserted into the radial artery of the non-dominant forearm before induction of anesthesia. The Vigileo/FloTrac system (Edwards Lifesciences, Irvine, CA, USA) was used to continuously monitor stroke volume (SV) and cardiac index (CI). Patients received 1 L of Ringer's lactate solution right before anesthesia induction. Then, fluid maintenance with crystalloid was set at 2~4 mL/kg/h for open procedures (maximum dose of 400 mL/h) and 1~2 mL/kg/h for laparoscopic procedures (maximum dose of 200 mL/h). Boluses of IV colloid were given to optimise SV using the GDFT protocol recommended by the National Institute for Health and Care Excellence (NICE) in the United Kingdom (NICE 2011) (Fig. 2). After incision for open cases and after pneumoperitoneum for laparoscopic cases, patients received a 200-mL colloid bolus (Voluven, Fresenius Kabi, Bad Homburg, Germany) over 5–10 min. If SV increased by > 10%, the bolus was repeated until it increased by < 10%. Once reached, the SV plateau value was used as a target value during the entire surgical duration. Additional colloid boluses were given only if SV dropped by > 10% below the plateau value. In case of hypotension [systolic arterial pressure (SBP) < 90 mmHg or mean arterial pressure

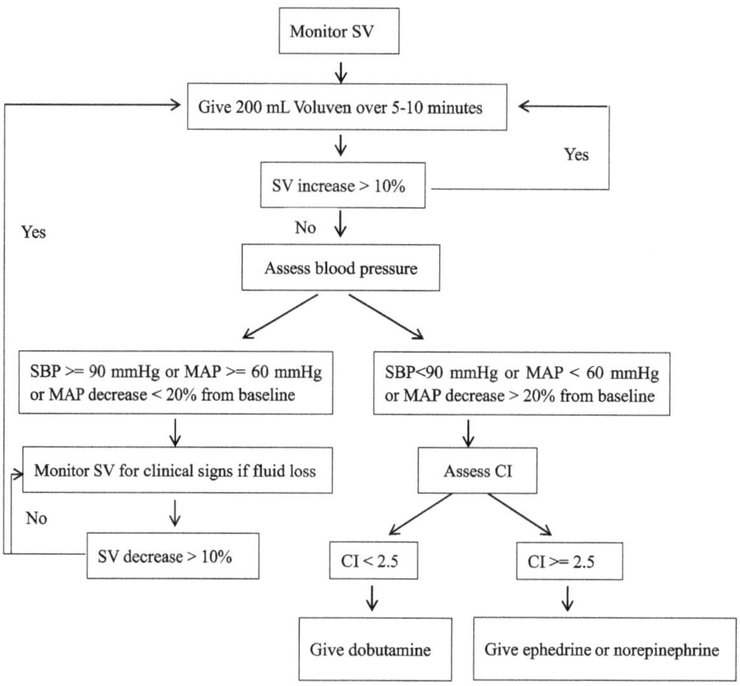

Fig. 2 Intraoperative goal-directed algorithm. SV stroke volume, SBP systolic blood pressure, MAP mean artery pressure. Maintained dose of infusion of crystalloid during surgery was 2~4 mL/kg/h for open procedure and 1~2 mL/kg/h for laparoscopic procedure. After incision for open cases and after pneumoperitoneum for laparoscopic cases, patients received a 200-mL colloid bolus over 5–10 min. If SV increased by > 10%, the bolus was repeated until it increased by < 10%. Once reached, the SV plateau value was used as a target value during the entire surgical duration. Additional colloid boluses were given only if SV dropped by > 10% below the plateau value. In case of hypotension (SBP < 90 mmHg or MAP < 60 mmHg or MAP decrease > 20% from baseline) in fluid non-responders, an infusion of dobutamine was recommended if CI was < 2.5 L/min/m^2, and ephedrine boluses of 5 to 15 mg or norepinephrine infusion were recommended if CI was > 2.5 L/min/m^2. Protocol should not influence blood product administration

(MAP) < 60 mmHg or MAP decrease > 20% from baseline] in fluid non-responders, an infusion of dobutamine was recommended if CI was < 2.5 L/min/m^2, and ephedrine boluses of 5 to 15 mg or norepinephrine infusion were recommended if CI was ≥ 2.5 L/min/m^2. Adherence to the GDFT protocol was strongly encouraged but not systematically confirmed during the implementation phase.

Outcome measures

The primary outcome measure was postoperative morbidity, defined as the percentage of patients with one or more complications within 30 days after surgery. Both postoperative in-hospital complications and complications that occurred after discharge and required ambulatory or in-hospital care up to day 30 after surgery were recorded. Postoperative complications included cardiac arrest (exclusive of death), myocardial infarction, stroke, pulmonary embolism, deep venous thrombosis, pneumonia, wound infection, wound dehiscence, urinary tract infection, ileus, anastomotic fistula, gastrointestinal bleeding, acute cardiac failure, acute respiratory failure, sepsis, unplanned reintubation, acute renal injury, hepatic dysfunction, and unplanned reoperation. Diagnosis and management of postoperative complications were undertaken by non-research staff according to our local practice. Secondary outcome measures included postoperative length of hospital stay, 30-day postoperative mortality, and total hospital costs. Costs are those associated with the actual procedures, as determined by the hospital using its accounting systems, and include both fixed and variable components. Both for the pre- and post-implementation periods, outcome data were extracted from our electronic medical records (EMR, Medicalsystem, Suzhou, Jiangsu, China). In order to guarantee that the data acquisition process was the same for the two study periods, data were collected retrospectively at the end of each period.

Statistical analysis

Based on previous literature (Benes et al. 2010, Salzwedel et al. 2013, Zakhaleva et al. 2013), we estimated that complications may appear in 50% of our patients. Assuming a decrease in morbidity rate from 50 to 35%, a study sample size of 185 patients in each group was calculated for two-sided tests with type I error of 5% and power of 90%. Owing to an anticipated loss of about 10% of patients entering the study, we proposed to include 200 patients in each group.

Continuous normally distributed variables are expressed as mean ± standard deviation (SD), and non-normally distributed continuous variables are expressed as medians (interquartile ranges). Categorical variables are expressed as numbers and percentages. An independent sample *t*-test was used to test differences between groups for continuous normally distributed variables; a chi-square test was used for categorical data to test for differences between groups. When data were not normally distributed, a Mann-Whitney *U* test was used to analyze differences between groups. A level of $p < 0.05$ was defined as statistically significant. The statistical analysis was performed with the use of SPPS 17.0 for Windows (SPSS Inc., Chicago, IL, USA).

Results

All eligible patients consented to participate in the study and thus 201 consecutive patients were prospectively recruited from July to November 2016 (GDFT group). They were compared with 200 patients who had surgery between January and May 2016 (control group). The relevant patient characteristics and surgical details are included in Table 1. There was no significant difference in age, gender, American Society of Anesthesiologists (ASA) physical status, surgical approach, surgical type, or duration of surgery between the two groups. A laparoscopic surgical technique was used in most of the cases.

The volume of fluid administered is shown in Table 2. Patients in the GDFT group received on average 102 mL more crystalloid than the control group but the total volume of intraoperative fluid was comparable in both groups. Surgical blood loss was slightly but significantly higher in the GDFT group, who received more blood products than the control group. During surgery, urine output was higher in the GDFT group, resulting in a significant reduction in the intraoperative fluid balance.

Table 1 Patient demographics and surgical characteristics

	GDFT (*n* = 201)	Traditional (*n* = 200)	*p* value
Sex (male/female, *n*)	116/85	125/75	0.328
Age (mean ± SD, year)	62.7 ± 12.2	62.2 ± 12.3	0.697
Height (mean ± SD, cm)	161.1 ± 7.3	162.0 ± 7.5	0.243
Weight (mean ± SD, kg)	57.1 ± 9.9	60.3 ± 10.9	0.002
ASA physical status (II/III/IV, *n*)	140/58/3	154/44/2	0.248
Comorbidities			
Coronary artery disease (yes/no, *n*)	12/189	14/186	0.675
Hypertension (yes/no, *n*)	50/151	48/152	0.838
Diabetes mellitus (yes/no, *n*)	22/179	18/182	0.516
Surgical type (gastric/small bowel/colonic/rectal, *n*)	34//3/70/94	46/1/67/86	0.228
Surgical approach (open/laparoscopic, *n*)	23/178	21/179	0.763
Arterial line inserted (yes/no, *n*)	201/0	183/17	< 0.001
Surgical duration (median (IQR), min)	219 (180–268)	220 (180–260)	0.327

Table 2 Intraoperative fluid administration and balance, use of vasoactive agents

	GDFT ($n = 201$)	Traditional ($n = 200$)	p value
Crystalloids (mean ± SD, mL)	1678 ± 361	1576 ± 466	0.014
Colloids (mean ± SD, mL)	672 ± 363	700 ± 289	0.390
Crystalloids + colloids (mean ± SD, mL)	2350 ± 572	2276 ± 612	0.210
Packed red blood cells (mean ± SD, mL)	48 ± 138	22 ± 90	0.022
Fresh frozen plasma (mean ± SD, mL)	13 ± 68	3 ± 24	0.047
Blood loss (mean ± SD, mL)	120 ± 162	90 ± 94	0.025
Urine output (mean ± SD, mL)	707 ± 466	467 ± 357	< 0.001
Net fluids balance (mean ± SD, mL)	1583 ± 562	1743 ± 571	0.005
Use of ephedrine (yes/no, n)	92/109	83/117	0.389
Use of norepinephrine (yes/no, n)	117/84	107/93	0.342
Use of dobutamine (yes/no, n)	44/157	14/186	< 0.001

More patients received dobutamine in the GDFT group (Table 2).

Postoperative morbidity was significantly lower in the GDFT group (30.8% vs. 44.0%, $p = 0.006$). Total hospital cost, postoperative length of hospital stay, and mortality within the 30 days following surgery were comparable in both groups (Table 3).

Discussion

This QIP study demonstrated that the implementation of GDFT was possible and effective in our institution. Indeed, it was associated with a significant reduction in postoperative morbidity and did not significantly increase costs.

Our findings are consistent with the results of several meta-analyses and randomized controlled trials which have demonstrated that GDFT is susceptible to improve postoperative outcomes in patients undergoing major abdominal procedures (Benes et al. 2010, Grocott et al. 2013, Zakhaleva et al. 2013, Zheng et al. 2013, Sun et al. 2017, Yuan et al. 2017, Calvo-Vecino et al. 2018). The beneficial effects of GDFT have been questioned in low-risk patients (Brandstrup et al. 2012) and during laparoscopic procedures (Senagore et al. 2009). Low-risk patients (ASA I) were excluded from our evaluation, but most of our patients had laparoscopic surgery, suggesting that GDFT may also have value in this context.

Before and after comparisons can provide valuable data regarding the effect of an intervention in real-life conditions, rather than under the stringent restraints of a randomized controlled trial (Saturni et al. 2014). A limited number of QIP studies have already investigated the effectiveness of GDFT implementation outside China (Cannesson et al. 2015, Habicher et al. 2016, Veelo et al.

Table 3 Postoperative morbidity and mortality, length of hospital stay, and total hospital costs

	GDFT ($n = 201$)	Traditional ($n = 200$)	p value
Cardiovascular complications	4 (2.0)	3 (1.5)	0.708
Cardiac arrest (exclusive of death, n, %)	0 (0)	0 (0)	–
Myocardial infarction (%)	0 (0)	1 (0.5)	0.315
Acute cardiac failure (%)	1 (0.5)	2 (1.0)	0.559
Stroke (%)	1 (0.5)	0 (0)	0.318
Pulmonary embolism (%)	1 (0.5)	0 (0)	0.318
Deep venous thrombosis (%)	1 (0.5)	0 (0)	0.318
Infectious complications	61 (30.3)	70 (35.0)	0.321
Pneumonia (%)	34 (16.9)	48 (24.0)	0.079
Wound infection (%)	23 (11.4)	17 (8.5)	0.325
Urinary tract infection (%)	3 (1.5)	4 (2.0)	0.698
Sepsis (%)	1 (0.5)	1 (0.5)	0.997
Gastrointestinal complications	12 (6.0)	15 (7.5)	0.541
Ileus (%)	6 (3.0)	3 (1.5)	0.315
Anastomotic fistula (%)	6 (3.0)	9 (4.5)	0.424
Gastrointestinal bleeding (%)	0 (0)	3 (1.5)	0.081
Respiratory complications	2 (1.0)	1 (0.5)	0.565
Acute respiratory failure (%)	1 (0.5)	1 (0.5)	0.997
Unplanned reintubation (%)	1 (0.5)	0 (0)	0.318
Other complications	11	17	0.234
Acute renal injury (%)	0 (0)	0 (0)	–
Hepatic dysfunction (%)	7 (3.5)	12 (6.0)	0.235
Wound dehiscence (%)	1 (0.5)	0 (0)	0.318
Unplanned reoperation (%)	3 (1.5)	5 (2.5)	0.471
Patients with one or more complications (%)	62 (30.8)	88 (44.0)	0.006
Readmission within postoperative 30 days (%)	5 (2.5)	9 (4.5)	0.430
Mortality within postoperative 30 days (%)	2 (1.0)	1 (0.5)	0.565
Postoperative length of hospital (median (IQR), day)	10 (8–14)	10 (8–13)	0.104
Total hospital cost (mean ± SD, RMB)	76,793 ± 26,522	74,444 ± 32,705	0.430
Total hospital cost (mean ± SD, $US*)	11,820 ± 4082	11,458 ± 5034	

*Exchange rate from June 22, 2018

2017). In Germany, Habicher et al. (Habicher et al. 2016) implemented GDFT in 130 patients undergoing hip revision arthroplasty and reported a significant decrease in postoperative morbidity. In the Netherlands, Veelo et al. (Veelo et al. 2017) compared the postoperative outcome of 100 patients undergoing esophagectomy before and after the implementation of a GDFT protocol. They observed a significant decrease in pneumonia, mediastinal abscesses, gastric tube necrosis, and ICU length of stay. In the USA, Cannesson et al. (2015) reported postoperative outcomes for 330 patients undergoing high-risk abdominal surgery and observed a decrease in postoperative morbidity from 39 to 25% after the implementation of GDFT. As of today, our study is therefore the largest QIP study investigating the effects of intraoperative GDFT on postoperative outcome. This is also the first one done in China, where surgical pathways and health care costs are different than in the USA and in Europe. Indeed, hospital costs reported in the manuscript are lower than those reported in the USA (Flynn et al. 2014, Michard et al. 2015) and in Switzerland (Vonlanthen et al. 2011).

Total intraoperative fluid volumes were not significantly different between the two groups, a finding consistent with the results of a meta-analysis of GDFT studies published in 2017 (Michard et al. 2017) and of the most recent multicenter GDFT randomized controlled trial (Calvo-Vecino et al. 2018). Our study design does not allow us to clarify why GDFT was more effective than our past practice. However, one may hypothesize that the individualization of fluid therapy is useful to ensure the right patients receive the right amount of fluid at the right time. Some patients likely received more fluid (because they were fluid responders) and others likely received less (because they were identified as non-responders) than they would have before the implementation of the GDFT protocol. This may explain why the average volume of fluid was comparable between groups (Michard et al. 2017). Differences in timing may also have played a role (Scheeren et al. 2013). However, because we did not study and record the timing of fluid boluses, we cannot draw any definitive conclusion regarding the influence of timing on postoperative outcome.

Interestingly, our study shows that implementing GDFT is a way to improve quality of surgical care without significantly increasing costs. Even if we did not specifically estimate the costs of complications, we can speculate that the cost for the hemodynamic equipment was offset by the reduction in postoperative morbidity and related costs. These findings are consistent with what has been reported by projection models (Bartha et al. 2012, Michard et al. 2015) and in prospective studies (Sadique et al. 2015), both in Europe and in the USA. This is an important message for hospitals that may be reluctant to invest in new technologies without knowing that it makes sense from a return on investment standpoint.

Our study has several limitations. First, given its "before and after" nature, we cannot claim causality between the GDFT intervention and the observed changes in postoperative outcome. Another potential disadvantage of such a design is the risk of imbalance between groups (Saturni et al. 2014). However, given the size of our study (> 400 patients), there was no significant difference at baseline between the GDFT and the control groups. A "before and after" study design also has advantages. It better represents daily clinical practice (Saturni et al. 2014). Indeed the control group is not influenced by the GDFT group. This is not the case in randomized controlled trials where the training and the Hawthorne effects inevitably affect the behavior of clinicians treating both groups (Habicher et al. 2016, Veelo et al. 2017). We believe that both randomized controlled trials and QIPs are useful and complementary, the former to demonstrate the value of new strategies, the later to confirm feasibility and efficacy in real-life conditions. Diagnosis of postoperative complications were undertaken by non-research staff according to our local practice, so that there was no official definition for each complication during the before implementation period. Proposing definitions for complications in the GDFT group only would have introduced a bias. Finally, if all patients from the GDFT group were equipped with a cardiac output monitor, we did not use—like in most GDFT studies—any tracking tools or target screens to optimize adherence to the hemodynamic protocol (Michard 2013). Therefore, we were unable to quantify the number of protocol violations, nor the time spent in target for hemodynamic variables, both factors that may have influenced our results.

Conclusion

In summary, our study showed that real-life implementation of an intraoperative GDFT protocol was doable in our tertiary medical center and was associated with a significant reduction in the incidence of complications following gastrointestinal surgery. Interestingly, the observed improvement in quality of surgical care was not associated with a significant increase in hospital costs.

Abbreviations

ASA: American Society of Anesthesiologists; CI: Cardiac index; EMR: Electronic medical records; GDFT: Goal-directed fluid therapy; MAP: Mean arterial pressure; NICE: National Institute for Health and Care Excellence; QIP: Quality Improvement Program; RCTs: Randomized controlled trials; SBP: Systolic blood pressure; SD: Standard deviation; SV: Stroke volume

Acknowledgements

We thank Dr. Frederic Michard, from MiCo, Denens, Switzerland (michardconsulting.com) for reviewing the manuscript.

Funding
Su Min has received a research grant for this study from Edwards Lifesciences. Funding was only for a part of the material costs (probes).The sponsor had no direct access to the data and no role in the design and conduct of the study, collection and management of the data, approval of the manuscript, and decision to submit the manuscript for publication. This work was also supported by grant of Integrated Demonstration Project of Chongqing Science and Technology Commission (Award No. cstc2015jcsf10008-1).

Authors' contributions
JJ participated in the design of the study, execution, and coordination and drafted the manuscript. MS was a site principal investigator and helped to revise the manuscript. LD and LL were involved in execution, coordination, and data acquisition. BX carried out statistical analyses. All authors read and approved the final manuscript.

Competing interests
The authors declare that they have no competing interests.

References

Bartha E, Davidson T, Hommel A, Thorngren KG, Carlsson P, Kalman S. Cost-effectiveness analysis of goal-directed hemodynamic treatment of elderly hip fracture patients: before clinical research starts. Anesthesiology. 2012;117(3):519–30.

Bellamy MC. Wet, dry or something else? Br J Anaesth. 2006;97(6):755–7.

Benes J, Chytra I, Altmann P, Hluchy M, Kasal E, Svitak R, Pradl R, Stepan M. Intraoperative fluid optimization using stroke volume variation in high risk surgical patients: results of prospective randomized study. Crit Care. 2010; 14(3):R118.

Bennett-Guerrero E, Welsby I, Dunn TJ, Young LR, Wahl TA, Diers TL, Phillips-Bute BG, Newman MF, Mythen MG. The use of a postoperative morbidity survey to evaluate patients with prolonged hospitalization after routine, moderate-risk, elective surgery. Anesth Analg. 1999;89(2):514–9.

Brandstrup B, Svendsen PE, Rasmussen M, Belhage B, Rodt SA, Hansen B, Moller DR, Lundbech LB, Andersen N, Berg V, et al. Which goal for fluid therapy during colorectal surgery is followed by the best outcome: near-maximal stroke volume or zero fluid balance? Br J Anaesth. 2012;109(2):191–9.

Brandstrup B, Tonnesen H, Beier-Holgersen R, Hjortso E, Ording H, Lindorff-Larsen K, Rasmussen MS, Lanng C, Wallin L, Iversen LH, et al. Effects of intravenous fluid restriction on postoperative complications: comparison of two perioperative fluid regimens: a randomized assessor-blinded multicenter trial. Ann Surg. 2003;238(5):641–8.

Bratzler DW, Dellinger EP, Olsen KM, Perl TM, Auwaerter PG, Bolon MK, Fish DN, Napolitano LM, Sawyer RG, Slain D, et al. Clinical practice guidelines for antimicrobial prophylaxis in surgery. Surg Infect. 2013;14(1):73–156.

Calvo-Vecino JM, Ripolles-Melchor J, Mythen MG, Casans-Frances R, Balik A, Artacho JP, Martinez-Hurtado E, Serrano Romero A, Fernandez Perez C, Asuero de Lis S, et al. Effect of goal-directed haemodynamic therapy on postoperative complications in low-moderate risk surgical patients: a multicentre randomised controlled trial (FEDORA trial). Br J Anaesth. 2018; 120(4):734–44.

Cannesson M, Ramsingh D, Rinehart J, Demirjian A, Vu T, Vakharia S, Imagawa D, Yu Z, Greenfield S, Kain Z. Perioperative goal-directed therapy and postoperative outcomes in patients undergoing high-risk abdominal surgery: a historical-prospective, comparative effectiveness study. Crit Care. 2015;19:261.

Corcoran T, Rhodes JE, Clarke S, Myles PS, Ho KM. Perioperative fluid management strategies in major surgery: a stratified meta-analysis. Anesth Analg. 2012;114(3):640–51.

Doherty M, Buggy DJ. Intraoperative fluids: how much is too much? Br J Anaesth. 2012;109(1):69–79.

Flynn DN, Speck RM, Mahmoud NN, David G, Fleisher LA. The impact of complications following open colectomy on hospital finances: a retrospective cohort study. Perioper Med (Lond). 2014;3(1):1.

Futier E, Constantin JM, Petit A, Chanques G, Kwiatkowski F, Flamein R, Slim K, Sapin V, Jaber S, Bazin JE. Conservative vs restrictive individualized goal-directed fluid replacement strategy in major abdominal surgery: a prospective randomized trial. Arch Surg. 2010;145(12):1193–200.

Grocott MP, Dushianthan A, Hamilton MA, Mythen MG, Harrison D, Rowan K, Optimisation Systematic Review Steering Group. Perioperative increase in global blood flow to explicit defined goals and outcomes after surgery: a Cochrane systematic review. Br J Anaesth. 2013;111(4):535–48.

Habicher M, Balzer F, Mezger V, Niclas J, Muller M, Perka C, Kramer M, Sander M. Implementation of goal-directed fluid therapy during hip revision arthroplasty: a matched cohort study. Perioper Med (Lond). 2016;5:31.

Hamilton MA, Cecconi M, Rhodes A. A systematic review and meta-analysis on the use of preemptive hemodynamic intervention to improve postoperative outcomes in moderate and high-risk surgical patients. Anesth Analg. 2011; 112(6):1392–402.

Holte K, Sharrock NE, Kehlet H. Pathophysiology and clinical implications of perioperative fluid excess. Br J Anaesth. 2002;89(4):622–32.

Luo J, Xue J, Liu J, Liu B, Liu L, Chen G. Goal-directed fluid restriction during brain surgery: a prospective randomized controlled trial. Ann Intensive Care. 2017; 7(1):16.

Michard F. Decision support for hemodynamic management: from graphical displays to closed loop systems. Anesth Analg. 2013;117(4):876–82.

Michard F, Giglio MT, Brienza N. Perioperative goal-directed therapy with uncalibrated pulse contour methods: impact on fluid management and postoperative outcome. Br J Anaesth. 2017;

Michard F, Mountford WK, Krukas MR, Ernst FR, Fogel SL. Potential return on investment for implementation of perioperative goal-directed fluid therapy in major surgery: a nationwide database study. Perioper Med (Lond). 2015;4:11.

Myles PS, Bellomo R, Corcoran T, Forbes A, Peyton P, Story D, Christophi C, Leslie K, McGuinness S, Parke R, et al. Restrictive versus liberal fluid therapy for major abdominal surgery. N Engl J Med. 2018;378(24):2263–74.

National Institute for Health and Clinical Excellence. Medical technologies guidance MTG3: CardioQODM oesophageal doppler monitor. 2011. https://www.nice.org.uk/guidance/MTG3.

Nisanevich V, Felsenstein I, Almogy G, Weissman C, Einav S, Matot I. Effect of intraoperative fluid management on outcome after intraabdominal surgery. Anesthesiology. 2005;103(1):25–32.

Pearse R, Dawson D, Fawcett J, Rhodes A, Grounds RM, Bennett ED. Early goal-directed therapy after major surgery reduces complications and duration of hospital stay. A randomised, controlled trial [ISRCTN38797445]. Crit Care. 2005;9(6):R687–93.

Sadique Z, Harrison DA, Grieve R, Rowan KM, Pearse RM, group Os. Cost-effectiveness of a cardiac output-guided haemodynamic therapy algorithm in high-risk patients undergoing major gastrointestinal surgery. Perioper Med (Lond). 2015;4:13.

Salzwedel C, Puig J, Carstens A, Bein B, Molnar Z, Kiss K, Hussain A, Belda J, Kirov MY, Sakka SG, et al. Perioperative goal-directed hemodynamic therapy based on radial arterial pulse pressure variation and continuous cardiac index trending reduces postoperative complications after major abdominal surgery: a multi-center, prospective, randomized study. Crit Care. 2013;17(5):R191.

Saturni S, Bellini F, Braido F, Paggiaro P, Sanduzzi A, Scichilone N, Santus PA, Morandi L, Papi A. Randomized controlled trials and real life studies. Approaches and methodologies: a clinical point of view. Pulm Pharmacol Ther. 2014;27(2):129–38.

Scheeren TW, Wiesenack C, Gerlach H, Marx G. Goal-directed intraoperative fluid therapy guided by stroke volume and its variation in high-risk surgical patients: a prospective randomized multicentre study. J Clin Monit Comput. 2013;27(3):225–33.

Senagore AJ, Emery T, Luchtefeld M, Kim D, Dujovny N, Hoedema R. Fluid management for laparoscopic colectomy: a prospective, randomized assessment of goal-directed administration of balanced salt solution or hetastarch coupled with an enhanced recovery program. Dis Colon Rectum. 2009;52(12):1935–40.

Sun Y, Chai F, Pan C, Romeiser JL, Gan TJ. Effect of perioperative goal-directed hemodynamic therapy on postoperative recovery following major abdominal surgery—a systematic review and meta-analysis of randomized controlled trials. Crit Care. 2017;21(1):141.

Thom O, Taylor DM, Wolfe RE, Myles P, Krum H, Wolfe R. Pilot study of the prevalence, outcomes and detection of occult hypoperfusion in trauma patients. Emerg Med J. 2010;27(6):470–2.

Veelo DP, van Berge Henegouwen MI, Ouwehand KS, Geerts BF, Anderegg MC, van Dieren S, Preckel B, Binnekade JM, Gisbertz SS, Hollmann MW. Effect of goal-directed therapy on outcome after esophageal surgery: a quality improvement study. PLoS One. 2017;12(3):e0172806.

Vonlanthen R, Slankamenac K, Breitenstein S, Puhan MA, Muller MK, Hahnloser D, Hauri D, Graf R, Clavien PA. The impact of complications on costs of major surgical procedures: a cost analysis of 1200 patients. Ann Surg. 2011;254(6):907–13.

Yuan J, Sun Y, Pan C, Li T. Goal-directed fluid therapy for reducing risk of surgical site infections following abdominal surgery—a systematic review and meta-analysis of randomized controlled trials. Int J Surg. 2017;39:74–87.

Zakhaleva J, Tam J, Denoya PI, Bishawi M, Bergamaschi R. The impact of intravenous fluid administration on complication rates in bowel surgery within an enhanced recovery protocol: a randomized controlled trial. Color Dis. 2013;15(7):892–9.

Zhang J, Chen CQ, Lei XZ, Feng ZY, Zhu SM. Goal-directed fluid optimization based on stroke volume variation and cardiac index during one-lung ventilation in patients undergoing thoracoscopy lobectomy operations: a pilot study. Clinics (Sao Paulo). 2013;68(7):1065–70.

Zheng H, Guo H, Ye JR, Chen L, Ma HP. Goal-directed fluid therapy in gastrointestinal surgery in older coronary heart disease patients: randomized trial. World J Surg. 2013;37(12):2820–9.

24

The effect of natural sounds on the anxiety of patients undergoing coronary artery bypass graft surgery

Mohammad Javad Amiri[1], Tabandeh Sadeghi[2,3*] and Tayebeh Negahban Bonabi[4,5]

Abstract

Background: This study aims to investigate the effect of natural sounds on the anxiety of patients undergoing coronary artery bypass graft surgery (CABG).

Methods: In this clinical trial, 90 patients, who were candidates for CABG in an urban area of Iran, were selected and randomly assigned to intervention and control groups by the minimization method. In the intervention group, natural sounds were broadcast through headphones for 30 min. In the control group, headphones connected to a silent device were used. The research instruments were a demographic questionnaire and the Spielberger State-Trait Anxiety Inventory (STAI). These were used before the intervention, 30 min after the music, and before the surgery in the waiting room for both groups. Data was analyzed using SPSS software.

Results: The mean anxiety level of the intervention group has been found to be significantly lower than that of the control group half an hour after the intervention as well as in the waiting room in the preoperative period ($p = 0.001$). Moreover, the mean anxiety of the intervention group decreases, while it increases for the control group over time ($p < 0.001$).

Conclusion: Natural sounds can be used as a non-pharmacological way to reduce the anxiety of patients undergoing CABG.

Keywords: CABG, Music therapy, Natural sounds, Anxiety

Background

Coronary artery bypass graft surgery (CABG) is one of the most valuable and effective methods for treating coronary artery diseases, but it is also one of the most stressful events that can occur during a person's lifespan (Smeltzer et al. 2012). Patients undergoing CABG may suffer from psychological problems such as anxiety, depression, worry, and fear. These problems start as early as CABG is selected as a therapeutic approach and continue until the moment of discharge (Dehghani et al. 2013).

* Correspondence: t.b_sadeghi@yahoo.com
[2]Non-Communicable Diseases Research Center, Rafsanjan University of Medical Sciences, Rafsanjan, Iran
[3]Department of Pediatric Nursing, School of Nursing and Midwifery, Rafsanjan University of Medical Sciences, Jomhori St., Rafsanjan 7718796755, Iran
Full list of author information is available at the end of the article

Symptoms such as fatigue, muscle weakness, palpitations, chest pain, headache, and sweating are negative effects of anxiety (Kipnis et al. 2016). Evidence suggests that candidates for surgery often worry about the procedure and fear the outcome (Thompson et al. 2014). Possible surgical pain, loss of control during surgery, changes in the body image, unpleasant diagnosis, worry about lack of rehabilitation, and worry for family members and occupation are among the preoperative anxiety-related factors (Kipnis et al. 2016).

With its risks, complications, and prognosis, cardiac surgery causes anxiety on a wider scale and sometimes causes patients to be defeated even before the surgery (Shojaee et al. 2014). Preoperative procedures, worry about the outcome, worry about lack of control over the situation, the risk of death, unfamiliar and unpleasant situations, and the expectation of undesirable results can contribute to anxiety in patients undergoing CABG (Padamanabhan et al. 2005). These issues cause postoperative pain, increase the need for analgesia, prolong hospital stay, delay discharge, have an overall effect on the induction and recurrence of anesthesia, and reduce the postoperative satisfaction in patients (Mirbagher et al. 2011). According to Krannich et al. (2007), patients undergoing CABG experience some degree of anxiety before and after surgery. These patients are very anxious due to the relationship between heart and life that exacerbates their excitement (Navarro et al. 2011).

Anxiety increases the heart rate, cardiac output, and the need for oxygen. It is necessary to reduce anxiety (Dehghani et al. 2013). One of the methods used in this field is music therapy (Sahmoddini et al. 2014), which is a complementary treatment that improves the patient's well-being by improving the threshold of stress and eliminating negative emotions, adjusting internal processes, and making them feel relaxed. Music with a slow, uniform, and repetitive rhythm may induce sleep or relaxation in the listener (Chang et al. 2008). Creating a therapeutic environment helps the patient to move from anxious and negative thoughts toward things that are pleasant and desirable (Fredriksson et al. 2009). In recent studies, music therapy has been found to reduce patient anxiety (Kipnis et al. 2016; Thompson et al. 2014; Lee et al. 2011; Motahedian et al. 2014; Maeyama et al. 2009; Han et al. 2010; Wakim et al. 2010). However, some other studies have reported no meaningful results for music therapy in terms of the level of anxiety and vital signs of patients (Dileo 2006; Ebneshahidi and Mohseni 2008; Bradt et al. 2013; Sendelbach et al. 2006; Nilsson et al. 2009).

One of the varieties of music is nature sounds. The use of natural sounds, such as the chirping of birds or the sound of rain and water, was introduced for the first time in 1984 to treat anxiety and pain in patients (Aghai et al. 2014). There is a vast body of research on the effects of music on the anxiety, pain, and vital signs of patients, but limited studies have been conducted on the effects of nature sounds. In Iran, no study has been conducted on this particular subject except the one by Aghaie et al. (2014), which investigated the effect of natural sounds on anxiety in CABG patients during the weaning of mechanical ventilation. Therefore, by considering the importance of the issue of anxiety in patients undergoing CABG and the contradictory results of studies on the effect of music, this study aims to investigate the effect of natural sounds on the anxiety of patients undergoing CABG.

Methods

This study was a clinical trial that was registered at the Iranian Registry for Clinical Trials with the code IRCT2017011723190N3. The research population included patients undergoing CABG hospitalization in an intensive care unit in an urban area of Iran. We calculated the study sample size by comparing two mean formulae with an effect size of 7 for anxiety and a standard deviation of 10 based on previous studies (McClurkin and Smith 2016). The level of significance was set at $p < 0.05$, while the study power was assumed to be 90%. We determined a sample size: $n = 43.82$. Considering the possibility of sample loss, 45 patients were allocated to each group. Alertness and being aware of the time and place, the age of over 18, undertaking heart surgery for the first time, having no pain, and having no evidence of organic fever during collection of information, taking no sedative, having no hearing problem, having no problem with the use of headphones, ability to participate in research and collaboration, signing the informed consent form, passing at least 2 h after admission, taking no beta blockers, and taking no narcotic drug in the morning before the surgery with any route of consumption such as oral, sublingual, injection, and inhalation were the inclusion criteria for this research study. The unwillingness to participate in research, interrupting music while performing the experiment, and the need to use sedative and narcotic drugs during voice playback or before completion of the second turn of the questionnaire formed the exclusion criteria.

As many as 90 candidates for CABG were selected based on inclusion and exclusion criteria by purposeful sampling. They were assigned to two intervention and control groups using the method of categorization through the minimization method (Pandis et al. 2011). In this method, the patients were initially categorized based on key variables such as anxiety score and gender. Afterward, the first participant was chosen from among those patients who met the inclusion criteria and then placed in the intervention or control group by the toss of a coin, while other participants were allocated to the study group with a lower number of variables (anxiety score and gender). In case of equality, random allocation was repeated.

The data collection tools comprise a demographic questionnaire for patients (age, sex, education, marital status, duration of disease) and the Spielberger State-Trait Anxiety Inventory (STAI). The reliability of the demographic questionnaire was determined by the content validity method as well as the opinion of professors and experts. The STAI is a commonly used measure of trait and state anxiety. Form Y, its most popular version, has 20 items for assessing trait anxiety and 20 for state anxiety. Internal consistency coefficients for the scale have ranged from 0.86 to 0.95, while test-retest reliability coefficients have ranged from 0.65 to 0.75 over a 2-month interval (Spielberger et al. 1983). In this study, we investigated state anxiety that relates to the apparent anxiety (expressing the patient's feelings at the current moment and at the time of filling in the questionnaire) by using 20 questions. Scoring this scale includes scores from 1 to 4. The scores are reversed for reverse questions (i.e., questions 1, 2, 5, 8, 10, 11, 15, 16, 19, 20) so that it includes from never (4) to many times (1). The range of the score remains between 20 and 80. In Mahram's study, the reliability of the research tool for the normal group (600 people) was 0.90 according to Cronbach's alpha, while it was estimated in the standard group (130 persons) as 0.94 (Mahram 1995).

The method was implemented in such a way that the researcher (first author) was referred to the hospital according to the cardiac surgery program in the night shift before the operation and following the selection of samples according to the inclusion and exclusion criteria. Consent was obtained from the participants, and the demographic data form and the Spielberger STAI were completed to assess the level of state anxiety through face-to-face interviews. The patients were then randomly assigned to the intervention and control groups. For the intervention group, nature sounds were played for 30 min via headphones in order to remove additional sounds. In the control group, headphones were connected to a silent device and were placed on the ears of the patients. Thirty minutes after the completion of the music playing and on the morning of the operation day in the waiting room, the anxiety questionnaires were completed by the members of the two groups. Nature sounds used in this study were the artwork "Sounds of Nature" recorded by Dr. Arnd Stein in 2011. The sounds included birds' chirping, roar of the sea, river and jungle sounds, and the sound of rain. The sound was broadcast by a 25–30-dB Sony MP3 player (as advised by the hearing aid) for 30 min for the intervention group. It should be noted that for preventing any transmission of infection from the headphones, they were disinfected after each use and disposable covers were used for them.

Finally, the data was analyzed using descriptive statistics, such as mean and standard deviation, and analytical statistics including the independent *t*-test and repeated measures ANOVA with SPSS software version 18. The significance level was less than 0.05.

Results

The demographic results indicate that in the intervention group, the mean age of patients was 58.61 ± 9.55 years and the mean duration of the disease was 9.51 ± 5.02 years. In the control group, the mean age of patients was 57.71 ± 9.88 years and the mean duration of their occurrence was 11.66 ± 3.99 years; they were homogeneous in terms of demographic characteristics (Table 1).

Based on the results, no significant difference was found between the two groups before the intervention (independent *t*-test, $p = 0.44$). However, there was a significant difference between the two groups after the intervention and the mean anxiety level in the intervention group was lower (independent *t*, $p < 0.05$). An intra-group analysis of variance with repeated measures was used: this resulted in no significant effect on the time ($p = 0.46$). The interactive effects of time and group were also evaluated using the repeated measures analysis of variance. While the result was significant and showed a decrease in the mean anxiety of the intervention group, the mean anxiety of the control group increased ($p < 0.001$) (Table 2). Normal distribution of data was confirmed by using the Kolmogorov–Smirnov statistical test ($p > 0.05$).

Discussion

Based on the results of this study, there was a significant statistical difference between the two groups in terms of playing natural sounds half an hour after and before surgery in the waiting room: the mean of anxiety in the intervention group was also lower. In the field of natural sounds, the results of the study by Aghaie et al. (2014) were consistent with the results of the present study—- this showed that playing natural sounds can reduce anxiety and restlessness in CABG patients during the weaning of mechanical ventilation. Although this study investigated the effect of natural sounds in CABG patients, the difference between this and the present study lies in the domain of time: this study was conducted before the surgery and the study by Aghaie et al. was conducted postoperation.

Although a similar study was not found in terms of the use of natural sounds before CABG, music intervention has been studied in several studies and various results have been reported. For example, the results of McClurkin et al. (2016) are consistent with the results of the present study which showed that listening to music for at least 15 min reduced the anxiety of patients undergoing surgery. But the difference with the present study was in the research procedure: in addition to the control group, there was a group hearing music for 15 min and one group for 30 min: all patients were candidates for various surgical procedures (orthopedics, general, neurological, plastic, urological), and based on their interest they selected classical, religious, or nature music. However, in the present study, the effect of natural sounds music was studied and patients were candidates for CABG. The results of the study by Thompson et al. (2014) and Maeyama et al. (2009) also showed that playing music before the surgery could reduce the anxiety of patients; these are consistent with the findings of the present study, although the type of music and patients of the aforementioned studies are different from the present study.

Despite the results of this study, the findings from Ebneshahidi and Mohseni (2008), Sendelbach et al. (2006),

Table 1 Comparison of demographic characteristics of patients in intervention and control groups

Demographic data		Intervention group number (%)	Control group number (%)	*p* value
Age (years)	>40	1(2.3)	4(8.9)	0.28[a]
	40–60	24(53.3)	14(31.1)	
	<60	20(44.4)	27(60)	
Gender	Man	27(60)	29(64.4)	0.66[b]
	Woman	18(40)	16(35.6)	
Marital status	Married	39(86.7)	34(95.6)	0.13[b]
	Single	6(13.3)	2(4.4)	
Disease duration (years)	>5	12(26.7)	9(20)	0.91[a]
	5–15	28(62.2)	34(75.6)	
	<15	5(11.1)	2(4.4)	

[a]Mann-Whitney *U* test
[b]Chi-square

and Nilsson et al. (2009) have no reported significant results from music intervention on the level of anxiety and vital signs of patients under surgery. Differences in the research population, type of music, patients' condition, and music playing time can be mentioned as the reasons for the differences between the present study and the aforementioned studies.

Based on the results of the present study, the mean anxiety of the intervention group decreased but the mean anxiety of the control group increased; in the preoperative waiting room, the intervention group had lesser anxiety than the control group. In this regard, the results of Kipnis et al. (2016) are consistent with the results of the present study, which shows that playing music in the waiting room can reduce the level of anxiety in patients. Considering that music intervention on the night before the surgery can be more convenient and has less interferences with preoperative care: based on the results of this study, playing music on the night before surgery can be considered as an intervention to reduce preoperative anxiety. This is the strength of the present study over all the aforementioned studies.

Music can facilitate anxiety reduction due to its physiological and neurological effects. After studying 23 studies on ischemic heart disease, Bardt and Dileo (2013) stated that music has beneficial effects on blood pressure, heart rate, respiration, anxiety, and pain in people with this disease. Han et al. (2010) also found that relaxing music can reduce patient anxiety: their results are consistent with the results of this study. In Iran, due to cultural and religious beliefs, any kind of music is not pleasant to people; therefore, the music of nature's sound, which is reminiscent of the natural habitats in the environment, is not in conflict with religious and cultural beliefs. Even in religious books such as the *Quran* and cultural books like *Divan Hafez*, thinking of nature and the consequences of thinking about it have been emphasized. These can help reduce this challenge.

Since the special environment of intensive care units increases the anxiety of patients due to factors such as sensory deprivation, severe medical noise, sleep deprivation, fear of diagnostic procedures, and separation from family members and friends (Rezaie et al. 2016), the results of this research can be used as a strategy by nurses to reduce the anxiety of patients undergoing CABG in intensive care units.

Physiological indices such as heart rates as well as blood pressure of these patients and the cortisol level taken at the time of the start of the surgery could have provided further evidence of the value of the administration of music to cardiac patients. These were not assessed in this study and are lost opportunities. Therefore, it is recommended

Table 2 Comparison of mean anxiety level in patients of both groups before and after the intervention

Groups	Time of intervention			Results of repeated measures ANOVA	
	Before intervention	30 min after the intervention	In the waiting room	*p* value[b]	*p* value[c]
	Mean ± SD	Mean ± SD	Mean ± SD		
Intervention group	4.37 ± 47.66	7.21 ± 43.68	7.11 ± 42.95	0.34	0.001
Control group	5.17 ± 48.44	6.69 ± 50.57	6.78 ± 51.28		
p value[a]	0.44	0.001	0.001		

[a]Independent *t*-test (inter-group comparison)
[b]Repeated measures ANOVA (intra-group comparison)
[c]Repeated measures ANOVA (interactive effect)

that future studies be conducted as to assess these variables. This study was limited to patients with CABG. Lack of similar research on natural sound music limited the possibility of comparing the results of this study. So, doing similar studies in people with a different age range and other illnesses, comparing this kind of music with other types of music, and comparing the duration of the music playback are recommended for future studies.

Conclusion

Natural sounds can be used as a way to reduce the anxiety of patients before surgery. Nurses can use this non-pharmacological approach along with other types of care to reduce the anxiety of patients before CABG.

Abbreviations

CABG: Coronary artery bypass graft surgery; STAI: State-Trait Anxiety Inventory

Acknowledgements

This study was extracted from a student's thesis (code: 20/1099) approved by Rafsanjan University of Medical Sciences. Hereby, we extend our gratitude to the authorities of the university for supporting this study. We would also like to thank all of patients for their cooperation in this research project.

Funding

This study was financially sponsored by Rafsanjan University of Medical Sciences.

Authors' contributions

MJA, TS, and TN conceived the study and contributed to study design. MJA performed the data collection. TS undertook the statistical analysis. MJA drafted the manuscript which underwent revision by all other authors. All authors read and approved the final manuscript.

Competing interests

The authors declare that they have no competing interests.

Author details

[1]School of Nursing and Midwifery, Rafsanjan University of Medical Sciences, Rafsanjan, Iran. [2]Non-Communicable Diseases Research Center, Rafsanjan University of Medical Sciences, Rafsanjan, Iran. [3]Department of Pediatric Nursing, School of Nursing and Midwifery, Rafsanjan University of Medical Sciences, Jomhori St., Rafsanjan 7718796755, Iran. [4]Social Determinants of Health Research Center, Rafsanjan University of Medical Sciences, Rafsanjan, Iran. [5]Deparment of Community Health Nursing, School of Nursing and Midwifery, Rafsanjan University of Medical Sciences, Rafsanjan, Iran.

References

Aghai B, Rejeh N, Heravi-Karimooi M, Ebadi A, Moradian T, Vaismoradi M, Jasper M. Effect of nature-based sound therapy on agitation and anxiety in coronary artery bypass graft patients during the weaning of mechanical ventilation: a randomized clinical trial. Int J Nurs Stud. 2014;51(4):526–38.

Bradt J, Dileo C, Potvin N. Music for stress and anxiety reduction in coronary heart disease patients. Cochrane Database Syst Rev. 2013;28(12):1–77.

Chang MY, Chen CH, Hauang KF. Effect of music therapy on psychological health of women during pregnancy. J Clin Nurs. 2008;17(19):2580–7.

Dehghani H, Dehghani K, Nasiriani K, Banaderakhshan H. The effect of familiarization with cardiac surgery process on the anxiety of patients undergoing coronary artery bypass graft surgery. Mod Care J. 2013;10(4):257–63.

Dileo C. Effect of music and music therapy on medical patients: a meta-analysis of the research and implications for the future. J Soc Integr Oncol. 2006;4(2):67–70.

Ebneshahidi A, Mohseni M. The effect of patient-selected music on early postoperative pain, anxiety, and hemodynamic profile in cesarean section surgery. J Altern Complement Med. 2008;14(7):827–31.

Fredriksson A, Hellstrom L, Nilsson U. Patients' perception of music versus ordinary sound in a post anaesthesia care unit: a randomized crossover trial. Intensive Crit Care Nurs. 2009;25(4):208–13.

Han L, Li JP, Sit JW, Chung L, Jiao ZY, Ma WG. Effects of music intervention on physiological stress response and anxiety level of mechanically ventilated patients in China: a randomized controlled trial. J Clin Nurs. 2010;19(7-8):978–87.

Kipnis G, Tabak N, Koton S. Background music playback in the preoperative setting: does it reduce the level of preoperative anxiety among candidates for elective surgery? J Perianesth Nurs. 2016;31(3):209–16.

Krannich JH, Weyers P, Lueger S, Herzog M, Bohrer T, Elert O. Presence of depression and anxiety before and after coronary artery bypass graft surgery and their relationship to age. BMC Psychiatry. 2007;12(7):47.

Lee KC, Chao YH, Yiin JJ, Chao YF. Effectiveness of different music-playing devices for reducing preoperative anxiety: a clinical control study. Int J Nurs Stud. 2011;48(110):1180–7.

Maeyama A, Kodaka M, Miyao H. Effect of the music-therapy under spinal anesthesia. Masui. 2009;58(6):684–91.

Mahram B. [Spielberger Test Standardization in Mashhad (Persian)]. MA Thesis. Tehran: Allameh Tabatabaei University; 1995.

McClurkin S, Smith C. Duration of self-selected music needed to reduce preoperative anxiety. J Perianesth Nurs. 2016;31(3):196–208.

Mirbagher N, Aghajani M, Shahshahani M. The effect of music and holly Quran on patients' anxiety and vital signs before abdominal surgeries. Evid Based Care J. 2011;1(1):63–76.

Motahedian E, Movahhedi Rad S, Lak M, Hajizadeh E. The effect of music therapy on anxiety and physiological variables in patients under spinal anesthesia. J Appl Environ Biol Sci. 2014;4(4):240–6.

Navarro MA, Fernandez BM, Alegre VC, Oroz AM. Preoperative mood disorders in patients undergoing cardiac surgery: risk factors and postoperative morbidity in the intensive care unit. Rev Esp Cardiol. 2011;64(11):1005–10.

Nilsson U, Lindell L, Eriksson A, Kellerth T. The effect of music intervention in relation to gender during coronary angiographic procedures: a randomized clinical trial. Eur J Cardiovasc Nurs. 2009;8(3):200–6.

Padamanabhan R, Hildreth AJ, Lawa D. A prospective, randomized, controlled study examining binaural beat audio and pre-operative anxiety in patients undergoing general anaesthesia for day case surgery. Anaesthesia. 2005; 60(9):874–7.

Pandis N, Switzerland B, Greece C. Randomization. Part 2: minimization. Am J Orthod Dentofacial Orthop. 2011;140:902–4.

Rezaie H, Sadeghi T, Abdoli F. The effects of scheduled visitation on the physiological indices of conscious patients admitted at intensive care units. Evid Based Care J. 2016;5(4):33–40.

Sahmoddini MA, Zamani Lari M, Rahimian MN, Danayi L, Beigi N, Habibi H. The effect of listening to the Quran on serum cortisol and anxiety in primiparous women during the first stage of labor. Iran J Obstet Gynecol Infertility. 2014;17(99):1–7.

Sendelbach SE, Halm MA, Doran KA, Miller EH, Gaillard P. Effects of music therapy on physiological and psychological outcomes for patients undergoing cardiac surgery. J Cardiovasc Nurs. 2006;21(3):194–200.

Shojaee A, Nehrir B, Naderi N, Zareyan A. Comparison of patient education and follow up by nurse on anxiety in heart failure patients. Med Surg Nurs J. 2014;3(1):52–60.

Smeltzer SC, Bare BG, Hinkle JL, Cheever KH. Brunner & Suddarth's textbook of medical-surgical nursing. 12th ed. London: Lippincott Williams & Wilkins; 2012. P: 284.

Spielberger CD, Gorsuch RL, Lushene R, Vagg PR, Jacobs GA. Manual for the state-trait anxiety inventory. Palo Alto: Consulting Psychologists Press; 1983.
Stein A. Available at: URL: http://dl.vmusic.ir/New%20Age/Dr.%20Arnd%20Stein%20-%20Sounds%20Of%20Nature%20. (2011). Accessed 12 Nov 2016.
Thompson M, Moe K, Lewis P. The effects of music on diminishing anxiety among preoperative patients. J Radiol Nurs. 2014;33(4):199–202.
Wakim JH, Smith S, Guinn C. The efficacy of music therapy. J Perianesth Nurs. 2010;25(4):226–32.

Permissions

All chapters in this book were first published in PM, by BioMed Central; hereby published with permission under the Creative Commons Attribution License or equivalent. Every chapter published in this book has been scrutinized by our experts. Their significance has been extensively debated. The topics covered herein carry significant findings which will fuel the growth of the discipline. They may even be implemented as practical applications or may be referred to as a beginning point for another development.

The contributors of this book come from diverse backgrounds, making this book a truly international effort. This book will bring forth new frontiers with its revolutionizing research information and detailed analysis of the nascent developments around the world.

We would like to thank all the contributing authors for lending their expertise to make the book truly unique. They have played a crucial role in the development of this book. Without their invaluable contributions this book wouldn't have been possible. They have made vital efforts to compile up to date information on the varied aspects of this subject to make this book a valuable addition to the collection of many professionals and students.

This book was conceptualized with the vision of imparting up-to-date information and advanced data in this field. To ensure the same, a matchless editorial board was set up. Every individual on the board went through rigorous rounds of assessment to prove their worth. After which they invested a large part of their time researching and compiling the most relevant data for our readers.

The editorial board has been involved in producing this book since its inception. They have spent rigorous hours researching and exploring the diverse topics which have resulted in the successful publishing of this book. They have passed on their knowledge of decades through this book. To expedite this challenging task, the publisher supported the team at every step. A small team of assistant editors was also appointed to further simplify the editing procedure and attain best results for the readers.

Apart from the editorial board, the designing team has also invested a significant amount of their time in understanding the subject and creating the most relevant covers. They scrutinized every image to scout for the most suitable representation of the subject and create an appropriate cover for the book.

The publishing team has been an ardent support to the editorial, designing and production team. Their endless efforts to recruit the best for this project, has resulted in the accomplishment of this book. They are a veteran in the field of academics and their pool of knowledge is as vast as their experience in printing. Their expertise and guidance has proved useful at every step. Their uncompromising quality standards have made this book an exceptional effort. Their encouragement from time to time has been an inspiration for everyone.

The publisher and the editorial board hope that this book will prove to be a valuable piece of knowledge for researchers, students, practitioners and scholars across the globe.

List of Contributors

Simon J Davies, James Francis, Jonathan Dilley and R Jonathan T Wilson
1Department of Anaesthesia, York Hospitals NHS Foundation Trust, Wigginton Road, York YO31 8HE, UK

Simon J Howell
Academic Unit of Anaesthesia, Leeds General Infirmary, Great George Street, Leeds LS1 3EX, UK

Victoria Allgar
Hull York Medical School, The University of York, Heslington, York YO10 5DD, UK

Chen-Fuh Lam, Shiu-Ying Hsieh,Hui-Shan Pan, Xiu-Zhu Liu and T sung-Ying Chen
Department of Anesthesiology, Buddhist Tzu Chi General Hospital and Tzu Chi University School of Medicine, No 707, Chung-Yang Road Section 3, Hualien 970, Taiwan, Republic of China

Jen-Hung Wang
Department of Medical Research, Tzu Chi General Hospital, Hualien, Taiwan

Yu-Ching Ho
Department of Health Administration, Tzu Chi University of Science and Technology, Hualien, Taiwan

Yussr M. Ibrahim, Nicole R. Marques, Carlos R. Garcia, Michael Salter, Christopher McQuitty and Michael Kinsky
Department of Anesthesiology, The University of Texas Medical Branch, Galveston, TX, USA

Mindy Juan
Department of Anesthesiology, Kadlec Regional Medical Center, Pasco, WA, USA

Achiau Ludomirsky
Department of Pediatrics, NYU Langone Health, School of Medicine, New York, NY, USA

Ben A. Goodman
Department of Perioperative Care, Royal Victoria Infirmary, Newcastle upon Tyne, UK

Alan M. Batterham
Health and Social Care Institute, Teesside University, Middlesbrough, UK

Gerard R. Danjoux
Health and Social Care Institute, Teesside University, Middlesbrough, UK
Department of Academic Anaesthesia, James Cook University Hospital, Marton Road, Middlesbrough TS4 3BW, UK

Elke Kothmann and Louise Cawthorn
Department of Academic Anaesthesia, James Cook University Hospital, Marton Road, Middlesbrough TS4 3BW, UK

David Yates
Department of Anaesthesia, York Hospital, York, UK

Helen Melsom
Department of Anaesthesia,University Hospital of North Durham, Durham, UK

Karen Kerr
Department of Anaesthesia, Northern General Hospital, Sheffield, UK

Rebecca M. Speck
Department of Anesthesiology and Critical Care, Center for Pharmacoepidemiology Research and Training, University of Pennsylvania, 3400 Spruce Street, Dulles 6, Philadelphia, PA 19104, USA
Evidera, 1417 4th Ave., Suite 510, Seattle, WA 98101, USA

Mark D. Neuman
Department of Anesthesiology and Critical Care, Leonard Davis Institute, University of Pennsylvania, 3400 Spruce Street, Dulles 6, Philadelphia, PA 19104, USA

Kimberly S. Resnick
Department of Psychiatry, University of Pennsylvania, 3535 Market St, Philadelphia, PA 19104, USA

Barbara A. Mellers
Department of Psychology, Department of Marketing, University of Pennsylvania, 3720 Walnut St, Philadelphia, PA 19104, USA

Lee A. Fleisher
Department of Anesthesiology and Critical Care, Center for Pharmacoepidemiology Research and Training, Leonard Davis Institute, University of Pennsylvania, 3400 Spruce Street, Dulles 6, Philadelphia, PA 19104, USA

Denise Weber, Silvia R Cottini, Pascal Locher, Urs Wenger, Paul A Stehberger, Mario Fasshauer, Reto A Schuepbach and Markus Béchir
Surgical Intensive Care Medicine, University Hospital of Zurich, Raemistrasse 100, CH-8091 Zurich, Switzerland

Sarka Moravcova and Bonnie Kyle
Royal Brompton & Harefield NHS Trust, London, UK

Hilary Shanahan, Savvas Giannaris, Andrew Smith and Colin Hamilton-Davies
Barts Health NHS Trust, London, UK

Zia Sadique and Richard Grieve
Department of Health Services Research and Policy, London School of Hygiene and Tropical Medicine, London, UK

David A. Harrison and Kathryn M. Rowan
Intensive Care National Audit & Research Centre, London, UK

Rupert M. Pearse
Queen Mary University of London, London EC1M 6BQ, UK
Adult Critical Care Unit, Royal London Hospital, Whitechapel, London E1 1BB, UK

Roman Melamed and Adnan Masood
Department of Critical Care Medicine, Abbott Northwestern Hospital, 800 East 28th Street, Minneapolis, MN 55407, USA

Lori L. Boland, James P. Normington, Rebecca M. Prenevost and Tyler G. Kinzy
Division of Applied Research, Allina Health, 2925 Chicago Ave South, Minneapolis, MN, USA

Lindsay Y. Hur
Department of Pharmacy, Abbott Northwestern Hospital, 800 East 28th Street, Minneapolis, MN, USA

Leslie F. Maynard and Molly A. McNaughton
Chronic Pain Team, Abbott Northwestern Hospital, 800 East 28th Street, Minneapolis, MN, USA

Mehdi Dastrange and Joseph A. Huguelet
Internal Medicine Residency Program, Abbott Northwestern Hospital, 800 East 28th Street, Minneapolis, MN, USA

Toby Richards
Division of Surgery and Interventional Science, University College London, 21 University Street, London WC1E 6DE, UK

James M Otto
Division of Surgery and Interventional Science, University College London, 21 University Street, London WC1E 6DE, UK
The Portex Unit, UCL Institute of Child Health, 30 Guilford Street, London WC1N 1EH, UK

Alasdair F O'Doherty and Philip J Hennis
The Portex Unit, UCL Institute of Child Health, 30 Guilford Street, London WC1N 1EH, UK

Michael PW Grocott
The Portex Unit, UCL Institute of Child Health, 30 Guilford Street, London WC1N 1EH, UK
Integrative Physiology and Critical Illness Group, Division of Clinical and Experimental Science, Faculty of Medicine, University of Southampton, University Road, Southampton SO17 1BJ, UK

Jackie A Cooper
Department of Medicine, Centre of Cardiovascular Genetics, University College London, 5 University Street, London WC1E 6JF, UK

Hugh E Montgomery
UCL Institute for Human Health and Performance, c/o 4th Floor, Rockefeller Building, 21 University Street, London WC1E 6DE, UK

Chris Snowdon
Newcastle Upon Tyne NHS Foundation Trust, Freeman Hospital, Freeman Road, High Heaton, Newcastle Upon Tyne NE7 7DN, UK

John B Carlisle and Michael Swart
Torbay Hospital, South Devon Healthcare NHS Foundation Trust, Torbay Hospital, Lawes Bridge, Torquay TQ2 7AA, UK

Takehiko Iijima
Department of Perioperative Medicine, Division of Anesthesiology, School of Dentistry, Showa University

Birgitte Brandstrup
Department of Surgical Gastroenterology, Hvidovre University Hospital, Copenhagen, Denmark

Peter Rodhe and Christer H Svensen
Karolinska Institutet, Department of Clinical Science and Education, Section of Anesthesiology and Intensive Care, Södersjukhuset, Stockholm, Sweden

Audrius Andrijauskas
Clinic of Anesthesiology and Intensive Care, Vilnius University, Vilnius, Lithuania

Kimberly L. Mei
Dartmouth College, Hanover, NH, USA

Jeannine B. Mills
Dartmouth-Hitchcock Medical Center, Lebanon, NH, USA

Stefan D. Holubar
Dartmouth-Hitchcock Medical Center, Lebanon, NH, USA
Geisel School of Medicine at Dartmouth, Hanover, NH, USA

John A. Batsis
Dartmouth-Hitchcock Medical Center, Lebanon, NH, USA
Geisel School of Medicine at Dartmouth, Hanover, NH, USA
The Dartmouth Institute for Health Policy & Clinical Practice, Lebanon, NH, USA

Elizabeth Ashby
Catterall Unit, Royal National Orthopaedic Hospital, Brockley Hill, Stanmore,Middlesex HA7 4LP, UK

Claire Matejowsky
Surgical Outcomes Research Centre, University College London Hospital, 235 Euston Road, Fitzrovia, London NW1 2BU, UK

Michael G Mythen
UCL Institute of Child Health, Surgical Outcomes Research Centre, Joint UCLH/UCL Comprehensive Biomedical Research Centre, Gower Street, London WC1E 6BT, UK

Michael PW Grocott
UCL Institute of Child Health, Surgical Outcomes Research Centre, Joint UCLH/UCL Comprehensive Biomedical Research Centre, Gower Street, London WC1E 6BT, UK
Integrative Physiology and Critical Illness Group, Clinical and Experimental Sciences, University of Southampton, University Road, Southampton SO17 1BJ, UK
NIHR Respiratory Biomedical Research Unit, University Hospital Southampton/University of Southampton, University Road, Southampton SO17 1BJ, UK

Fares S Haddad
University College London Hospital, 235 Euston Road, Fitzrovia, London NW1 2BU, UK

David N Flynn
Department of Anesthesiology and Critical Care, Perelman School of Medicine, University of Pennsylvania, 3400 Spruce Street, Philadelphia, PA 19104, USA

Rebecca M Speck
Department of Anesthesiology and Critical Care, Perelman School of Medicine, University of Pennsylvania, 3400 Spruce Street, Philadelphia, PA 19104, USA
Center for Pharmacoepidemiology Research and Training, Center for Clinical Epidemiology and Biostatistics, Perelman School of Medicine, University of Pennsylvania, 423 Guardian Drive, Philadelphia, PA 19104, USA

Lee A Fleisher
Department of Anesthesiology and Critical Care, Perelman School of Medicine, University of Pennsylvania, 3400 Spruce Street, Philadelphia, PA 19104, USA
Center for Pharmacoepidemiology Research and Training, Center for Clinical Epidemiology and Biostatistics, Perelman School of Medicine, University of Pennsylvania, 423 Guardian Drive, Philadelphia, PA 19104, USA

Senior Fellow, Leonard Davis Institute of Health Economics, University of Pennsylvania, Colonial Penn Center, 3641 Locust Walk, Philadelphia, PA 19104, USA

Najjia N Mahmoud
Department of Surgery, Hospital of the University of Pennsylvania, 3400 Spruce Street, Philadelphia, PA 19104, USA

Guy David
Department of Health Care Management, The Wharton School, University of Pennsylvania, Colonial Penn Center, 3641 Locust Walk, Philadelphia, PA 19104, USA
Senior Fellow, Leonard Davis Institute of Health Economics, University of Pennsylvania, Colonial Penn Center, 3641 Locust Walk, Philadelphia, PA 19104, USA

Jason B. O'Neal and Andrew D. Shaw
Department of Anesthesiology, Vanderbilt University Medical Center, Nashville, TN, USA

Jaap Jan Vos, Marieke Poterman, Laura N Hannivoort, Michel MRF Struys and Thomas WL Scheeren
Department of Anesthesiology, University of Groningen, University Medical Center Groningen, Groningen, The Netherlands

Alain F Kalmar
Department of Anesthesiology, University of Groningen, University Medical Center Groningen, Groningen, The Netherlands
Department of Anaesthesiology and Intensive care medicine, Maria Middelares hospital, Ghent, Belgium

Victor W Renardel De Lavalette
Department of Ophthalmology, University of Groningen, University Medical Center Groningen, Groningen, The Netherlands

Cathrine Tadyanemhandu, Rufaro Mukombachoto, Clement Nhunzvi and Farayi Kaseke
Department of Rehabilitation, College of Health Sciences, University Of Zimbabwe, Avondale, Harare, Zimbabwe

Vasco Chikwasha
Department of Community Medicine, College of Health Sciences, University Of Zimbabwe, Avondale, Harare, Zimbabwe

Samson Chengetanai
Division of Basic Medical Sciences, Faculty of Medicine, National University of Science and Technology,Ascot, Bulawayo, Zimbabwe

Shamila Manie
Division of Physiotherapy, Department of Health and Rehabilitation Sciences, Faculty of Health Sciences, University of CapeTown, Anzio Road, Observatory, CapeTown, South Africa

Elena J. Koepke, Timothy E. Miller, David G. A. Williams and Michael W. Manning
Division of General, Vascular and Transplant Anesthesiology, Department of Anesthesiology, Duke University, 2301 Erwin Road, Durham, NC 27710, USA

Erin L. Manning
Division of Regional Anesthesiology, Department of Anesthesiology, Duke University, Durham, USA

Arun Ganesh
Division of Pain, Department of Anesthesiology, Duke University, Durham, USA

Robert G. Hahn
Research Unit, Södertälje Hospital, SE-152 86 Södertälje, Sweden

Hans Bahlmann and Lena Nilsson
Department of Anaesthesiology and Intensive Care, Linköping University, Linköping, Sweden
Department of Medical and Health Sciences, Linköping University, Linköping, Sweden

Owain Thomas
Department of Anaesthesiology and Intensive Care Medicine, Institute of Clinical Sciences, Lund, Medical Faculty, University of Lund, 221 00 Lund, Sweden
Department of Paediatric Anaesthesia and Intensive Care, SUS Lund University Hospital, 22185 Lund, Sweden

Per Flisberg
Department of Anaesthesiology and Intensive Care Medicine, Institute of Clinical Sciences, Lund, Medical Faculty, University of Lund, 221 00 Lund, Sweden
Department of Anaesthesia and Intensive Care, Helsingborg Hospital, Södra Vallgatan 5, 254 37 Helsingborg, Sweden

Ulf Schött
Department of Anaesthesiology and Intensive Care Medicine, Institute of Clinical Sciences, Lund, Medical Faculty, University of Lund, 221 00 Lund, Sweden
Department of Anaesthesia and Intensive Care, SUS Lund University Hospital, 221 85 Lund, Sweden

Emanuel Lybeck
Oskarshamn Hospital, 572 28 Oskarshamn, Sweden

Stephen T. McSorley, Campbell S. D. Roxburgh, Paul G. Horgan and Donald C. McMillan
Academic Unit of Surgery, School of Medicine, University of Glasgow, R2.06, Level 2, New Lister Building, Glasgow Royal Infirmary, Alexandra Parade, Glasgow G31 2ER, UK

C. Michael Dunham and Gregory S. Huang
Trauma, Critical Care, and General Surgery Services, St. Elizabeth Youngstown Hospital, 1044 Belmont Ave., Youngstown, OH 44501, USA

Barbara M. Hileman and Elisha A.Chance
Trauma and Neurosciences Research Department, St. Elizabeth Youngstown Hospital, 1044 Belmont Ave., Youngstown, OH 44501, USA

Amy E. Hutchinson and Gregory Szmaj
Department of Anesthesiology, St. Elizabeth Youngstown Hospital, 1044 Belmont Ave., Youngstown, OH 44501, USA

Tamara Antonaccio
OR Nursing Staff, St. Elizabeth Youngstown Hospital, 1044 Belmont Ave., Youngstown, OH 44501, USA

Kristen Calabro
Department of Surgery, St. Elizabeth Youngstown Hospital, 1044 Belmont Ave., Youngstown, OH 44501, USA

Cynthia Bishop
Surgical and Perioperative Services, St. Elizabeth Youngstown Hospital, 1044 Belmont Ave., Youngstown, OH 44501, USA

Tyson T. Schrickel
Department of Orthopedic Surgery, St. Elizabeth Youngstown Hospital, 1044 Belmont Ave., Youngstown, OH 44501, USA

Juying Jin, Su Min, Dan Liu, Ling Liu and Bixiao Lv
Department of Anesthesiology, the First Affiliated Hospital, Chongqing Medical University, 1 Youyi Road, Chongqing 400016, China

Mohammad Javad Amiri
School of Nursing and Midwifery, Rafsanjan University of Medical Sciences, Rafsanjan, Iran

Tabandeh Sadeghi
Non-Communicable Diseases Research Center, Rafsanjan University of Medical Sciences, Rafsanjan, Iran
Department of Pediatric Nursing, School of Nursing and Midwifery, Rafsanjan University of Medical Sciences, Jomhori St., Rafsanjan 7718796755, Iran

Tayebeh Negahban Bonabi
Social Determinants of Health Research Center, Rafsanjan University of Medical Sciences, Rafsanjan, Iran
Deparment of Community Health Nursing, School of Nursing and Midwifery, Rafsanjan University of Medical Sciences, Rafsanjan, Iran

Index

CPSIA information can be obtained
at www.ICGtesting.com
Printed in the USA
BVHW011503190820
586704BV00025B/300